Healthcare Delivery in the Information Age

Epworth Chair Health Information Management

Series Editor:
Nilmini Wickramasinghe

For further volumes:
http://www.springer.com/series/8783

Nilmini Wickramasinghe · Rajeev K Bali
Reima Suomi · Stefan Kirn
Editors

Critical Issues for the Development of Sustainable E-health Solutions

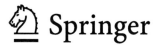 Springer

Editors
Nilmini Wickramasinghe
Epworth Chair Health Information
Management
School of Business Information Technology
RMIT University
Melbourne, VIC, Australia
nilmini.wickramasinghe@rmit.edu.au

Reima Suomi
University Turku, Finland
reima.suomi@utu.fi

Rajeev K. Bali
Biomedical Computing and Engineering
Technologies (BIOCORE) Applied
Research Group, Health Design and
Technology Institute (HDTI),
Coventry University , Coventry , UK
e-mail: r.bali@ieee.org

Stefan Kirn
The University of Höhenheim,
Germany
Stefan.kirn@uni-hohenheim.de

ISBN 978-1-4614-1535-0   e-ISBN 978-1-4614-1536-7
DOI 10.1007/978-1-4614-1536-7
Springer New York Dordrecht Heidelberg London

Library of Congress Control Number: 2011940830

Printed on acid-free paper

Springer is part of Springer Science+Business Media (www.springer.com)

For Our Families

Foreword

Health services are under hard pressure everywhere in the world and increasingly a topic of public and international discussions. Health and well-being are issues that have endless demand. With increasing standard of living health, and well-being in general, are higher and higher as a value. At the same time the possibilities of treatment – even of milder problems – are rapidly increasing and many of the treatment modalities are more and more costly.

In this situation a crucial issue is how to spend – both the public and also individual's – resources wisely. Both the public and the individual should get value for money. The interventions should be effective and efficient. Health gain is the key issue.

Information technology can be a key component in these endeavors, but it is of course not an end in itself. Well-thought of structures and fluent and efficient processes, supported by adequate and good-quality knowledge, information and data, are cornerstones of a well-functioning health care system. Information technology can help in developing and maintaining these valuable resources. Information technology is often the clue and structure that keeps best practices together and gives them operational frames.

Digging deeper into the world of e-health is an interesting journey. Health care is a very regulated industry, and things are slow and difficult to change. Information technology, on the other hand, is changing fast, and the big trend goes towards environments such as social media, virtual worlds, peer-to-peer contacting and networking and web 2.0 or even web 3.0. Common to all these is self-organization and low hierarchy and control by some external party. When these two different worlds meet, confrontations can emerge, but hopefully also fruitful innovations.

The concept of health is multidimensional, so even in this book. Caring for physical health is one cornerstone, but health and well-being materialize in many other, even more complex, dimensions too. Especially useful computer-based communication can be in maintaining social, societal and mental health. For example, patients in institutional care might be much better of, if they would be given possibilities to contact with their friends and relatives through the means modern information technology allows.

The e-health innovations are crucial for both the health services and the patients/individuals. For the health services the great change in public health form an important background. Most patient visits are no more for acute problems – infections or accidents – but due to chronic conditions, often among older people.

Chronic, non-communicable diseases determine much contemporary public health. These diseases, like cardiovascular, cancer, diabetes, chronic lung diseases, mental health problems or musculoskeletal diseases – or their risk factors like obesity, high blood pressure or high blood cholesterol – are not treated at one visit, demand years of or often lifelong visits to health services. This calls for completely new ways to organize the services. "Chronic care model" is the concept often mentioned. This means evidence-based treatment schemes, multiprofessional team work, agreed follow-up system and – well supporting IT and e-health solutions.

Also for the patients and individuals e-health opens completely new horizons – together with increasing educational level of the population. These issues deal with access to electronic health information (both prevention & health promotion and treatment of diseases), electronic risk assessments, easy personal monitoring, health service contact arrangements and all kind of e-health services.

Information technology is also a tool to bring services to many disadvantaged: vision or hearing impaired, or people living in distant geographical areas. Telemedicine, also contacting between care personnel and the patient over telecommunication networks is already routine in many places. New computer interfaces allow for efficient communication even for vision and hearing impaired, that would have little means to communicate without these new innovations.

The book at hand has collected contributions from leading experts from all around the world. One of the strengths of the book is its wide international scope. Worldwide we have many different arrangements and governance structures for national health care systems, and we can widely learn from the best practices around the world. Facilitating knowledge transfer and dissemination, of which process this book is also a part, is a crucial and important activity.

I wish all readers good and educative moments in reading of this book.

Chancellor, University of Turku   Pekka Puska
Director General, National institute for Health
and Welfare (THL)

Preface

Healthcare delivery globally is at a cross roads. In particular, the U.S. healthcare system has been noted as being significantly more costly than any other OECD country (Wickramasinghe et al. 2008a). Moreover, the use of healthcare services in the U.S. is below the OECD median by most measures and it is predicted that healthcare costs will be over 20% of GDP before 2020 (Wickramasinghe et al. 2008a). Given this, most experts are in agreement that the current healthcare system in the US is in crisis. In response to the current untenable situation, the Obama government has made healthcare reform a priority (Wickramasinghe et al. 2008b). Integral to such reform is the need to redesign inefficient and out dated processes and transition to a patient centric technology enabled healthcare delivery system.

While the situation appears to be less drastic in Europe, cost increases and ineffective healthcare delivery is apparent (Wickramasinghe et al. 2008a; Gronlund 2002; European commission 2008), which in turn has led to similar sentiments having been voiced by the European leaders (The Oslo Declaration on Health 2003; Global Medical Forum Foundation 2005) and the World health organization (World Health Organization 1998; WHO-EMRO http://www.emro.who.int/his/ehealth/ehealthPlan.htm). Both European and US authorities define their initiatives primarily in terms of medical information technology centering on computerized patient record [CPR] or, in more acceptable parlance, the [EHR] electronic health record (Brailer and Terasawa 2003; Gronlund 2002). WHO's platform statement (Global Medical Forum Foundation 2005) speaks of "health telematics policy", an all inclusive term that incorporates not only HER but essentially all healthcare services provided at a distance and based on the use of information communications technologies [ICT]. While implementation of these concepts is preeminently realistic in the context of EU and USA, the WHO plan appears, for many reasons, a combination of a list of good ideas and delineation of significant obstacles that make the good ideas seem almost futuristic.

Effective conduct of healthcare operations is not only extremely expensive, but it is also extremely complex, particularly when executed at the global scale. Most healthcare problems affecting the world have multiple roots involving social, economical, political, and even geographical factors whose combination provides fertile grounds for the spread of illnesses, prevalence of trauma, enhanced mortality, etc.

In the current debates of healthcare economy, ICT use then is heralded as the silver bullet. Healthcare is an information rich, knowledge intensive environment. In order to treat and diagnose even a simple condition a physician must combine many varied data elements and information. Such multispectral data must be carefully integrated and synthesised to allow medically appropriate management of the disease. Given the need to combine data and information into a coherent whole and then disseminate these findings to decision makers in a timely fashion, the benefits of ICT to support decision making of the physician and other actors throughout the healthcare system are clear (Wickramasinghe et al. 2005). In fact, we see the proliferation of many technologies such as HER (health electronic records), PACS (picture archive computerized systems) systems, CDSS (clinical decision support systems) etc. However and paradoxically, the more investment in ICT by healthcare the more global healthcare appears to be hampered by information chaos which in turn leads to inferior decision making, ineffective and inefficient operations, exponentially increasing costs and even loss of life (Wickramasinghe et al. 2005).

Recognizing the need for technology solutions does not in and of itself translate into realising the full potential afforded by the technology. To truly realise the full potential it is imperative to understand the healthcare technology paradigm, develop a sustainability model for the effective use of technology in a specific context and then successfully design and implement the patient centric technology solution (Suomi et al. 2007). Many of the problems with technology use are connected to the platform centric nature of these systems and the fact that they cannot support seamless transfer of data and information. This, on top of already inferior healthcare processes leads to the realizing of inferior, not superior healthcare delivery. Hence, it is of paramount importance to focus on designing effective and efficient healthcare processes enabled with technology to support the delivery of superior healthcare and thus better access, quality and value. An essential aspect then becomes identifying the barriers and facilitators to move from idea generation to concept realization and application.

In order to understand the role for technology in healthcare delivery, it is first important to understand the unique aspects of the healthcare industry, the key challenges and the components of the healthcare value proposition. Irrespective of the specific healthcare model, unlike most other industries, healthcare has the unique structure that the receiver of the services (i.e. the patient) is often not the predominant payer for those services (i.e. the insurance company). Moreover, any healthcare intervention is complex and typically involves directly or indirectly a multiplicity of players including providers, payers, patients and regulators (Heikkinen et al. 2009). This then leads to many economic dilemmas such as moral hazard, orthogonal considerations pertaining to cost versus quality and information asymmetry which in turn have the potential to create obstacles in an attempt to deliver efficient and effective healthcare (Wickramasinghe and Bali 2008; Wickramasinghe 2008; Wickramasinghe et al. 2007). In order to ameliorate these problems, relevant data, pertinent information and germane knowledge play a vital role and can only be obtained via the prudent structure and design of technology (WHO-EMRO http://www.emro.who.int/his/ehealth/ehealthPlan.htm; Brailer and Terasawa 2003; Gronlund 2002). Of equal significance are the major challenges facing today's healthcare organizations; i.e., demographic challenges, technology challenges, and finance challenges (Wickramasinghe and Goldberg 2007; Wickramasinghe and Lichtenstein 2006; Sharmaet al. 2006; Von Lubitz and Wickramasinghe 2006; Wickramasinghe 2006).

Demographic challenges are reflected by longer life expectancy and an aging population; technology challenges include incorporating advances that keep people younger and healthier; and finance challenges are exacerbated by the escalating costs of treating everyone with the latest technologies. Healthcare organizations should respond to these challenges by focusing on three key solution strategies, which taken together form the healthcare value proposition (Wickramasinghe and Goldberg 2007); namely:

1. Access – caring for anyone, anytime, anywhere;
2. Quality – offering world class care and establishing integrated information repositories;
3. Value – providing effective and efficient healthcare delivery.

These three components are interconnected such that they continually impact on the other and all are necessary to meet the key challenges facing healthcare organizations today. In such a context it is yet again only through the judicious application of technology solutions that effect superior healthcare delivery (Wickramasinghe and Goldberg 2007; Wickramasinghe and Lichtenstein 2006).

Healthcare to date has been shaped by each nation's own set of cultures, traditions, payment mechanisms and patient expectations. Therefore, when looking at health systems throughout the world it is possible to place them on a continuum from high to essentially 100% government involvement at one extreme to little or essentially 0% government involvement at the other extreme. However, given the common problem facing healthcare globally; i.e., exponentially increasing costs, no matter which particular health system one examines, the future of the healthcare industry will be shaped by commonalties based on this key unifying problem and the common solution; namely, the embracing of ICT and thereby developing an e-health focus. In turn, this common problem and application of the common solution will bring with it three key future trends, including; (a) empowered consumers, (b) e-health adaptability and (c) shift to focus on healthcare prevention, as well as four key implications, including; (a) health insurance changes, (b) workforce changes and changes in the roles of stakeholders within the health system, (c) organizational changes and standardization and (d) the need to make difficult choices.

Currently, most if not all countries begin to analyse and evaluate what is essential to reform their own healthcare delivery system. The common solution appears to focus on the embracing of ICTs in particular some type of electronic medical record system (Suomi 2009). However, in order for such a solution to be truly beneficial it is necessary to critically evaluate the fundamental elements that must be considered to ensure sustainability and key metrics to ensure it does indeed support value driven patient centric healthcare. To date no such book (to the best of our knowledge) has attempted to do this. Thus, we set out to bring together a collection of articles that focus on the key issues, critical success factors, barriers and facilitators related to sustainable electronic health records and thereby superior healthcare delivery. Moreover we invited experts in these respective areas and disciplines to contribute thereby making this compilation a collection of discussions and discourses on the state of the art from leading scholars.

Specifically, this book, presents various chapters that investigate the impact of adopting and implementing ICT in various health systems globally, and thus serves to (a) provide an understanding of the impact of ICT in healthcare delivery and how adapting to e-health impacts the healthcare industry and the various organizations within the healthcare industry, (b) identify the major barriers and facilitators related to ICT design, development and diffusion in the healthcare sector and (c) identify the major drivers and key success factors as well as to determine the implications on the healthcare industry at both the macro and micro level of the use of ICT to support value driven healthcare delivery.

The book consists of four sections: Innovation & Process, Design & Organisation, People and Information Systems and Information Technology. After a brief section introduction, the chapters in each section serve to discuss past, present and future implications; thus taken together they describe key issues necessary for the sustainability of prudent e-health solutions. This book then provides a thorough and far reaching analysis of key areas that must be considered when designing and developing superior e-health solutions. The book is as relevant for academics and scholars, the myriad of healthcare practitioners, consultants, graduate students and anyone who is desirous to have a complete understanding of the drivers, barriers and facilitators of successful e-health solutions. We hope our readers enjoy this book at least as much as we have enjoyed compiling it for you. We know you will find it a most invaluable resource.

Nilmini, Raj, Reima & Stefan
The Editors

References

Wickramasinghe, N., Bali, R., &Schaffer, J. (2008a). The health care intelligence continuum: Key model for enabling KM initiatives and realizing the full potential of SMT in healthcare delivery. *International Journal of Biomedical Engineering and Technology (IJBET)*, *1*(4), 415–427.

Wickramasinhge, N., Bali, R., Gibbons, C., & Schaffer, J. (2008b). Realizing the knowledge spiral in healthcare: The role of data mining and knowledge management. *Studies in Health Technology and Informatics*, *137*, 147–162.

The Oslo Declaration on Health, Dignity and Human Rights (2003). 7th Conference of European Health Ministers, Oslo, Norway 12–13 June 2003, http://odin.dep.no/hod/norsk/aktuelt/taler/monister/042071-990209/dpk-bn.html.

Global Medical Forum Foundation (2005). GMF IV: New Frontiers in healthcare 4–6 April 2005. http://www.globalmedicalforum.org/gmf_iv/session3.asp.

World Health Organization (1998). A health telematics policy in support of WHO's health-for-all strategy for global health development: Report of the WHO Group Consultation on Health Telematics, 11–16 Dec 1997. Geneva: World Health Organization.

E-Health in the eastern Mediterranean, WHO-EMRO, http://www.emro.who.int/his/ehealth/ehealthPlan.htm.

Brailer, D. J., & Terasawa, A. B. (2003). Use and adoption of computer-based patient records, California HealthCare Foundation (pp. 1–42).

Gronlund, T. (2002). ERDIP: HER issues and lessons learned report: Notes for the national workstreams (Final Version), National Health Service Information Authority, Birmingham (pp. 1–37).

Wickramasinghe, N., Geisler, E., & Schaffer, J. (2005). Realizing the value proposition for healthcare by incorporating KM strategies and data mining techniques with the use of information communication technologies. *International Journal of Healthcare Technology and Management*, in press.

Wickramasinghe, N., & Bali, R. (2008). Controlling Chaos through the application of smart technologies and intelligent techniques. *International Journal of Risk Assessment and Management*, *10*(1–2), 172–182.

Wickramasinghe, N. (2008). Building a learning healthcare organisation by fostering organisational learning through a process centric view of knowledge management. *International Journal of Innovation and Learning*, *5*(2), 201–216.

Wickramasinghe, N., Puentes, J., Bali, R.K., & Naguib, R. (2007). Telemedicine trends and challenges: A technology management perspective. *International Journal of Biomedical Engineering and Technology (IJBET)*, *1*(1), 59–72.

Wickramasinghe, N., & Goldberg, S. (2007). Adaptive mapping to realisation methodology (AMR) to facilitate mobile initiatives in healthcare. *International Journal of Mobile Communications*, *5*(3), 300–318.

Wickramasinghe, N., & Lichtenstein, S. (2006). Supporting knowledge creation with E-Mail. *International Journal of Innovation and Learning*, *3*(4), 416–426.

Sharma, S., Wickramasinghe, N., Xu, B., & Ahmed, N. (2006). Electronic healthcare: Issues and challenges. *International Journal of Electronic Healthcare*, *2*(1), 50–65.

Von Lubitz, D., & Wickramasinghe, N. (2006). Networkcentric healthcare: Applying the tools, techniques and strategies of knowledge management to create superior healthcare operations. *International Journal of Electronic Healthcare (IJEH)*, *4*, 415–428.

Wickramasinghe, N., Geisler, E., & Schaffer, J. (2006). Realizing the value proposition for healthcare by incorporating KM strategies and data mining techniques with the use of information communication technologies. *International Journal of Healthcare Technology and Management*, *7*(3/4), 303–318.

European commission (2008). White paper together for health: A strategic approach for the EU 2008–2013.

Suomi, R. (2009). Governing health care with IT. In J. Tan (Ed.) *Medical informatics: Concepts, methodologies, tools and applications*. Information Science Reference, Hershey, USA, 1658–1668. ISBN 978-1-60566-050-9.

Heikkinen, K., Suomi, R., Jääskeläinen, M., Kaljonen, A., Leino-Kilpi, H., & Salanterä, S. (2009). The creation and evaluation of an ambulatory orthopaedic surgical patient education website to support empowerment. Computers in Nursing. Forthcoming.

Suomi, R., Serkkola, A., & Mikkonen, M. (2007) GSM-based SMS time reservation system for dental care. *International Journal of Technology and Human Interaction*, *3*(3), 54–68.

Acknowledgements

This book would not have been possible without the cooperation and assistance of numerous people: the contributors, reviewers, our respective institutions, our colleagues, students and the staff at Springer. In today's networked environment when we are not co-located but distributed across various continents and continually meeting the challenges of the respective local demands on our time, we are especially appreciative to all the contributors and reviewers for not only your timely responses but also the high quality of your submissions and feedback. Finally, we would especially like to thank the production staff at Springer, in particular Khristine Queja and Kathryn Hiller, for all their efforts in helping us to make this book possible.

Contents

Contributors

Nilmini Wickramasinghe who currently holds the Epworth Chair Health Information Management was appointed in Dec 2009 as a Professor to RMIT University's School of Business IT and Logistics after being a professor in the US for 15 years. She researches and teaches in several areas within information systems including knowledge management, e-commerce and m-commerce, and organizational impacts of technology with particular focus on the applications of these areas to healthcare and thereby effecting superior healthcare delivery. Professor Wickramasinghe is well published with more than 200 referred scholarly articles, several books and an encyclopedia. She has collaborated with many large organizations such as NASA and GE as well as leading healthcare organizations such as the Cleveland Clinic, Johns Hopkins, Kaiser and NorthWestern Memorial Hospital. In addition, she regularly presents her work throughout North America, as well as in Europe and Australia. Professor Wickramasinghe is the editor-in-chief of two scholarly journals: *International Journal of Networking and Virtual Organisations* (IJNVO – www.inderscience.com/ijnvo) and *International Journal of Biomedical Engineering and Technology* (IJBET- www.inderscience.com/ijbet) and the Springer Series editor for Healthcare Delivery in the Information Age.

Dr. Rajeev K. Bali is a Reader in Healthcare Knowledge Management at Coventry University. His main research interests lie in clinical and healthcare knowledge management (from both technical and organisational perspectives). He founded and leads the Knowledge Management for Healthcare (KARMAH) research subgroup (working under BIOCORE). He is well published in peer-reviewed journals and conferences and has been invited internationally to deliver presentations and speeches. He serves on various editorial boards and conference committees and is the Associate Editor for the International Journal of Networking and Virtual Organisations as well as the International Journal of Biomedical Engineering and Technology.

Reima Suomi is a professor of Information Systems Science at Turku School of Economics and Business Administration, Finland since 1994, and a part-time professor at Huazhong Normal University, Wuhan, Hubei, China. He is a docent for the universities of Turku and Oulu, Finland. Years 1992–93 he spent as a "Vollamtlicher Dozent" in the University of St. Gallen, Switzerland, where he led a research project on business process re-engineering. Currently he concentrates on topics around management of telecommunications, including issues such as management of networks, electronic and mobile commerce, virtual organizations, telework and competitive advantage through telecommunication-based information systems. Different governance structures applied to the management of IS and are enabled by IS belong too to his research agenda, as well as application of information systems in health care. Reima Suomi has together over 300 publications, and has published in journals such as Communications of the Association for Information Systems, CIN: Computers, Informatics, Nursing, Information & Management, Information Services & Use, Technology Analysis & Strategic Management, The Journal of Strategic Information Systems, Behaviour & Information Technology, Journal of Management History, Orthopaedic Nursing and Information Resources Management Journal. For the academic year 2001–2002 he was a senior researcher "varttunut tutkija" for the academy of Finland. With Paul Jackson he has published the book "Virtual Organization" and workplace development with Routhledge, London.

Stefan Kirn holds diploma degrees in management science from the "Universität der Bundeswehr München" (1976–1980), and in computer science (1984–1989) from the "Fern Universität Hagen", Germany. Since 2003, Stefan Kirn holds a chair on information systems at University Hohenheim at Stuttgart, Germany. His fields of research are software technology, information systems, and agent-based economics. Over the last 20 years, Stefan Kirn and his group have edited and co-edited 17 books, and they have published about 200 scientific articles, mainly in international journals, international conferences, and edited books. They have won several prices and awards from scientific institutions, from research funding organizations, from professional bodies, from conferences, and from industry. In addition, Stefan Kirn has also a high commitment to professional activities. Currently, he is CEO of the Hohenheim Research Center on Innovation Management and Service Industries. He is member of the board of several national and international scientific journals, a former Vice President of the German Computer Association, and one of the founders of the German Special Interest Groups in Computer Supported Cooperative Work, and in Distributed Artificial Intelligence. He is intensively involved in European research, in the organization of conferences, and he acts as a reviewer for numerous research funding organizations, for national and international governmental authorities, and for industry.

Mark Dominik Alscher is a graduate of the University of Freiburg (M.D. *magna cum laude*, 1990). He is Professor of Internal Medicine, the University of Tuebingen, Germany and director, department of Internal Medicine and Nephrology, Robert Bosch Krankenhaus (RBK), Stuttgart, Germany. He is the chief medical director of the RBK. He is a recognized authority in nephrology and internal medicine. His scientific interests center on peritoneal dialysis, clinical pharmacology, acute kidney failure and medical expert systems. He has led organizational projects at RBK such as reorganization of the ER, integration of medical IT into patient care and clinical research area. He is author or coauthor of more than 70 scientific articles and several book chapters in standard medical texts.

Dr. Vikram Baskaran is an Assistant Professor in the Ted Rogers School of Information Technology Management at Ryerson University. He is an engineer by profession with an interest in biomedical computing. His research interest is on finding a viable application of the KM paradigm in healthcare. His special interest in developing HL7 messaging and healthcare informatics has provided opportunities to excel in these fields. His current activities overlap KM, e-health, AI and healthcare informatics. He has been previously engaged in a wide area of industrial projects (software and engineering at the senior level).

Juerg P. Bleuer, MD, MPH Dr. Bleuer is Senior Consultant for healthcare knowledge and information management and general manager of Healthevidence GmbH, Berne, Switzerland and General practitioner FMH. He graduated in medicine with doctorate (1983) at the University of Berne; further training as general practitioner FMH (1994), Master of Public Health (2005). Scientific expert for medical IT at the Federal Office of Public Health (1987–90). Senior physician at the Institute of Social and Preventive Medicine, University of Berne and coordinator of an international Chernobyl research project (1994–97). Head of the evidence-based medicine department at the documentation service of the Swiss Academy of Medical Sciences DOKDI (1997–2000). Medical director of Mediscope AG (2000–02). Own consulting company for healthcare knowledge and information management. Various publications in the fields of medical IT and epidemiology.

Lodewijk Bos After a short career in the arts, Lodewijk Bos received an M.A., and had a career as an international conference organiser. In 2003 he started the International Congress on Medical and Care Compunetics. In 2004 he was founder of the International Council on Medical and Care Compunetics, ICMCC. Since 2006 Drs Lodewijk Bos is member of the Administrative Council of the WABT-ICET-UNESCO, charged with Strategic Planning and Programs. In 2010 he was appointed Editor-in-Chief of the Springer journal Health and Technology. Drs Lodewijk Bos is member of the advisory board of the Dutch diabetes web portal Mijn DVN; the IFMBE working Group on "Medical and Biological Engineering Contributions to the Safety and Security of Individuals and Society"; the IFMBE Ethics Committee; Member of the advisory board of the World Health Care Congress Middle East; Member of the advisory board of the World Health Care Congress Europe; the NEN normcommissie "Informatievoorziening in de zorg"; the advisory board of the European Privacy Institute. He is co-editor of the series on Medical and Care Compunetics (IOSPress) and series editor of "Communications in Medical and Care Compunetics" (Springer-Verlag).

Kurt Bösch Kurt is Head of the Competence Centre ECMS, Suva, Lucerne, Switzerland. He trained as a primary school teacher (1975–80), trained secondary technical teacher (1984–86), business data processing specialist with Federal diploma (2001), IT trainer, in charge of office automation, planning, implementation and management of RAD programming, IT project management (including InWiM). Head of the Competence Centre ECMS since May 2006.

Jan vom Brocke holds the Hilti Chair in Business Process Management at the University of Liechtenstein. He is Director of the Institute of Information Systems and President of the Liechtenstein Chapter of the AIS. Jan has more than 10 years of experience in BPM projects and has published more than 170 refereed papers in the proceedings of internationally perceived conferences and established IS journals, including the Business Process Management Journal (BPMJ), the Communications of the Association for Information Systems (CAIS) and Management Information Systems Quarterly (MISQ). He is author and co-editor of 15 books, including Springer's International Handbook on Business Process Management. He is a member in the EU Programme Committee of the 7th Framework Research Programme on ICT and serves as an advisor to a wide range of institutions. Jan is a visiting professor e.g. at the University of Muenster in Germany, the LUISS University in Rome, the University of Turku in Finland, and the University of St. Gallen in Switzerland.

Caroline De Brún (née Papi) graduated from University of North London in 1998, with an MA in Library and Information Studies. She has worked in various medical libraries, both physical and virtual, and gained experience in mental health, primary care, knowledge and health mangement, consumer health information literacy, and information skills training. She has co-written a book called Searching Skills Toolkit: Finding the Evidence and also a chapter for Healthcare Knowledge Management: Issues, Advances, and Successes. Caroline is currently working at the Royal Free Hampstead NHS Trust on the NHS Evidence Neurological Conditions and Gastroenterology and Liver Diseases Specialist Collections.

H. Czap born in 1945, studied Mathematics at Univ. of Wuerzburg (Germany), SUNY (Oneonta, NY, USA), Dundee (Scotland) and graduated 1974 with Ph-D. 1983 he became professor for Business Information Systems and 1985 chair for Business Information Systems at University of Trier (Germany). He was president and member of the board of directors of diverse international and national scientific associations. His scientific interests cover a broad range: systems theory, cost accounting, information systems, neural networks and multi-agent systems. He is author, editor or co-editor of 15 monographs and has published more than 100 papers.

S. Duennebeil is a research associate and PhD student at the Chair for Information Systems at the Department of Informatics, Technische Universität München (TUM) in Munich, Germany. He holds a Bachelor's Degree in Computer Science and Master's Degree in Information Systems. He worked in the Embedded Systems Industry, located in Thailand, Taiwan, The Netherlands and Germany, between 2004 and 2008. His research interests include e-health, Telemedicine, Market Engineering and IT-Security.

Julia Fernandes is a research assistant at the Chair of Information Systems 2, University of Hohenheim, Germany. She holds a diploma in economics from the

University of Hohenheim. Her research interest includes business process engineering and the application of information systems in health care, especially the field of ubiquitous and mobile computing.

Michael C. Gibbons, MD, MPH is an Associate Director of the Johns Hopkins Urban Health Institute and is an Assistant Professor at the Johns Hopkins' Schools of Medicine and Public Health. Dr. Gibbons' is an Urban Health expert and informatician who works primarily in the area of Consumer Health informatics where he focuses on using Health Information and Communications Technologies to improve urban healthcare disparities. He is an advisor and expert consultant to several state and federal agencies and policymakers in the areas of urban health, eHealth, minority health and healthcare disparities. Dr. Gibbons has been named a Health Disparities Scholar by the National Center for Minority Health and Health Disparities at the National Institutes of Health.

Dr. Chris Gonzalez is an Associate Professor and Director of the Genitourinary Reconstructive surgery fellowship program with the Northwestern University Department of Urology. He obtained his medical degree from the University of Iowa in 1994 and completed his general surgery and urologic residency training with the Northwestern University Medical School in 2000. He obtained his MBA degree from the Kellogg Graduate School of Management in 2006, and he currently serves as the Clinical Practice Director for the Northwestern Department of Urology. He also serves as the Administrative Chief for the Northwestern residency training program at the Jesse Brown Veterans Administration hospital in Chicago. In the area of hospital administration Dr. Gonzalez is a member of the Northwestern Medical Faculty Foundation Investment Committee, the Northwestern Memorial Hospital (NMH) Medical Executive Committee, Medical Director of the Surgical Unit Leadership model, and he is a Co-Chairman for the NMH Surgical Quality Oversight Committee. He recently completed a 3 year term as a member of the Northwestern University Feinberg School of Medicine Admissions Committee.

R. Halonen currently acts as a University Lecturer in the Department of Information Processing Science in the University of Oulu, Finland. She has worked both in the public sector and in private IT enterprises. She did her PhD about challenges in an inter-organisational information system implementation. After receiving her PhD she acted as a Postdoctoral Fellow in the Centre of Innovation & Structural Change, National University of Ireland Galway where she continues as a Research Associate while working in Finland. Lately she has studied ICT and social inclusion while continuing research on information systems.

Dr Amir Hannan is a full-time general practitioner in Hyde, UK. Developing a "Partnership of Trust" between patient and clinician, he has enabled over 800 citizens to access their GP electronic health record on-line, helping them to self care and become eMPOWERed. Presently he is Information Management & Technology lead for NHS Tameside & Glossop as well as Primary Care IT lead and Map of Medicine clinical lead for NHS North-West. He is a member of the Clinical Leaders Network, a member of the National Clinical Reference Panel for the Summary Care

Record, NHS Connecting for Health and an editorial board member for the Journal of Communication in Healthcare. Recently he set up an innovative health 2.0 website for his practice, www.htmc.co.uk putting patients and clinicians at the heart of healthcare and enabling "Real-time Digital Medicine".

Anna Heidebrecht is a research associate in the in the Department of Information Systems 2 at the University of Hohenheim. She obtained a Bachelor of Science degree in business administration and economics. Her research interests focus on agency theory and game theory in economics.

Wilfred Huang received the M.S. and Ph.D. degrees in Industrial Engineering from State University of New York at Buffalo, and B.S. degree in Industrial Engineering from Purdue University. He has been a faculty of Alfred University since 1983.Wil is the George G. Raymond Chair in Family Business and Professor of Management Information Systems at Alfred University. He is the director of Confucius Institute at Alfred University and the coordinator of SAP Program in Alfred University. He is also a certified quality engineer (CQE) of American Society of Quality and Cisco certified academy instructor (CCAI). His research interests include e-business and entrepreneurship. He has published articles in *Information & Management, IEEE Transactions on Engineering Management, International journal of Organizational Analysis, Family Business Review, European Journal of Operations Research, International Journal of Computers and Industrial Engineers, Decision Support Systems, etc.* He is the associate editor of the *International Journal of Modeling and Simulation (IJMS)* and *International Journal of Information Systems and Social Change.* He has been guest editor of *International Journal of Network and Virtual Organisations (IJNVO), Electronic Markets The International Journal, International Journal of Information Technology and Management (IJITM)* and *International Journal of Entrepreneur and Innovation Management (IJEIM).* Wil has been co-chairing the Wuhan International Conference on e-Business which takes place in Wuhan, China every summer since 2000.

Alexandra Karagiozis is a bachelor student of business education at the University of Hohenheim, Germany.

Prof. Dr. H. Krcmar is a full professor of Information Systems and holds the Chair for Information Systems at the Department of Informatics, TUM since 2002. He worked as Post Doctoral Fellow at the IBM Los Angeles Scientific Center, as assistant professor of Information Systems at the Leonard Stern School Business, NYU, and at Baruch College, CUNY. From 1987 to 2002 he held the Chair for Information Systems, Hohenheim University, Stuttgart. His research interests include Information and Knowledge Management, IT-enabled Value Webs, Service Management, Computer Supported Cooperative Work, and Information Systems in Health Care and eGovernment.

Irene Krebs born in 1951, received her M.Sc. degree in Computer Science from the Technical University of Dresden, she obtained her PhD degree in Engineering sciences from the Technical University of Cottbus, works as an academic staff member in the Chair of Information Systems in Enterprises at the Technical University of

Cottbus and as an Honorary Professor at the University of Potsdam; her research interests focus on computer applications in administration and eGovernment.

Vincent Lampérière is an ECMS specialist and solution architect at Suva, Lucerne, Switzerland. He graduated in mechanical engineering (1996). IT consultant (1997–2009). Senior software engineer (2001–2009). Certified in IBM FileNet P8 administration 4.5 and IBM FileNet P8 platform installation 4.5.

Tuomas Lehto is a PhD student (Information Systems) at the Department of Information Processing Science, University of Oulu, Finland. He has a versatile background in information systems and digital media. His main research interests lie within persuasive design and technology, (health) behavior change, and Web- and mobile-based information systems. He is a part of the OASIS (Oulu Advanced Research on Software and Information Systems) research group. His forthcoming doctoral dissertation is supervised by Professor Harri Oinas-Kukkonen.

J. Leimeister is a full professor, holding the Chair for Information Systems at Kassel University in Germany. He is furthermore a research group manager at the Computer Science Department at TUM. He runs research groups on Virtual Communities, eHealth, Ubiquitous/Mobile Computing and manages several publicly funded research projects. His teaching and research areas include IT Innovation Management, Service Science, Ubiquitous and Mobile Computing, Collaboration Engineering, eHealth, Online Communities, and IT Management.

Dr. Joerg Leukel is a senior researcher in the Department of Information Systems 2 at the University of Hohenheim. He obtained his doctoral degree in business information systems from the University of Duisburg-Essen. His research interests are in the areas of inter-organizational information systems, supply chain management, semantic interoperability, business ontologies, and service-oriented computing.

Christian A. Ludwig, M.D., M.H.A. is Chief Medical Officer, Suva, Lucerne, Switzerland. He graduated in medicine (1981) with doctorate (1982) at the University of Zurich; further training as internist FMH (1989), senior physician at Baden Cantonal Hospital (1989–1996), chief of staff at Berne's Inselspital (University Hospital, 1996–2001); Master of Health Administration (M.H.A., University of Berne, 1999); certificate in 'medical IT' from the German Association for Medical Informatics, Biometry and Epidemiology (GMDS) and the German Society of Informatics (DGI) (1999). Since 2001 Chief Medical Officer and Head of the Insurance Medicine Department at Suva, the Swiss National Accident Insurance Fund. In addition, lectureships at the medical faculty of the University of Berne. Various publications and book contributions in the fields of medical IT, healthcare management as well as social and insurance medicine.

Marco De Marco is full professor of Organization and Information Systems at the Università Cattolica in Milan. He also teaches the Business Organization course at the LUISS Guido Carli University in Rome. Before embarking upon his academic career he worked as a research engineer and product planning manager in the aerospace (Boeing) and computer (IBM, GE, and Honeywell) industries. He is the author of four books and numerous essays and articles; mainly on the development of information systems and the impacts of technology on organizations. Marco De Marco has worked as a consultant for a wide range of important public institutions, such as the Venice City Council, the Rome City Council, the Lombardy Regional Government, the Hospital Administration Authority, and the Ministry of Justice as well as the Italian Parliament. He has also been a consultant to the major trades unions of Italian bank employees. He is a member of the editorial board of several academic journals, including the *Journal of Information Systems, the Journal of Digital Accounting Research, Banking and Information Technology, Information Systems and e-Business Management.*

Fatemeh Moghimi is currently a PhD student in Information Systems in the RMIT University. Through her work experience in different industries as a system developer and analysis, she has acquired skills in fields such as implementing Business Intelligence, Data Mining, Data Warehouse, OLAP, ERP as well as IT solution selection for enterprises. Her academic research interests are in the area of health informatics, intelligent solutions and e-services. She has published in some national and international conference (HICSS, IITA, ICTM, EGMM, e-health symposium Hoehenheim) and journal (Economic & Management Journal, knowledge management) papers. Recently, she received IPRS (international postgraduate research scholarship) award from the Australian government.

Ulli Münch holds a diploma degree of information systems from the Georg-Simon-Ohm University of Applied Science in Nuremberg. Since October 2008 he works as research assistant at the Fraunhofer-Working Group for Supply Chain Services SCS a department of the Fraunhofer Institute of integrated circuits IIS. On the associated Center for Intelligent Objects ZIO he worked in the laboratory "Application Design and Implementation". Since middle of 2010 he leads the laboratory "Integration Platforms", which integrated RFID, WSN and RTLS into existing IT infrastructures.

Raouf N.G. Naguib is Professor of Biomedical Computing and Head of BIOCORE. Prior to this appointment, he was a Lecturer at Newcastle University, UK. He has published over 240 journals and conference papers and reports in many aspects of biomedical and digital signal processing, image processing, AI and evolutionary computation in cancer research. He was awarded the Fulbright Cancer Fellowship in 1995–1996 when he carried out research at the University of Hawaii in Mānoa, on the applications of artificial neural networks in breast cancer diagnosis and prognosis. He is a member of several national and international research committees and boards.

Apl. Prof. Dr.-Ing. habil. Arnim Nethe born 1963, studied at the Technical University Berlin electro-technology, after his graduation he came to the Brandenburg Technical University Cottbus, where he get his venia legendi in 1999 in the subject theoretical electro-technology. He has researches in electromagnetic field theory and is specialized in medical technology. He is action field representative of the federal state government for the master plan health region Berlin Brandenburg in the action field medical technology and telemedicine.

Pirkko Nykänen is professor in health informatics at the University of Tampere, School of Information Sciences and Technology (www.cs.uta.fi). She has been working as a senior researcher in VTT Medical Engineering Laboratory (1975–2000), as a development manager in the National Institute for Health and Welfare (2000–2003). She has been a visiting researcher in Lille University, Medical Informatics, France (1994) and in the Pennsylvania State university, School of Information Science and Technology USA (2000–2001). Her major research topics cover eHealth systems, ontologies and interoperability aspects of Health IT, evaluation theories and methods for e-Health systems and services. She has been involved in many international research activities, in review of international journal articles and conference papers, and she has more than 150 publications in the medical and health informatics domain.

Michael L. Popovich has over 37 years of applied engineering and information technology consulting in support of health, environmental, transportation, and defense planning projects. He is the founder and CEO of Scientific Technologies Corporation, established in 1988, which provides health information technology strategic planning, solutions, and services to local, state, federal and international governments. Mr. Popovich was instrumental in developing standards and Health Information Technology solutions for population-based immunization registries, working closely with the U.S. CDC, private foundations, and state governments. Mr. Popovich received his MS in Systems Engineering and BS in Engineering Mathematics from the University of Arizona.

Professor Pekka Puska is currently the Director General of the National Public Health Institute of Finland (KTL). KTL is a comprehensive national public health institute under Ministry of Health in Finland. Prior to his present position professor Puska was the Director for Noncommunicable Disease Prevention and Health Promotion at the World Health Organization Headquarters in Geneva. His previous work in Finland and nternationally was strong background when he helped WHO to upgrade its work to respond to the rapid increase of chronic noncommunicable diseases (NCDs) in many parts of the world. At WHO, Pekka Puska directed the work on integrated prevention of NCD targeting the main risk factors (tobacco, unhealthy diet and physical inactivity) through broad health promotion, national programmes, policy measures and regional networks. Professor Puska's Department also worked on school health & youth health promotion, ageing and life-course, health behaviour surveillance, oral health, evidence in health promotion etc. Professor Puska's Department was the focal point of this work that culminated in adoption of the Global Strategy on Diet, Physical Activity and Health by the World Health Assembly in 2004. Practical programmes at WHO included the global QUIT AND WIN (Smoking cessation campaign), coordinated by KTL in Finland. Before joining WHO, professor Puska has, for most of his career, worked at the National Public Health Institute as Director of the Department of Epidemiology and Health Promotion. He was, for 25 years, the Director and Principal Investigator of the North Karelia Project: prevention of cardiovascular diseases in the province and later on in all Finland.Professor Puska has, internationally, been involved in a number of scientific, expert and public health functions e.g. scientific conferences, WHO's expert work, international consultations, multinational research projects etc. He has over 500 scientific publications in the field of epidemiology, preventive medicine, health promotion and public health. Professor Puska has served as a Member of the National Parliament of Finland, as well as the Elector of the President of the Republic. In his current position as Director General of the National Public Health Institute (KTL) professor Puska has a central position in Finnish public health work and health policy, while he also maintains a number of international commitments. Among other things, he is currently the chair of National Nutrition Council, the President of Finnish Heart Association and chair of the Board of the UKK Institute for health promotion. Internationally, Professor Puska is the President elect of World Heart Federation and the Vice-President of the International Association of National Public Health Institutes (IANPHI). The association links the national public health institutes of the world and helps countries to establish or develop their institutes to strengthen the national public health infrastructure. Professor Puska also represents Finland in the Governing Council of the WHO International Agency for Cancer Research (IARC).Professor Puska has M.D and M.Pol.Sc. degrees and PhD in epidemiology and public health. Among several honours are Honorary Doctorate at St. Andrew's University (Scotland) and Academician of Russian Academy of Natural Sciences. He has received, among other things, WHO's annual Health Education Award in 1990, WHO Tobacco Free World Award in 1999, the Nordic Award for Public Health in 2005, and the Rank Prize in 2008.

Reetta Raitoharju has her Doctoral degree in Economics and business administration. Her main research interests are in the field of health informatics, especially in adoption of IS in health care. She has worked in various teaching and research positions and published several articles in the field of health informatics. She currently works as a principal lecturer in Turku University of Applied Sciences, Finland.

Francesca Ricciardi is a lecturer in "ICTs and the Information Society" at the Catholic University, Milan, Italy.Her research interests span themes such as e-health, e-government, territorial networks, network ecology and ecology of knowledge.As for e-health, she wrote in particular on the possible role of Information Systems to address the challenge of population ageing; in the e-government field, she focused on the relationship between technological and organizational innovation within PA bodies; as for territorial networks, she published writings on destination management mainly; her interest in network ecology results in works on inter-firm cooperation and supply chain management; her last work in the field of ecology of knowledge is: "The ecology of learning-by-building: bridging design science and natural history of knowledge", in Global Perspectives on Design Science Research, Springer 2010. Before dedicating herself to research and teaching, she has been working as a consultant in the fields of processes re-engineering in health care and facility management, Information Systems analysis, organizational innovation and Human Resources.

Simone Schillings is research assistant at the University of Hohenheim, Chair for Information Systems 2, Germany. After working for an international automobile group between 1999 and 2001 she studied economics at the University of Hohenheim following her diploma in 2007 on process oriented calculation of outpatient services. Her research interests are in the field of service production and engineering in ehealth as well as business process modeling.

Dr. Martin Sedlmayr is senior researcher at the Chair of Medical Informatics at the University of Erlangen-Nuremberg. He studied computer science at the University of Ulm. Following his diploma on process-adequate visualization for integrated anesthesiological workplaces in 1999 he worked at the Research Institute for Applied Knowledge Processing (FAW, Ulm) until 2002 and at the Fraunhofer-Institute for Applied Information Processing (FIT, Sankt Augustin). Focusing on weakly structured domains, he developed concepts and tools for process- and knowledge-management in which process knowledge synergizes with ICT and usability. He was developer, software architect and technical coordinator in various European and national multidisciplinary projects. After receiving a Ph.D. for his thesis on modeling and automating clinical guidelines in intensive care in 2008 he moved to Erlangen to develop a clinical service platform based on wireless sensor networks.

Juergen Seitz received his diploma in business administration and business information systems from the University of Cooperative Education Stuttgart, nowadays, Baden-Wuerttemberg Cooperative State University Stuttgart, Germany, and in economics from the University of Stuttgart-Hohenheim. He received his Ph.D. from Viadrina European University, Frankfurt (Oder), Germany. He is professor for business information systems and finance, and chair of the business information systems department at Baden-Wuerttemberg Cooperative State University Heidenheim, Germany. Dr. Seitz is editor, associate editor and editorial board member of several international journals. He is member of Gesellschaft für Informatik (German association) and an executive council member of Information Resource Management Association, USA. He was and is member of the program or organizing committee of several international conferences, e. g. the 10th Wuhan International Conference on E-Business 2011.

Antto Seppälä, M.Sc. Is a PhD student in at the University of Tampere, School of Information Sciences and Technology (http://www.cs.uta.fi/). His PhD work focuses on citizen-centred care paradigms, personal wellness systems development, information modeling and ontology development. He has also worked as a research in the University of Tampere, e-Health research group since 2006. His major research topics are health information systems development, personal health systems, interoperability aspects of health IT and ontologies. He has been involved in some national and international research and development projects, and publications related to the medical and health information domain.

Hidayah Sulaiman is currently undertaking her PhD at Royal Melbourne Institute of Technology – RMIT University, Melbourne, Australia on the assimilation of Healthcare Information Systems in a Malaysian hospital context. She was a software engineer in one of Malaysia's leading telecommunication service provider before changing her career path from industry to academia in 2002 at Tenaga Nasional Universiti Malaysia (UNITEN). She earned her MSc in Computer Science-Software Engineering from Universiti Putra Malaysia (UPM). Her research areas of interest include healthcare information systems, e-health, IT Governance and organization best practices.

Daniele Talerico is a coftware engineer at Suva, Lucerne, Switzerland and graduated in computer science with master of science (2003) at the University of Berne.. Consultant at Deadalos Consulting AG, Zurich (2001–03). Software-engineer at Bison Schweiz AG, Sempach (2004–08). Since 2008 software engineer at Suva.

Dr. Say Yen Teoh is a lecturer of Business Information Technology in the RMIT University, Australia. Dr. Teoh's primary research interest is to explore the effective and efficient use of medical informatics relating to the strategic innovative development, promotion and use of the system. Currently, her publications have appeared in the *Information Systems Frontiers,* Journal of Systems and Information Technology, Journal of Enterprise Information Management, Journal of Information Technology Management, with a few book chapters published with ICEG Publisher, World Scientific Publisher, IRM Press, and other conferences such as European Conference on Information Systems (ECIS); Pacific Asia Conference on Information Systems (PACIS).

Dr. L. Waehlert Personal data: born on 11.07.1967 in Herborn.Academic career: study of economics at the University of Trier (Diploma 1992), Graduation with PhD (1996) and Habilitation with venia legendi for economics (2004). Since 2004 she works as Private Lecturer for economics at the University of Trier and since 10/2008 as research associate in a scientific project at the University of Trier. Scientific interests: Organizational research, Systems Theory, Business Ethics, Healthcare Management.

Yu Yun is a student of successive postgraduate and doctoral programs in Resources Economics from China University of Geosciences (Wuhan) in China. From October, 2009 to April, 2010, she was a Visiting Scholar at Alfred University in USA. Her research interests include mineral resource economics and e-business. She has published 13 articles in the chinese core learned periodicals in China, include in China Population Resources & Environment, Theory Monthly, Hubei Social Sciences, etc.

Hossein Zadeh holds the position of Senior Lecturer and Program Director at RMIT University. He has researched and published in Multicrew Optimisation and Decision Support Systems, linking the diverse fields of engineering, management, and IT, attracting over $1,000,000 in grants, awards, scholarships and contracts, from organisations such as the Australian Research Council and the Australian Department of Defence.Hossein has taught in Australia, Hong Kong, Vietnam, Singapore, and Sweden, and is the recipient of 2008 University Team Teaching Award and 2009 Certificate of Achievement in innovative teaching. Hossein's current research focuses on educational and healthcare services as pillars of most modern (service) economies.in 2004, Hossein was a visiting scholar at Linkoping University, Sweden, and in 2009/2010, was a Distinguished Visiting Scholar at IBM Almaden Research Labs, USA. Hossein is the recipient of the prestigious 2010 IBM Faculty Award.

David Zakim is a graduate of Cornell University [B.A. chemistry, 1956] and The State University of New York, Brooklyn, N.Y. [M.D. *summa cum laude*, 1961]. He trained in internal medicine and gastroenterology at The New York Hospital- Cornell Medical Center. After 3 years in the U.S. army, he began his academic career at the University of California San Francisco [1968] and moved in 1983 to Cornell University Medical College as Vincent Astor Distinguished Professor of Medicine and Director of the Division of Digestive Disease at The New York Hospital. He is the founding editor of *Hepatology: A Textbook of Liver Disease*, now in its 5th edition. He is author or co-author of more than 160 articles in biochemistry and biophysics of drug metabolism. He holds several patents for applications of spectroscopy and computing to diagnosis and management of human disease. DZ is Professor of Medicine emeritus from Cornell.

Xiaohui Zhang, PhD, MS Chief Scientist, Scientific Technologies Corporation, has led the scientific effort in the development of infectious disease surveillance systems, disease outbreak early detection and early warning systems, information systems supporting organized population-based screenings, public health emergency preparedness and response systems, and information systems for supporting comprehensive health care management for children enrolled in Medicaid. Dr. Zhang holds a PhD in resource management focusing on high performance modeling and simulation, and an MS in systems engineering, both from the University of Arizona. He has a BS in Electrical Engineering from the Beijing University of Aeronautics and Astronautics.

Manuel Zwicker (MBA, Diploma in Business Information Systems) is a PhD student at Royal Melbourne Institute of Technology (RMIT University), Australia. His research is in the area of business information systems, especially in the area of e-health. He received his MBA from ESB Business School, Reutlingen, Germany and his diploma degree from University of Cooperative Education Heidenheim, Germany (nowadays Baden-Wuerttemberg Cooperative State University Heidenheim, Germany). During his studies, he decided to participate in different exchange programs with universities in USA, Poland, Denmark and Mexico. Furthermore, he worked in a German financial institute for several years.

Section I
Innovation and Process Considerations in the Role of IS/IT in e-Health

Nilmini Wickramasinghe

Without IS/IT e-health would not be possible, in fact it is the advances in computers and computing capability that have been the genesis of e-health while the continued advances in IS/IT capabilities keeps fuelling the growth in the plethora of e-health possibilities. Thus, to understand e-health it is essential and of paramount importance to understand appreciate the role and potential of IS/IT to facilitate the delivery of superior healthcare hence this section is devoted to an examination of the role of innovation and process at both the macro and micro levels. Naturally, in a book of this size it is not possible to come close to covering all the possibilities and issues regarding IS/IT in e-health but this section provides a miscellany of chapters that address some very key areas.

Chapter 1 "Improving e-performance management in healthcare using intelligent IT solutions" by Moghimi and Wickramasinghe discusses the issue of e-performance in e-health services and the opportunities enabled through the incorporation of business intelligences and business analytic tools.

Chapter 2 by Mogihim, Zadeh and Wickramasinghe examines the issues of using an intelligence risk detection framework to improve decision efficiency in healthcare contexts. In their chapter they discuss the benefits of such an approach in the orthopaedic operating room.

Chapter 3 "Healthcare Information Systems Design Using a Strategic Improvisation Model" by Theoh and Wickramasinghe changes focus form IT issues to predominantly IS considerations. In particular this chapter proposes how taking a resource-based view coupled with techniques of bricolage can facilitate better HIS design, implementation and usage.

Chapter 4 by Sulaiman and Wickramasinghe continues to explore important issues regarding design, implementation and use of HIS. In particular this chapter discusses the key aspects that contribute to successful HIS assimilation.

Chapter 5 "e-health in China" by Yun, Huang, Seitz and Wickramasinghe presents a macro analysis of the level of e-health preparedness in China. In particular an area of importance that is currently weak for China, as discussed in the chapter, pertains to the level of ICT infrastructure.

Chapter 6 "improving the process of healthcare delivery in an outpatient environment: the case of the urology department" by Gonzalez and Wickramasinghe introduces the issues of process and design as critical for the ultimate realisation of superior healthcare operations. Process and design issues are so critical that later sections of this book are respectively devoted to them. This chapter serves to introduce some of these key issues and how they impact IS/IT considerations.

Chapter 7, the final chapter of this section, "adaptations for e-kiosk systems n Germany to develop barrier-free terminals for handicapped persons" by Zwicker, Seitz and Wickramasinghe introduces the human aspect into IS/IT considerations for e-health developments. People considerations and the human element is also of such significance, some would argue the most critical issue, that Sect. 3 in this book serves to delve deeper into various aspects of the human angle with regard to e-health. Chapter 7 serves to highlight that a well functioning IS/IT solution that doesn't take people issues into consideration can have significant consequences especially concerning use and acceptance.

Taken together these chapters then serve to provide illustrative insights into some of the critical aspects of IS/IT for e-health and more especially the role of process and innovation in order to develop superior healthcare solutions.

Chapter 1
Improving e-Performance Management in Healthcare Using Intelligent IT Solutions

Fatemeh Hoda Moghimi and Nilmini Wickramasinghe

Abstract Leading healthcare organizations are discovering the power of a performance management approach, driven by intelligent solutions (Hurst and Jee-Hughes 2001). Moreover, IT solution providers are nowadays developing and providing internet based electronic services (e-services) featuring various intelligent functions. This then necessitates the development of an e-performance management application to improve performance management efficiency in the healthcare area by using such intelligent e-services. Specifically, this chapter examines how a web based performance management application, will transform healthcare as hospitals strive to become more efficient in the way they manage their resources and deliver quality service. Through our proposed application, some services are being put into electronic form at an exponential rate with the result that information can be managed as never before. Such applications provide the possibility to engage clinical staff and patients and their families in decision-making, giving them greater responsibility for their own health. Thus, this chapter explores such technologies as business intelligence (BI) led realtime performance management, both as a concept and as a technology, and defines some of the associated knowledge driven health solutions followed by an e-performance management application.

Keywords Healthcare performance management • Business intelligence • Data mining • e-services • e-performance management

1.1 Introduction

The popularity of the web has made it a prime vehicle of disseminating information (Vaughan-Nichols 2002). The relevance of increasing performance management in the healthcare area using intelligent tools and web based services has led to a

F.H. Moghimi • N. Wickramasinghe (✉)
School of Business IT and Logistics, RMIT University, Melbourne, VIC, Australia
e-mail: nilmini.wickramasinghe@rmit.edu.au

N. Wickramasinghe et al. (eds.), *Critical Issues for the Development of Sustainable E-health Solutions*, Healthcare Delivery in the Information Age, DOI 10.1007/978-1-4614-1536-7_1, © Springer Science+Business Media, LLC 2012

3

significant body of recent research addressing some issues related to performance management efficiency. In this chapter, we try to review some issues regarding current performance management systems and suggest a web-based application using business intelligence to introduce some e-service into the healthcare context.

Although through this chapter we focus on identifying the role of business intelligent/analytics to enhance online and real time performance management efficiency, it is envisaged that in future we can find some more services or tools to improve performance management. When healthcare organizations look at making investments to improve patient care, they tend to look at funding staff or equipment-an MRI machine for example-rather than IT (Hope 2008). However, performance management solutions include activities to ensure that goals are consistently being met in an effective and efficient manner. Performance management can focus on performance of the organization, a department, processes to build a product or service, employees, etc. Information in this topic will give some sense of the overall activities involved in performance management.

In this chapter, healthcare performance management is presented after an introduction on business intelligence and its importance to improve performance management. Then, after reviewing current performance management issues, the role of an online and real-time solution is presented and a technical framework to designing an intelligence e-performance management is demonstrated.

1.2 Background

1.2.1 How Healthcare Manages Information

The proliferation of databases in every quadrant of healthcare practice and research is evident in the large number of claims databases, registries, electronic medical record data warehouses, disease surveillance systems and ad hoc research database systems (Wickramasinghe et al. 2008a). Pattern-identification tasks such as detecting associations between certain risk factors and outcomes, ascertaining trends in healthcare utilisation, or discovering new models of disease in populations of individuals rapidly become daunting even to the most experienced healthcare researcher or manager (Holmes et al. 2002).

From Fig. 1.1, we can see the central role of the ICT architecture as well as the far-reaching implications of data and information flows throughout this web and thus the importance of such data and information for the various key players. Maximizing these data and information assets then becomes a key need for healthcare organizations in order to realize their value proposition. This then is where the techniques of knowledge management, data mining and business intelligence become strategic necessities for healthcare (Wickramasinghe et al. 2008a).

Fig. 1.1 The web of primary
healthcare information flows
(Source: Wickramasinghe
et al. 2008b)

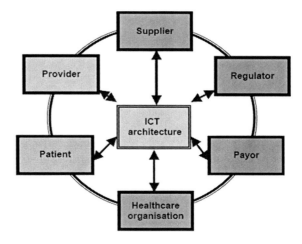

1.2.2   Business Intelligence/Analysis

Perhaps the biggest single evolutionary driver in the expansion of modern data
warehouse management is the democratization of business Intelligence. Where BI
was once the purview of specially trained business analysts who used sophisticated
software to slice-and-dice highly complex data sets, the advent of easy to use, multidimensional analytical applications have extended BI to the farthest corners of the
enterprise. Online Analytical Processing (OLAP), Google Docs, Service Oriented
Architecture (SOA) implementations and other developments have given-in some
cases mandated- BI availability to nearly everyone whose job description involves
some level of business management.

With the shift from backroom strategic application to essential daily management
tool comes the need for real-time, or near real-time, data collection (Friedman 2006).

It is important to note that true real-time, or instantaneous, data availability is
oftentimes more an ideal driven by perceived competitive pressures, than a necessary or even desirable goal (ASCI 2010). While many enterprises report that users
are demanding data refresh rates down to the millisecond, only those individuals
who depend on "business-aware" applications, in fields like production management or transactional processing, are likely to need such immediate and fluid information. Most operational applications, and nearly all BI tools, can fulfill their tasks
with periodic or near real-time data.

1.2.2.1   On-Line Analytical Processing (OLAP)

Typical manufacturing OLAP applications as a part of Business Intelligence/
Analytic solution include production planning and defect analysis. Important to all

of the mentioned tasks is the ability to provide managers with the information they need to make effective decisions about an organization's strategic directions. The key indicator of a successful OLAP application is its ability to provide information as needed, that is, its ability to provide "just-in-time" information for effective decision-making. This requires more than a base level of detailed data (Baragoin Corinne et al. 2001).

Just-in-time information is computed data that usually reflects complex relationships and is often calculated on the fly. Analyzing and modeling complex relationships are practical only if response times are consistently short. In addition, because the nature of data relationships may not be known in advance, the data model must be flexible. A truly flexible data model ensures that OLAP systems can respond to changing business requirements as needed for effective decision making.

Although OLAP applications are found in widely divergent functional areas, they all require the following key features (Baragoin Corinne et al. 2001):

- Multidimensional views of data
- Calculation-intensive capabilities
- Time intelligence

1.2.3   A Survey of Web Service Management Systems

Given the high rate of growth of the volume of data available on the WWW, locating information of interest in such an anarchic setting becomes a more difficult process every day. Thus, there is the recognition of the immediate need for effective and efficient tools for information consumers, who must be able to easily locate disparate information in the web, ranging from unstructured documents and pictures to structured, record-oriented data (Bhowmick Sourav. et al. 2004).

Web services are at a higher level of abstraction with respect to conventional middleware services, and therefore directly impact business-level metrics and need to be guided by them (Alonso et al. 2003). Management of Web services can be classified based on its scope. It's distinguished between infrastructure-level, application-level, and business-level (or business-oriented) management. Infrastructure-level management focuses on the Web services platform (Casati Fabio et al. 2003). So, to analyze Web services from Infrastructure-level management in a business perspective it is important to define and correlate metrics through interfaces, conversations, and compositions. The other important thing is that simplicity and flexibility in managing the manager are crucial. In fact, metrics and reports are not "static," and there is the frequent need to modify them to perfect the analysis and cope with changes (Casati Fabio et al. 2003). This means the best solution to increase the efficiency of the Web services is using a flexible report generator or business

Fig. 1.2 The performance measurement and management (Adapted from Nutley and Smith 1998)

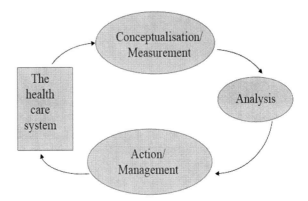

analysis in the back front. Data warehousing and business Intelligence are some effective solutions that can enhance the web services utilities.

1.2.4 Healthcare Performance Management

There are similarities and differences across many countries in performance management institutions, using "performance management" in a broad sense (Hurst and Jee-Hughes 2001). All countries rely heavily on professional licensure, self-regulation and peer review for controlling the quality of medical and nursing care. That is not surprising in view of the asymmetry of knowledge referred to above. Apart from that, the institutions of 'external' performance management differ widely between countries. The optimal role for external scrutiny is not yet well defined. Questions remain about who should be the recipients of performance indicators and what incentives there should be to act upon them (Hurst and Jee-Hughes 2001). Figure 1.2 depicts the key aspects.

There are signs that providers may be more responsive than other actors in the health care system are to such publication. However, publication can also have unintended and unwanted side effects. That is probably an inevitable consequence of the fact that the available measures of health outcomes and responsiveness are frail and incomplete. A possible implication is that 'external' review and peer review should be seen as complementary and used in a climate of co-operation (Hope 2008). Meanwhile, it is clear that the searches both for better indicators of the 'quality' of health care, and for a better understanding of what determines the behavior of the key actors in health systems, should go on. Based on literature review, although some countries are trying to apply performance management, they are faced with some limitations and challenges with on line and real time access usually being the most important of them.

1.3 Challenges Currently Facing Performance Management in Healthcare Area

1.3.1 Performance Indicators/Measures

A selective review of the performance indicators/measures being developed by WHO, OECD and each of the four OECD Member[1] countries, suggests that the development of indicators is proceeding at different speeds, in different areas of performance measurement (Hurst and Jee-Hughes 2001). Relatively slow progress is being made in the area of health outcomes. Moreover, such measures as do exist at a population level are usually proxies. Faster progress is being made with the development of indicators of the responsiveness of health services to consumers. There is slow progress with the development of equity indicators. There is also slow progress with the compilation of overall measures of the efficiency of health systems of a kind that command widespread confidence. The asymmetry of knowledge between health-care professionals, on the one hand, and health-care consumers and lay managers, on the other, seems here to stay for some time to come. Nevertheless, given the effort now being put into collecting performance indicators in many OECD Member countries, there seem to be good prospects for improving coverage of such indicators in OECD Health Data within the next few years. However, there may be a need for international harmonization of measures if comparative work is to proceed at an international level.

1.3.2 Controllable and Uncontrollable Variations

A key issue is how to discriminate between controllable and uncontrollable variations in performance (Hurst and Jee-Hughes 2001). As we have seen, that arises particularly in the area of health outcome measures, when health status measures are used as proxies for health outcomes. There is likely to be less of a problem with process 'measures' of outcomes or with measures of responsiveness. However, even here it may be require investigation and analysis to identify what levers must be pulled to improve performance. For example, poor quality in the service provided by a department in a globally budgeted public hospital may be due to inefficient working practices (which are the responsibility of local management), shortages of resources (which are the responsibility of the relevant funding body) or inappropriate national wage scales (which are likely to be the responsibility of central government).

---

[1] US, UK, Canada, Australia.

1.3.3 Aggregate the Indicators

Another issue, which faces all who devise sets of performance indicators, is whether or not to aggregate the indicators to provide composite or summary measures (Hurst and Jee-Hughes 2001). The main argument in favor of aggregation is that without it, those trying to monitor performance may drown in a sea of detail. The main argument against aggregation is that to the extent indicators reflect performance against different goals; aggregation requires adding 'apples' and 'pears'. Value judgments are required to weight different objectives, unless market prices or average unit costs can be used as weights. Moreover, if only summary indicators are published, the origin of variations in performance tends to be concealed. However, it is possible to publish both summary measures and their components.

1.3.4 Setting Standards or Benchmarks for Performance

The other issue is how to set standards or benchmarks for performance. One possibility – adopted recently by the UK – is to adopt certain ambitious but achievable targets for key areas of care, combined with a 'traffic light' system (Hurst and Jee-Hughes 2001). The national standards will include targets for key conditions and diseases, waiting times, the quality of care and efficiency. All NHS organizations will be classified as 'green', 'yellow' or 'red' on the basis of their performance. Red organization will be those failing to meet a number of the core national targets. 'Yellow' organizations will be those meeting all or most national core targets but would not be in the top 25% of performance. Green organization will be those meeting all targets and scoring in the top 25% of organizations on performance, taking account of 'value added'. The benchmarks will be reviewed periodically.

1.4 Using Business Intelligence as a Solution to Solve the Current Issues

There are three critical concepts of performance management: monitoring, analytics, and planning. With BI all three are brought together to help give everyone in the health organization the information they need to make informed decisions.

1.4.1 Monitoring

Quickly and easily enables the creation of dashboards and scorecards with its functional soft wares, so that everyone can align with departmental and organizational goals.

In addition, other aspects include: enabling automating the supporting processes, displaying process metrics and KPIs in Office Performance Point Server business intelligence software, and managing the workflow with Office SharePoint Server. Office SharePoint Server also lets the hospital share reports and analysis, and collaborate with colleagues.

1.4.2 Reporting and Analysis

This involves equipping the people with reporting and analysis tools and technologies that will help capture the structured and unstructured information they use to make decisions. In addition easy creation of reports and perform analysis with BI Reporting Services I supported. Moreover, pivot functionality and slice and dice techniques enables hospitals to look at data in different ways and drill down to explore trends. Of course, users can always count on Office Excel to manipulate data and create reports.

1.4.3 Data Warehouse

Features within the data warehouse support the obtaining of insights into the data needed through an integrated, centrally managed, and trusted data source. Many healthcare organizations are using data warehouses for data and records management, and so are already familiar with how easy it is to manage data in such a setting. In addition it is possible to combine data from multiple sources into one location and provide access to information, and even create an integrated data base.

1.5 Proposed Intelligent e-Performance Management Application

Today we are seeing the emergence of a powerful distributed computing paradigm, broadly called web services (Vaughan-Nichols 2001). In the healthcare domain, using web services will play a key role in dynamic performance management.

1.5.1 A Set of e-Services Recommended by Our Intelligent e-Performance Management Application

There are many ways BI can help clinical organizations manage their performance. Whether it's early detection of illness trends, understanding lab turnaround times, or meeting compliance and accreditation standards, having easy access to real-time information can help the organization take their progress to the next level. Below are some specific examples that show how healthcare organizations can use BI to better manage their organization's performance. (These services are recommended based on some provided tools by Microsoft business intelligence tools).

1.5.1.1 Service Line Analysis and Reporting

Healthcare organizations can use BI tools to conduct service line analysis and reporting. Analyzing and reporting on service lines allows the organization to accurately- and in real time-understand service inefficiencies, and improve the coordination of services, patient satisfaction, and the quality of care. Health organizations typically track and analyze performance metrics for health and wellness service lines (for example: weight management and nutrition), women and infant services, traditional lines of service (for example: musculoskeletal, orthopedic, and emergency), and chronic disease lines (for example: cancer, heart, and diabetes).

By using BI, organizations can analyze and report on service lines to help improve the quality and efficiency of medical service delivery, align with organizational goals, reduce costs, and improve margins.

1.5.1.2 Health and Wellness Service Line Management

BI can help healthcare organizations manage performance at all levels of operation, including the health and wellness service line. This service line includes wide-ranging programs such as those that build awareness about disease prevention and healthy lifestyles or that help individuals cope with specific health and well-being issues. Within the health and wellness service line, organizations look to improve disease prevention testing and adherence, analyze demographic information and trends to align service offerings, analyze recurring episodes of illness, and track immunization rates and disease outbreaks. Effective tracking and analysis of these indicators can help healthcare organizations reduce episodes of illness, improve outcomes, reduce costs, and improve patient satisfaction.

BI can help organizations better understand and track trends in health issues and health programs with easy access to real-time information. Healthcare professionals can drill down into the data to explore details behind the trends, allowing them to quickly respond and to adjust efforts.

1.5.1.3 Balanced Scorecard

Healthcare organizations are motivated to make performance management a part of their culture. BI tools help healthcare organizations use the Balanced Scorecard as a strategic management system to track organizational performance across financial, clinical, business process, and learning and growth measures. Once performance metrics are set, organizations identify the key drivers, or desired outcomes, and then define indicators to gauge progress.

By using BI to manage to key indicators, healthcare organizations can achieve consistent strategy execution and monitor performance. By tracking patient satisfaction, quality of care, financial performance, and enhanced learning and growth metrics, the Balanced Scorecard can provide a complete view of the organization. BI enables organizations to link together all the key elements of the Balanced Scorecard with easy-to-use templates and a single interface for viewing KPIs. Decision makers can track operational performance drivers and analyze financial, operational, and clinical KPIs across the organization with customizable scorecards for groups and individuals.

1.5.2 Technical Aspects of an Intelligent e-Performance Management Application

The intelligent e-performance management application (Fig. 1.3), technically, has three main components that they are:

- Information System Infrastructure
- A service based framework
- On-line data Access

Further, Data staging area, Data presentation area, Web based protocols and e-services are four different layer of the second component.

Through the intelligence e-performance application, data will be sent electronically from each GP's local systems to data warehouse. It will integrate with information from the both administrative and clinical sides, and arranged using online analytical processing cubes for rapid analysis. The results were then presented as a series of scorecards and key performance indicators on the authority's intranet by some dashboards, sharepoint or office performance points.

In the web based layer, we use gateways to controls the amount of server resources allocated to each traffic class. By dynamically changing the amount of resources it can control the response time experienced by each traffic class (Pacifici Giovanni et al. 2003).

In such an environment, a web service provider may provide multiple web services, each in multiple grades, and each of those to multiple customers. The provider will thus have multiple classes of web service traffic, each with its own characteristics and requirements.

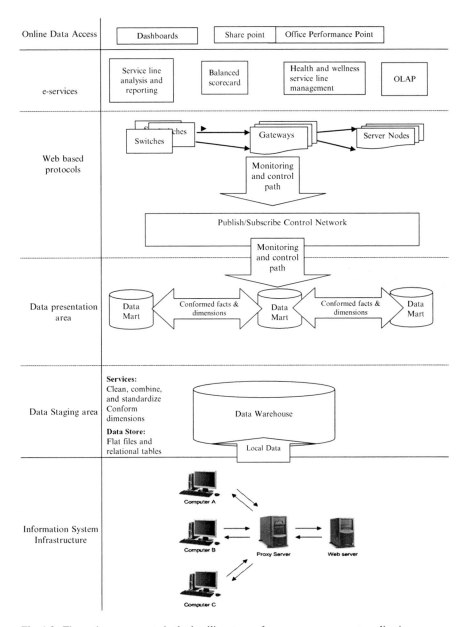

Fig. 1.3 The main components in the intelligent e-performance management application

1.6 Research Issues

We now summarize the research issues raised by the literature review and initial modelling and present only a brief description of the issue here, with details deferred to later publications.

First of all, we know that data in the web are typically semi structural (Buneman 1997). So, this nature of data may introduce a serious challenges to reiterative a data through a real-time and on-line data warehouse.

The other important issue is different between type and efficiency of such intelligence services in order to their solution providers. It means choosing a vendor is very important as well as choosing a solution. However, already some research is published in regard to this issue, although they are not completely relevant to choose such intelligence services providers. Designing some security levels and permissions through this application is the other significant issue in this research.

Moreover, although participants believed that the Internet could and should play an important role in the delivery of health services, there was a concern about the lack of evidence about the effectiveness of Internet delivered services. Our own review of the literature on e-health and e-mental health sites largely supports these concerns.

1.7 Conclusions and Future Research

Our chapter has served to identify the key role for business intelligence tools in healthcare. Our discussion of these intelligent solutions served to demonstrate an intelligence e-performance application enables the realisation of the performance management.

Hence, we believe that if healthcare organisations apply some e-services by data mining and business intelligence as some techniques, strategies and protocols, it will be possible for healthcare delivery to realise its value proposition of superior access, quality and value.

In future work, we will focus on developing an algorithm and model for online and real-time mining useful information for patients as well as clinical staffs from the proposed application with respect to knowledge discovery. We will try to improve our application to make it more intelligent and efficient to apply for remote disease management control using e- intelligent services.

References

Alonso, G., Casati, F., Kuno, H., & Machiraju, V. (2003). *Web services: Concepts, architectures, and applications*. Berlin: Springer Verlag.

ASCI (Advanced System Concept) Online Computer Library Center, (2010), ASCI Enterprise Job Scheduling Software white paper on A Strategic Pathway for Improved Data Warehouse/Business Intelligence Performance, [White paper]. Retrieved from http://whitepapers.technologyevaluation. com/view_document/21262/job-scheduling-a-strategic-pathway-for-improved-data-warehousebusiness-intelligence-performance.html.

Baragoin, C., Andersen, C., Bayerl, S., Bent, G., Lee, J., & Schommer, C. (2001). Business intelligence architecture: Mining your own business in telecoms using DB2 Intelligent Miner for Data,first edition, California, IBM Corp., chapter 2:p.17

Bhowmick, S., Madria, S., & Keong Ng, W. (2004). *Web data management*. New York: Springer.

Buneman, S. (1997), Semistructured data, Proceedings of the sixteenth ACM SIGACT-SIGMOD-SIGART symposium on Principles of database systems, New York, U.S.

Casati, F., Shan, E., Dayal, U., & Ming-Chien, S. (2003). Business-oriented management of web services. *Communications of the ACM, 46*(10), 55–60.

Friedman, T. (2006). Data integration identifies key usage trends. Gartner Inc, ID Number: G00138812, p. 3

Holmes, J., Abbott, P., Cullen, P., Moody, L., Phillips, K., & Zupan, B. (2002). Clinical data mining: Who does it, and what do they do? *AMIA, 9*(13), 62–65

Hope, J, (2008). Performance management in healthcare: Why Management Tools Don't Work, Cognos Innovation Center for Performance Management, p.7

Hurst, J., & Jee-Hughes, M. (2001). Performance measurement and performance management in OECD health systems. OECD publishing, 47(8). P. 27–31.

Pacifici, G., Spreitzer, M., Tantawi, A., & Youssef, A. (2003). *Performance management for cluster based web services.* IBM TJ Watson Research Center.

Vaughan-Nichols, S. (2001). Web services: Beyond the hype. *IEEE Computer, 35*, 18–21.

Vaughan-Nichols, S. (2002). Web services: Beyond the hype. *IEEE Computer, 35*, 18–21.

Wickramasinghe, N., Bali, R., & Schaffer, J. (2008a). The healthcare Intelligence Continuum: key model for enabling KM initiatives and realising the full potential of SMT in healthcare delivery. *Biomedical Engineering and Technology, 1*(4), 415–426.

Wickramasinghe, N., Geisler, E., & Schaffer, J. (2008b). Realising the value proposition for healthcare by incorporating KM strategies and data mining techniques with the use of information and communication technologies. *International Journal of Healthcare Technology and Management, 9*(3), 213–230.

Chapter 2
An Intelligence e-Risk Detection Model to Improve Decision Efficiency in the Context of the Orthopaedic Operating Room

Fatemeh Hoda Mogihim, Hossein Zadeh, and Nilmini Wickramasinghe

Abstract Decision making in healthcare is unstructured, complex and critical. Today, given the healthcare professionals are continually under immense time pressure to make appropriate treatment decisions. Moreover, in order to make such decisions it is necessary for them to process large amounts of disparate data and information. We contend that such a context is appropriate for the application of real time intelligent risk detection decision support system. To illustrate the benefits of risk detection to improve decision efficacy in healthcare contexts we focus on the case of the orthopaedic operating room for hip and knee replacements. In the orthopaedic operating room complex high risk decisions must be made which have for reaching implications on the success of the surgery and ongoing quality of life of the patient.

Keywords Data mining • Decision support system • Healthcare systems • Intelligent risk detection decision ˙ Knowledge discovery

2.1 Introduction

Effective decision making is vital in all healthcare activities. While this decision making is typically complex and unstructured, it requires the decision maker to gather multi-spectral data and information in order to make an effective choice when faced with numerous options (Wickramasinghe et al 2009a). Unstructured decision making in dynamic and complex environments is challenging and in almost every situation the decision maker is undoubtedly faced with information inferiority. The need for germane knowledge, pertinent information and relevant data are critical and hence the value of harnessing knowledge and embracing the tools, techniques, technologies and tactics of knowledge management are essential to

F.H. Mogihim • H. Zadeh • N. Wickramasinghe (✉)
School of Business IT and Logistics, RMIT University, Melbourne, VIC, Australia
e-mail: nilmini.wickramasinghe@rmit.edu.au

N. Wickramasinghe et al. (eds.), *Critical Issues for the Development of Sustainable E-health Solutions*, Healthcare Delivery in the Information Age,
DOI 10.1007/978-1-4614-1536-7_2, © Springer Science+Business Media, LLC 2012

ensuring efficiency and efficacy in the decision making process. Recognizing this Wickramasinghe and Schaffer (Wickramasinghe et al. 2009a) developed the Intelligent Continuum, a systematic approach that enables the application of knowledge management (KM) principles and tools necessary for improving the decision making processes in healthcare and to ensure that the healthcare decision making process outcomes are optimized for maximal patient benefit. The following research-in-progress attempts to extend this idea, specifically focusing on the case of hip and knee replacements in orthopaedic operating rooms, an area that is not only of significance but also involves multiple risks and critical decision making processes and hence an appropriate environment to demonstrate the benefits of our approach. This work focuses on answering the research question of how to incorporate real time intelligent risk detection into healthcare decision support systems.

2.2   Background

Hip and knee replacements are procedures performed frequently to relieve pain and improve function in patients with advanced hip and knee joint destruction (Davidson et al. 2008). The Australian Orthopaedic Association National Joint Replacement Registry (AOANJRR) (Davidson et al. 2008) categorizes hip replacements as either primary or revision procedures. Primary hip procedures are further categorized as partial or total hip replacements. Partial hips are further sub-categorized depending on the type of prostheses used; these are monoblock, unipolar modular and bipolar procedures. Similarly, there are a number of different categorizations for knee replacement procedures. What is important is that these categorizations are made correctly and this requires a correct evaluation and assessment of various multi spectral data and information (Wickramasinghe and Schaffer 2006).

In general, knee replacement is more common in females (56.0%). There are however gender variations depending on the type of procedure. The indication for almost all primary knee replacement procedures is osteoarthritis (partial resurfacing 90%, unispacer 100%, patella/trochlear 98.9%, uni-compartmental 98.8%, bicompartmental 100% and primary total 96.8%). The principal cause for revision knee replacement is loosening (36.5%) (Davidson et al. 2008).

The most common knee procedure is a primary total knee replacement (78.7% of all knee procedures recorded by the Registry). The proportion of other knee procedures is 12.2% for unicompartmental, 0.5% for patella/trochlear and 8.5% for revision procedures. There are a small number of procedures recorded for the other types of primary knee replacement, partial resurfacing (90), unispacer (39) and bicompartmental.

The mortality associated with hip replacement varies as shown at Table 2.1, depending on the category and there has been little change in mortality trends over the 2007. As would be anticipated, crude cumulative mortality of primary partial hip replacement is high (45.4%) compared to primary total hip (6.6%) (Davidson et al. 2008).

On the other hand, trends previously reported for mortality following knee replacement remain unchanged. The cumulative mortality varies according to the extent of the procedure. There were no deaths recorded for unispacer, partial resurfacing and

Table 2.1 Mortality following primary hip replacement by type (Based on Davidson et al. 2008)

Type of hip replacement	Number deaths	Number patients	Cumulative mortality (% deaths)	Standardised mortality	Person years	Rate per 100 person years	Exact 95% Cl
Bipolar	2,789	7,749	36.0	26.2	20,176	13.8	13.32, 14.35
Unipolar monoblock	9,048	15,810	57.2	14.5	32,973	27.4	26.88, 28.01
Unipolar modular	2,013	6,924	29.1	18.8	12,242	16.4	15.73, 17.18
Partial resurfacing	0	8	0.0	0.0	12	0.0	0.00. 30.76
Total resurfacing	83	9,143	0.9	0.6	29,291	0.3	0.23, 0.35
Thrust plate	2	140	1.4	0.5	581	0.3	0.04, 1.24
Conventional total	7,580	106,540	7.1	2.6	349,195	2.2	2.12, 2.22
Total	21,515	146,314	14.7	3.8	444,469	4.8	4.78, 4.91

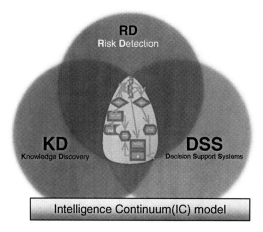

It is important to note that the proposed IRD model draws primarily from 3 significant bodies of literature, RD, KD and DSS and its foundations are derived from the IC model.

Fig. 2.1 The proposed IRD model

bicompartmental replacement. The cumulative mortality for patella/trochlear replacement is 2.3%, unicompartmental is 3.5% and primary total is 5.4% (Davidson et al. 2008). Hence, what on the surface seems to be simply a knee replacement is in reality much more complex. Table 2.1 summarises their issues.

In general total hip and total knee replacement surgeries are successful and very frequent procedures in the orthopedic or for people experiencing pain associated with degenerative joints. However the other types of partial hip and knee replacements are complex and involve with many different risk factors.

Since these risk factors are associated with decrease in quality of life (Dijkman et al. 2008), the importance of the decision making processes have increased significantly through hip and knee replacement.

In addition, Hip and knee implants are undergoing a constant state of innovation and improved technology (Wickramasinghe et al. 2009b). As can be seen, the critical decisions need to be made by both for orthopaedic surgeons and their patients.

Recognizing these risk factors, we have categorized the orthopaedic operating room issues, particularly hip and knee replacement, into four key components:

- Physiological issues followed by importance of quality of life.
- Technological issues based on new technologies and their performance.
- Biomechanical issues on conditions of patients' bones to do the surgery.
- Financial issues regarding the costs of these high-quality technologies and type of surgery.

We content therefore, that an Intelligence Risk Detection (IRD) model in support of better treatment decision making for this population of patients during and after surgery can provide superior healthcare outcomes for the patients and their families. In developing such a solution, it is necessary to combine three key areas of knowledge discovery, risk detection with decision support systems (Fig. 2.1). This is an important contribution to both theory and practice in healthcare.

2.3   Literature Review

The following section will outline the major issues pertaining to the key areas of decision support systems, risk detection and knowledge discovery and their importance to the design of our proposed real time intelligence risk detection model to improve healthcare decision making processes.

2.3.1   *Knowledge Discovery in Data Bases (KDD)*

Knowledge discovery in data bases (KDD) is defined as the nontrivial process of identifying valid, novel, potentially useful, and ultimately understandable patterns in data (Cios et al. 2007). One of the most relevant applications of KDD for healthcare contexts is the model of the Intelligence Continuum (IC) (Wickramasinghe et al. 2006). The IC model includes but is not limited to applying the techniques of data mining, business intelligence/business analysis (BI/BA) and knowledge management (KM) to facilitate superior healthcare delivery add here on IC model. In order to maximize the value/utility of our IRD model and because the combined techniques of DM, BA/BI and KM are essential in the present context, we use the IC model as the foundation for our model as shown in Fig. 2.1.

2.3.2   *Decision Support Systems (DSS)*

Even though research in decision support systems in healthcare is relatively established, the use of DSSs in medical diagnosis and clinical practice is set to increase tenfold within the next decades (Miller 1994). Fundamentally this research covers clinical and medical aspects typically focusing on how information technology emulates and improves decision-making effectiveness for individual physicians (Fieschi et al. 2003). Specifically, computer based decision support systems focus on any software designed to directly aid in clinical decision making in which characteristics of individual patients are matched to a computerized knowledge base for the purpose of generating patient-specific assessments or recommendations that are then presented to clinicians for consideration (Hunt et al. 1998). In addition, the computer-based patient record, the Internet, shared decision-making processes, and new regulations also facilitate medical decision support systems (Fieschi et al. 2003). Therefore, for the purpose of our research the literature pertaining to Clinical Decision Support Systems (CDSS) and Medical Decision Support Systems (MDSS) is equally relevant as integral to both is the use of computer systems to promote decision support to healthcare professionals.

Decision-making regarding surgery for patients who needs hip or knee replacements is especially multi-faceted and complex. Patients may have a variety of symptoms, but are often quite functional. It is appealing to lean towards a complete

Fig. 2.2 Decision making framework across orthopaedic operating room

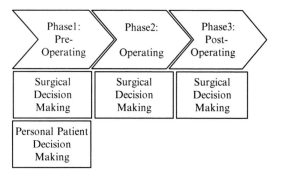

anatomical repair (Reddy et al. 1997). However, if the decision is for late repair, risks and benefits of surgery must be weighed against potential risks not proceeding with the surgery (Stamatis 2010). Moreover, the decision to treat replacement with either drugs, or surgery, or a combination of both depends on (Roy and Brunton 2008) a large number of factors.

The decision making process in the context of orthopaedic operating room can be divided into three phases (Fig. 2.2). In the first phase, or pre-operation phase, the surgeon, having received enough information about the patient and his/her medical condition, makes a decision relating to whether surgery is the best medical option. Once this decision has been made, and before surgery, the patients must decide whether to accept or reject the surgeon's decision in consideration of the predicted surgery outcomes. Once patients and surgeons have agreed to proceed, in phase 2, ad-hoc decisions pertaining to the unique situations during the surgery must be addressed. Finally, in the post operating phase, or phase 3, decision making is primarily done at two levels; level a, strategies to ensure a sustained successful result for the patient during aftercare and beyond, and level b, lessons to apply for future cases.

To capture this complexity, we define two steps of decision making in three different and key phases of the decision making process across orthopaedic surgery. The first type of decision making is called "surgical decision making" as it is primarily associated with the surgeons and the second type is called "personal decision making" as it is primarily associated with the patients because some surgery outcomes are related to "quality of life" that patients' decision is critical. Figure 2.2 shows the decision making framework we have developed based on the key phases in the orthopaedic operating room decision making process that it is required for our IRD model.

Although DSSs in the healthcare area is generally well discussed, unfortunately acceptance of such solutions tends to be low because doctors (the primary users) are reluctant to use computers (Baldwin 2001). Close consideration must also be paid to ensuring the clinical utility of any proposed solution. We contend that by incorporating real time risk detection the system is likely to then become more relevant and helpful which in turn will enhance its utility and thus adoption.

2.3.3 An Intelligence Risk Detection Framework in Healthcare Area

Surgical performance is usually indirectly measured by postoperative outcome of the initial hospital stay by means of risk-adjusted audits (Lacour-Gayet 2002). Although risk adjustment is important to assess performance and compare outcomes amongst individuals or institutions (Kang et al. 2004), statistical inferences alone cannot be used to determine what is considered acceptable performance (Gayet et al. 2005). Today's available methods look at the "big picture," from diagnosis to surgery and postoperative care (Larrazabal et al. 2007b). It is somewhat misleading, however, to judge an individual surgeon's performance by using postoperative outcome data such as 30-day survival or hospital survival (Larrazabal et al. 2007b). A poor outcome can be the result of a technical error, a nursing mistake, a drug error, or substandard intensive care monitoring (Larrazabal et al. 2007b).

Regarding to literature review, we find risk adjusters that meet these criteria have been under development since the 1980s and have been implemented by Medicare Choice program, numerous states, employer coalitions, and health plans (Keenan et al. 2001). Such systems have been based on many factors, including diagnosis, prior utilization, demographics, persistent diseases, and self-assessments of health and/or functional status. At Table 2.2, a review of selected risk adjustment systems in healthcare area is provided.

Table 2.2 A review of selected risk adjustment systems in healthcare area

Systems	Descriptions
ACG	This system was originally developed as a case-mix adjustment measure for ambulatory populations (Weiner et al. 1996). Later, it was extended to incorporate inpatient diagnoses as well. The system categorizes diagnoses based on duration, severity, etiology, diagnostic certainty and the likelihood that specialty services will be needed. ICD-9-CM codes are assigned to 32 ADGs (Adjusted Diagnostic Groups). The ACG system explains about 40–60% of the variation in concurrent health costs, and less for prospective health costs. The ACG system has been implemented by the Minneapolis Buyers Health Care Action Group. They reported a relatively smooth experience with the ACG system (Dunn 1998)
DCG	This system was developed as a health adjuster for HMOs that enroll Medicare populations (Pope et al. 2000; Ash et al. 2000). DCGs are clinically oriented and resource-based, and use demographic and diagnostic information. Initially, the model was calibrated on the Medicare population. It was later extended to commercial and Medicaid populations. This model estimates beneficiary health status (expected cost next year) from demographics and the worst principal inpatient diagnosis (principal reason for inpatient stay) associated with any hospital admission. The Washington State Health Care Authority also incorporated a DCG model

(continued)

Table 2.2 (continued)

Systems	Descriptions
CMS-HCC	CMS (Centers for Medicare and Medicaid Services) was required by Congress's BIPA (2000) to use ambulatory diagnoses in Medicare risk-adjustment, to be phased in from 2004 to 2007. To this end, CMS evaluated several risk-adjustment models that use both ambulatory and inpatient diagnoses, including ACGs (Weiner et al. 1996), the chronic disease and disability payment system (CDPS) (Kronick et al. 2000), clinical risk groups (CRGs) (Hughes et al. 2004), the clinically detailed risk information system for cost (CD-RISC) (Kapur et al. 2003), and DCG/HCCs (Pope et al. 2000). CMS chose the DCG/HCC model for Medicare risk adjustment, largely on the basis of transparency, ease of modification, and good clinical coherence
CDPS	The Chronic Illness and Disability Payment System was developed specifically to compensate more fairly for individuals with disabilities. It is a primarily resource-based system that is based on detailed clinical information for the disabled. The system has been developed for Medicaid and Medicare populations (Kronick et al. 2000, 2004). The system uses demographics and diagnostic information, and also used the length of enrollment, dates of services, type of provider, procedural information, and category of service. The model has over 700 diagnostic groups that are combined into over 50 diagnostic subcategories. The system predicts between 30% and 50% of the variance in a population with disability. However, it is important to note that this population is likely to have costs that easier to predict than the general population. The CDPS was implemented for the Medicaid population in Colorado. Plans did suffer from some selection, and required rates to be adjusted over time (Dunn 1998)
GRAM	The Global Risk Assessment Model is a clinically based, hierarchical model of health care use (Hornbrook and Goodman 1996). The model was developed on 100,000 individuals who were randomly selected from several HMOs. The model uses data on demographics, eligibility, diagnoses, and costs. The system uses Kaiser Permanente Clinical Behavioral Disease Classification System, which groups diseases by their clinical attributes and the expected responses to the disease. There are 350 diagnostic categories that are further grouped into 19 categories. The model explains 17% of the variance, or 70% of the explainable variance in prospective costs. This model has not been implemented to date
CRG	This system was developed to predict costs for individuals with congenital and chronic health conditions (Hughes et al. 2004). CRG is a categorical clinical system that classifies individuals into mutually exclusive categories and assigns each person to a severity level if he or she has a chronic health condition. The system uses demographic, diagnostic, and procedural information. The CRG grouper assigns each individual to a hierarchically defined health status group, and then to a specific CRG category and severity level if they are chronically ill. There are nine health status groups, and over 250 CRG categories. Unlike most other risk adjustment systems, the CRG is a categorical clinical model and not a regression model. The testing and refinement of CRGs included three large data sets representing different populations – Medicare, Medicaid, and an employer based population. Prediction performance varied depending on the population tested. For a Medicaid population, the CRG yielded a predictive power of 30%. CRG was implemented for several pediatric populations in Ohio and Maryland

An analytical review on these systems shows some limitations, most important of which are listed below:

- Focus on some risk factors related to cost management and financial issues rather than surgical issues.
- Applying such risk adjustment frameworks rather than risk detection frameworks.
- Without any function to apply some new risk factors.
- Having no look at on some procedures to evaluation the system.

Therefore, regarding these limitation through current systems, with an in depth review of risk detection in healthcare area, particularly in orthopaedic operating room, we find that applying some IT based techniques such as knowledge discovery followed by data mining would increase the performance of current risk adjustment methods significantly.

In order to find the relationships between the risk factors as well as relationships between these factors and surgery results, an intelligent model will be more effective and efficiency. It means, improving performance of surgery by applying the effect of the risk factors on surgery results is a significant advantage of an intelligence risk detection model.

Risk adjustment for hip and knee replacement operations, in itself, is challenging due to the great diversity of the patient population in terms of the diagnoses, indications for operation, the operation performed, the age at which an operation is deemed necessary and feasible, and other factors (Kang et al. 2004).

Regarding this issue, surgery-driven validated risk-adjusted outcome analysis can indeed lead to improvements in performance by both individual orthopaedic surgeons and orthopaedic surgery centres (Mavroudis and Jacobs 2002).

Although risk detection is an essential part of healthcare decision making, to the best of the authors knowledge there exist very few intelligence systems in healthcare with specific real-time risk detection component.

Table 2.3 serves to summarise the relevant studies. Given the importance of risk detection for the context of hip and knee replacement and the fact that real-time risk detection has not been significantly incorporated into healthcare decision support to date we believe this is an essential aspect of our proposed model.

2.4   Conceptual Model

Figure 2.3, depicts, the first stage in risk assessment. The output of the risk assessment process will help in determining important surgery risk factors and also predicting anticipated results based on the those risk factors.

The anticipated results enable the surgeons making informed decision whether to proceed with the surgery. If the decision is indeed to proceed with the surgery, all relevant information is passed on to the patients in order to allow them to make the final decision regarding the surgery. Any conflict in decision of the surgeon and that of the patients is an indication of high-levels of risk or some negative outcome of

Table 2.3 A list of relevant previous works in using knowledge discovery in healthcare area

Title	Technologies	Objectives
Analysis of health care data using different data mining techniques (Kumar and Gosain 2009)	The potential use of classification based data mining techniques such as decision tree and association rule to massive volume of health care data	In this study, our objective are to: (1) present an evaluation of techniques such as decision tree and association rules to Predict the occurrence of route of transmission based on treatment history of HIV patients; (2) demonstrate that data mining method can yield valuable new knowledge and pattern related to the HIV patient; (3) assesses the utilization of healthcare resources and demonstrate the socioeconomic, demographic and medical histories of patient
Intelligent heart disease prediction system using data mining techniques (Palaniappan and Awang 2008)	Data mining techniques, namely, decision trees, naïve bays and neural network	This research has developed a prototype Intelligent Heart Disease Prediction System (IHDPS) using medical profile such as age, sex, blood pressure and blood sugar it can predict the likelihood of patients getting a heart disease
Knowledge discovery approaches for early detection of decomposition conditions in heart failure patients (Candelieri et al. 2009)	Several KD algorithms have been applied on collected data	They propose an innovative knowledge based platform of services for effective and efficient clinical management of heart failure within elderly population

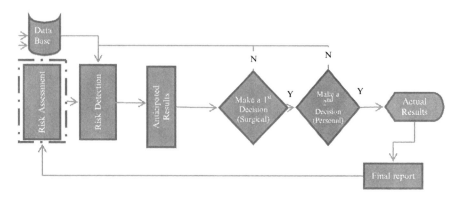

Fig. 2.3 The conceptual model

Fig. 2.4 The risk assessment process

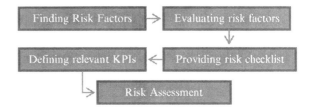

surgery. Any such conflicts are fed back into the system for future risk assessments for the same or other patients.

After the surgery, actual outcomes are compared to the anticipated results. This comparison is an evaluation procedure for the model to ensure continual improvement of its predicting capabilities.

2.4.1   Risk Assessment

To assess hip and knee replacement surgery improvement, detecting risk factors is a useful method (Larrazabal et al. 2007a). To detect the risk factors, we will need to develop a multidimensional risk model to apply risk assessment.

Therefore, to address this issue, across our research, after finding some critical risk dimensions and factors from the literature, we use two experimental approaches, which required different degrees of the orthopaedic specialists' involvement in risk assessment.

In first approach, the orthopaedic specialists in a focus group are presented with certain risk factors based on the available literature. Then experts identify some main risk dimensions that should be used on the surgical decision making and the levels of these risk factors to provide a risk assessment checklist. In the second approach, the surgeons are asked to complete this risk assessment checklist to assess the risk factors and also define the relationships between these factors or between these factors and some actual and anticipated results and risk ranges to define some relevant KPIs (key performance indicators). Moreover, we document the surgeons' and specialists' recommended additional procedures and ask them to assess the responses provided by our subjects. The risk assessment process is shown in Fig. 2.4.

2.4.2   Risk Detection Using Knowledge Discovery

To incorporate an intelligent technology into the proposed risk assessment process, we suggest a data mining process followed by knowledge discovery. In the research case, the data types have a significant impact on the data mining tasks. Hence, after finishing the data collecting phase, the suitable tasks will extract such as neural networks and association rules. To apply the necessary data mining techniques, developing and then implementing the model, after the risk assessment process, we created a small database that included patients' data and also some data to show risk factors. Then we move through step 1 to step 6 (below).

The steps are:

Step 1. Understand business requirements, dataset structure and data mining task Knowledge-Rich Data Mining in healthcare Risk Detection. Designing a dimensional data mart will be more effective to apply data mining tasks on this data mart.

Step 2. Prepare target datasets: select and transform relevant features; data cleaning; data integration. Communicate any findings during data preparation to domain experts.

Step 3. Train multiple data mining models in randomly sampled partitions using Clementine[1] or Rapid miner.[2]

Step 4. Evaluate data mining models using a set of performance metrics.

Step 5. Discuss the data mining results with domain experts. Explore potential patterns from data mining results. If new risk factors or patterns are identified, communicate the findings with decision makers and determine appropriate actions.

Step 6. Go back to Step 1 if new business questions are raised during the process or new KPI, rule(s) or risk factor are discovered after comparing the actual and anticipate results. Otherwise, finish and exit the process.

Data from a large hospital in Melbourne, Australia will be used to operate the procedure described above. Input to the system will be a dataset of hip and knee replacement surgery risk factors, and the outcome will be decision functions results of performance metrics; new and revised risk factors.

2.4.2.1 On-Line or Realtime Outputs to Create an e-Risk Detection Model

The mining process in not time-limited (Ting and Hui-Ju 2009), this risk detection process typically takes hours or days. So, choosing a real time processing technique should be a critical step to design a high performance application based on IRD model.

Services with more than a critical amount of user access traffic need to apply highly efficient, real-time processing techniques that are constrained both computationally and in term of memory requirements (Ting and Hui-Ju 2009). Web Usage Mining (WUM) is a great technique that provides solution to create a real-time intelligent model.

As shown in Fig. 2.5, user interaction with a web server are pre-proceed continuously and fed into online WUM systems that process the data and update the models in real-time.

Ting and Hui-Ju 2009, have stated that the out puts of this model are used to support online decision making as well as detecting some changes. They proposed a system to online monitor and improve website connectivity based on the site topology and usage data.

So, based on literature review, we find that using WUN technique is the best relevant and effective solution to create a realtime or online model to monitor decision

---

[1] A commercial software for data mining.

[2] An open source software for data mining.

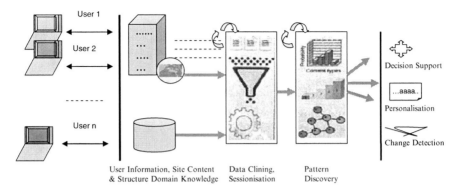

Fig. 2.5 An overview of online WUN (Source: Ting and Hui-Ju 2009)

making results. However, this technique still has some challenges to develop a novel web usage mining system.

2.4.3 Applying Anticipated and Actual Results

The decision making process for patient surgery is presented in Sect. 2.3.2. Based on this framework, two types of decision making, surgical and personal, are defined. Our model (Fig. 2.3) will enable contemporaneous and real time detection of risks factors and prediction of surgery results. The results will be a significant importance in forming surgical and personal decisions.

In the proposed conceptual model, to evaluate a risk detection process, the actual results will be compared to the anticipated results. This is because sometimes actual results present some new risk factors or new measurement to assess the risk factors. The business intelligence reporting tools would be the best solution to create a final report to show some important items, and finally apply them to the risk assessment process, for next iterations of evaluations.

2.5 Discussion

The above outlines a research in progress that is examining the merits of combining real time intelligent risk detection with decision support in a healthcare context. The case of orthopaedic operation room was chosen because of the complex nature of the decision making in this context as well as the many risks inherent with these decisions.

The lack of interaction between healthcare industry practitioners and academic researchers makes it hard to discover implant risks, and limits opportunities for the application of data mining techniques, and hence weakens the value that knowledge discovery and data mining methods may bring to healthcare risk detection.

The hip and knee replacement risk detection has many dimensions and perspectives that their main focuses are usually on pathological process, physiological variables, some general health perceptions, social paradigm and also quality of life

(Wilson and Cleary 1995). So, detecting risk factors in all of these dimensions is not easy but based on our two approaches to assess the risks, with contribution of some orthopaedic specialists, we try to cover some main dimensions.

To best of our knowledge, this is the first study that directly examines the benefits of real time risk detection and outcome prediction in order to augment decision making process in healthcare area.

Also, using KPIs (key performance indicators) as a set of metrics is a novel idea to control the risk factors, finding its level and defining their relationships together, also with the other factors in such healthcare context. Furthers, KPIs will be so effective to monitor some key items during surgery for surgeons. It will be one of the valuable outcomes through this research that will be effective for orthopaedic specialist during all stages of patients' treatments.

Moreover, this research has the potential to contribute to understanding of the usefulness of involving orthopaedic specialists in designing an intelligent model when they has identified risk factors during the planning stages of the risk assessment and risk detection.

Additionally, it should reduce the burden of hip and knee replacement on its patients, their family and society is the other strategic benefits that will examined.

Being continuous is yet another advantage of this model. By comparing anticipant results and actual outcomes, risk factors will be amended to improve future predictions.

An important feature of our IRD model is the integration of the three IT solutions to solve a clinical issue in the definition and assessment of "outcomes" in patients, combined by some assessment measures. It is noted that the theoretical framework developed in this work needs to be tasted in a future research. However, empirical testing of the framework is likely to face a number of challenges such as:

1. The IRD model developed here will be used to identify common metrics for measuring the risk factors.
2. We have found a few instances where hospitals have well developed capabilities to develop and implement an intelligent model. However, our field research to date has found that the majority of hospitals who have implemented an IT infrastructure are employing some computerised clinical decision support systems (CDSSs) mainly to improve practitioner performance (Garg et al. 2005).

The transformation of the healthcare domain to develop capabilities to apply intelligence models to detect risks is likely to occur over an extended period of time and may be evident only in case studies. The willingness of hospitals to provide the required access for conducting such in-depth case studies is another challenge that needs to be overcome.

2.6 Conclusions

In this paper, we propose an intelligence risk detection model using knowledge discovery methods. Intelligent risk detection is a particularly challenging area for the healthcare industry while relatively common for fraud detection in finance, diagnosis in industry, and affect analysis in chemistry. This not only because building cases of training sets is difficult, but also because the cases may have many forms, causes, and unknown relations. We propose the application of knowledge discovery to high-level surgery risk detection and outcome prediction. The model designed is based on two steps of decision making process (surgical and personal) and, includes a decision support system which is suitable for high concentration prediction. Continual model update inherent in the proposed system results in adaptive and more accurate risk detection and outcomes prediction capabilities compared to fixed model. This study confirms that the selection of the risk detection, prediction by knowledge discovery and then decision making are also very important for hip and knee replacement surgical decision making process. The next phases for this research are to trial the model in appropriate clinical settings.

In closing, we contend that real time intelligent risk detection appears to be critical for many areas in healthcare where complex, high risk decision must be made and thus call for more research in this area.

References

Ash, A.S., Ellis, R.P., Pope, G.P., Ayanian, J.Z., Bates, D.W., Burstin, H., Iezzoni, L.I., MacKay, E. and Yu, V. (2000) "Using Diagnoses to Describe Populations and Predict Costs," Health Care Financing Review, 21(3), spring.

Baldwin, J. (2001) Automating patients' records. MD computing [cited May 2010]; Available from:www.technologyinpractice.com.

Candelieri, A., Conforti, D., Sciacqua, A., & Perticone, F. (2009). Knowledge discovery approaches for early detection of decompensation conditions in heart failure patients. In *Ninth international conference on intelligent systems design and applications*. IEEE.

Cios, K. J., Pedrycz, W., Swiniarski, R. W. & Kurgan, R. A. (2007) Date mining and knowledge discovery approach, Springer

Davidson, D., de Steiger, R., Ryan, P., Griffith, L., McDermott, B., Pratt, N. et al. (2008). Hip and knee arthroplasty. In *Annual report*. Adelaide: Data Management & Analysis Centre and University of Adelaide.

Dijkman, B. A., Kooistra, B. A., Ferguson, T. B., & Bhandari, M. A. C. (2008). Decision making open reduction/internal fixation versus arthroplasty for femoral neck fractures. *Techniques in Orthopaedics, 23*(4), 288–295.

Dunn DL. (1998) Applications of health risk adjustment: what can be learned from experience to date? Inquiry. Summer; 35,132–147.

Fieschi, M., Dufour, J. C., Staccini, P., Gouvernet, J., & Bouhaddou, O. (2003). Medical decision support systems: Old dilemmas and new paradigms? Tracks for successful integration and adoption. *Methods of Information in Medicine, 42*(3), 191–198.

Garg, A. X., Adhikari, N. K. J., McDonald, H., et al. (2005). Effects of computerized clinical decision support systems on practitioner performance and patient outcomes a systematic review. *JAMA, 293*(10), 1223–1238.

Gayet, F. L., Jacobs, J. P., et al. (2005). Performance of surgery for congenital heart disease: Shall we wait a generation or look for different statistics? *The Journal of Thoracic and Cardiovascular Surgery, 130,* 234.

Hornbrook M.C. & Goodman M.J. (1996) Chronic disease, functional health status, and demographics: a multi-dimensional approach to risk adjustment. *Health Service Research Journal.* 1996 August; 31(3), 283–307.

Hughes, J.S., Averill, R.F., Eisenhandler, J. (2004) Clinical Risk Groups (CRGs): A Classification System for Risk-Adjusted Capitation-Based Payment and Health Care Management. Medical Care 42, 81–90.

Hunt, D. L., Brian Haynes, R., Hanna, S. E., et al. (1998). Effects of computer-based clinical decision support outcomes: A systematic review systems on physician performance and patient. *JAMA, 280*(15), 1339–1346.

Kang, N., Tsang, V., Cole, T., Elliott, M., & de Leval, M. (2004). Risk stratification in paediatric open-heart surgery. *European Journal of Cardio-Thoracic Surgery, 26*, 3–11.

Keenan, P., Buntin Beeuwkes, M., McGuire, T., & Newhouse, J. P. (2001). The prevalence of formal risk adjustment in health plan purchasing. *Inquiry, 38*, 245–259.

Kronick, R., Gilmer, T., Dreyfus, T. and Ganiats, T. (2002)"CDPS-Medicare: The Chronic Illness and Disability Payment System Modified to Predict Expenditures for Medicare Beneficiaries" Final Report to CMS, June 24, 2002.

Kumar, A. and Gosain A. (2009) Analysis of Health Care Data Using Different Data Mining Techniques., International Conference on Intelligent Agent & Multi-Agent Systems(IAMA), Chennai, Print ISBN: 978-1-4244-4710-7. P1–6.

Lacour-Gayet, F. (2002). Risk stratification theme for congenital heart surgery. *Seminars in Thoracic and Cardiovascular Surgery. Pediatric Cardiac Surgery Annual, 5*, 148–152.

Larrazabal, L. A., del Nido Pedro, J., Jenkins Kathy, J., & Gauvreau, K. (2007a). Measurement of technical performance in congenital heart surgery: A pilot study. *The Annals of Thoracic Surgery, 83*, 179–184.

Larrazabal, L. A., Jenkins, K. J., Gauvreau, K., Vida, V. L., Benavidez, O. J., Gaitán, G. A., et al. (2007b). Improvement in congenital heart surgery in a developing country: The Guatemalan experience. *Circulation, 116*, 1872–1877.

Mavroudis, C. & Jacobs, J. P. (2002) Congenital heart disease outcome analysis: Methodology and rationale. *The Journal of Thoracic and Cardiovascular Surgery, 123*(7), 35–47.

Miller, R. A. (1994). Medical diagnostic decision support systems – past, present, and future: A threaded bibliography and brief commentary. *Journal of the American Medical Informatics Association, 1*, 8–27.

Palaniappan, S. and Awang R. (2008). Intelligent Heart Disease Prediction System Using Data Mining Techniques, International Conference on Computer Systems and Applications (AICCSA). IEEE/ACS, Doha, Print ISBN: 978-1-4244-1967-8, p. 108–115

Pope, G.C., Ellis, R.E, Ash, A.S., (2000) Principal Inpatient Diagnostic Cost Group Model for Medicare Risk Adjustment. Health Care Financing Review 21(3):93–118, Spring.

Reddy, V. M., McElhinney, D. B., Silverman, N. H., & Hanley, F. L. (1997). The double switch procedure for anatomical repair of congenitally corrected transposition of the great arteries in infants and children. *European Heart Journal, 18*(9), 1470–1477.

Roy, C. B., & Brunton, S. (2008). Managing multiple cardiovascular risk factors. *The Journal of Family Practice, 57*(3), 13–20.

Stamatis, G. (2010). Intensively lowering glucose: Possible benefits must be weighed against risks. ed. University Hospitals Case Medical Center.

Ting, I.-H., Hornbrook Hui-Ju, W. (2009). *Web mining applications in e-commerce and e-services.* Berlin: Springer.

Wickramasinghe, N., Bali, R. K., Capt. James Choi, J. H., & Schaffer, J. L. (2009a). A systematic approach optimization of healthcare operations with knowledge management. In *HIMSS*, USA.

Wickramasinghe, N., Bali, R., Gibbons, C., Choi, C., & Schaffer, J. (2009b). Optimization of health care operations with knowledge management. *JHIMS, 3*(4), 44–50.

Wickramasinghe, N., & Schaffer, J. (2006). Creating knowledge-driven healthcare process with the intelligence continuum. *Int J.Electronic Healthcare, 2*, 164–174.

Wilson, I. B., & Cleary, P. D. (1995). Linking clinical variables with health-related quality of life: A conceptual model of patient outcomes. *Journal of the American Medical Association, 273*, 59–65.

Weiner, J.P., Dobson, A., Maxwell, S.L., (1996) Risk-Adjusted Medicare Capitation Rates Using Ambulatory and Inpatient Diagnoses. *Health Care Financing Review* 17, 77–100, Spring.

Chapter 3
Healthcare Information Systems Design: Using a Strategic Improvisation Model

Say Yen Teoh and Nilmini Wickramasinghe

Abstract As globally governments start to move forward with regard to their respective healthcare reform policies, the role for HIS (healthcare information systems) will become ever more critical in the attainment of healthcare-value strategies. This in turn places pressure to hospitals to identify appropriate and superior design strategies. Drawing on the research pertaining to improvisation and IS design, a model of strategic improvisation is proffered as suitable in the context of HIS design. Multiple case study data from Singapore and the United States – countries with different and distinctive healthcare systems – are presented to illustrate the benefits of such an approach.

Keywords Bricolage and resource-time-effort • Case study • Healthcare information systems (HIS) • Improvisation • Resource-based view (RBV)

3.1 Introduction

Healthcare organizations worldwide currently face multiple challenges such as demographic – coping with an increasing aging population reflected in longer life expectancy; technological – incorporating advances in providing optimal use of health-related information for decision-making and problem-solving processes; and financial – the difficulty in attempting to provide value-based healthcare treatment being exacerbated by escalating costs; and labour issues – dealing with an industry

S.Y. Teoh • N. Wickramasinghe (✉)
School of Business IT and Logistics, RMIT University, Melbourne, VIC, Australia
e-mail: nilmini.wickramasinghe@rmit.edu.au

N. Wickramasinghe et al. (eds.), *Critical Issues for the Development
of Sustainable E-health Solutions*, Healthcare Delivery in the Information Age,
DOI 10.1007/978-1-4614-1536-7_3, © Springer Science+Business Media, LLC 2012

shortage of doctors and nurses. A suitable response to these challenges lies in the formulation of healthcare-value strategies created by focusing on three key solutions (Wickramasinghe et al. 2009), namely:

1. Access – caring for anyone, anytime, anywhere;
2. Quality – offering world-class care and establishing integrated information repositories;
3. Value – providing effective and efficient healthcare delivery systems.

In today's dynamic and complex world of healthcare operations, IS/IT (information systems/information technology) play a critical, if not key, role in effecting the successful realization of any healthcare-value strategy (Wickramasinghe et al. 2007). Further, the design of HIS to enable the realisation of the healthcare-value proposition for any healthcare organization is subjective, complex, and dynamic. Sound improvisation 'involves the reworking of pre-composed materials and designs in relation to unanticipated ideas conceived, shaped, and transformed under the special conditions of performance, thereby adding unique features to every creation' (Weick 1998, p. 554). This has been shown as effective in complex and dynamic contexts (Ash et al. 2004).

Generally research on improvisation remains relatively underdeveloped (Vendelo 2009; Cunha et al. 2009) and this is particularly the situation in regard to the formation of HIS design (Heeks 2006). Hence, we contend that given the need for healthcare organizations to develop appropriate HIS in order to realize their value proposition, it is useful to understand how strategic improvisation contributes to the formation of superior HIS design. Specifically in this research, we attempt to fill this present void in the literature by examining the resource-based view and the bricolage literature to understand the recombination and transformation of existing resources and, thereby, how strategic improvisation might give rise to superior HIS design, which in turn leads to the delivery of valuable and quality patient-centric healthcare delivery.

Qualitative data from multiple case studies in the United States and Singapore are analyzed to show how strategic improvisation with regard to HIS design can lead to better patient care. In this way, our study serves to contribute to the theoretical discourse on HIS design improvisation and provides insights on how to improvise HIS design (Aktas et al. 2007).

3.2 Theoretical Background

This section presents an overview of the relevant literature including a summary of HIS improvisation, a resource-based view and bricolage. In addition, a summary of each of the healthcare systems in which the respective case studies are situated is provided to highlight key criteria of these healthcare systems – both their similarities and unique aspects.

3.2.1   Healthcare Information Systems Improvisation

Recognizing the potential of transforming societal health and wellness quality, the study of HIS design and improvisation research has slowly gained interest in the healthcare industry.

Technically, improvisation is referred to as a situational, embodied, and temporal process (Oliver 2009) that shifts the emphasis to incorporate the social, cultural, and embodied context (Burner 1993) that is iterative and cyclical (Oliver 2009). The process of improvisation typically occurs between the conception and execution of ideas, with a specific purpose being to enable a suitable and successful final outcome (Cunha et al. 1999). In particular, improvisation is viewed as 'a situated performance where thinking and action emerge simultaneously and on the spur of the moment' (Ciborra 1999, p. 78); often 'time' and 'people' play a crucial role in improving the system (Vendelo 2009). In view of this we propose to conceptualize improvisation with 'resource–time–effort', drawing upon the resource-based view (RBV) literature to suggest how resources might be managed within the context of healthcare. We believe this is an appropriate approach, especially given that few studies exist which specifically address this aspect (Sirmon et al. 2007). In an extension to RBV, bricolage literature is used to understand where resource-seeking occurs (Levi-Strauss 1966), in particular the interaction and involvement of time and effort in co-shaping the IS design (Garud and Karnoe 2003).

In this study, improvisation is defined as an iterative process to transform ideas through the incorporation of the hospital social context with the support of resource–time–effort as valuable features in the design of IS. The conceptualization of IS design improvisation is presented in Fig. 3.1.

3.2.2   Resource-Based View

Limited healthcare funding requires hospitals to find more effective ways to manage and utilize their resources (Aktas et al. 2007). In this study, hospital resources is valuable, rare, imperfectly imitable, and (or) non-substitutable. Typically, in literature, resources are managed by organizations in three processes – structuring the resources (includes acquiring, accumulating, divesting), bundling (includes stabilizing, enriching,

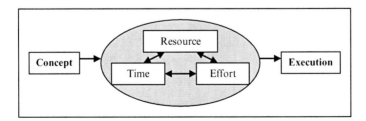

Fig. 3.1 Conceptualization of IS design improvisation

pioneering), and leveraging (includes mobilizing, coordinating, and deploying) (Sirmon et al. 2007) to analyze the effect and applicability of the available technologies to enhance IS deign for higher performance.

3.2.3 Bricolage

Since the concept of bricolage has been adopted by improvisational theorists (Innes and Booher 1999; Weick 1993), it is useful to turn to it in order to develop a deeper understanding of improvisation. Bricolage serves to complement reasoning and collective creativity that is fundamentally different, so as to introduce new options and new combinations (Innes and Booher 1999) to enable appropriate designs to ensue. This approach also complements the strengths of deploying modest resources to prevail over superior ones, such as from aspects of intellectual and financial perspectives (Garud and Karnoe 2003). This would prove especially useful in a hospital context, where there is always competition for superior resources. Hospital operations and IT management must maximize modest resources, which are normally allocated to core business functions, such as medical, laboratory and pharmacological research, and equipment to achieve optimal results. To do so, bricoleurs use resources with which they are familiar to address new tasks and challenges (Ferneley and Bell 2006).

In designing HIS one requires a combination of 'bricolage materials', that is information technology hardware and software artefacts, and 'network bricolage' which allows the bricoleurs to use pre-existing contacts and networks for strategic improvisation (Baker et al. 2003). An examination of bricolage will not only facilitate a better understanding of the operationalization of the improvisation concept, but it will also enable a deeper understanding from the strategic perspective (Baker et al. 2003; Mintzberg 1994).

3.2.4 Background of the Singapore and US Healthcare Systems

Singapore, with a population of almost five million (Straits Times 2009), that is renowned for having one of the highest-ranking healthcare systems in the world (WHO 2000; National Center for Policy Analysis 2004). In prioritizing the healthcare standards for its populace, the Singapore government focuses on its objective of developing the world's most cost-effective healthcare system. Three approaches are the key to attempting to achieve this objective: (1) promoting good health and lifestyle, (2) ensuring access to good and affordable healthcare, and (3) pursuing medical excellence (WHO 2006).

In contrast to Singapore, the United States is a large country with a population of over 307 million. Key features that make the US healthcare system stand apart from other OECD countries include its essentially private healthcare model, the fact that healthcare services are at least three times more expensive than in any other OECD country and the significant amount of funds expended each year on healthcare

(Wickramasinghe and Silvers 2003). Given that the US healthcare industry is in a state of flux (Von Lubitz and Wickramasinghe 2006), with the most recent large-scale change to affect this industry being the passing of the Healthcare Reform Bill proposed by the Obama government in March 2010,[1] the redesign of the healthcare process enabled through IS/IT is an important nationwide priority.

Table 3.1 summarises the key issues of each healthcare system under observation.

3.3   Research Methodology

Multiple case study methodology is adopted in this study to unveil the 'how' question (Walsham 1995) that delves into the process of developing strategic IS improvisation. The process of unveiling strategic IS improvisation is a complex, multi-faceted phenomenon that is inextricably connected to the specific organizational context (Pentland 1999) which comprises technological and complex human/social components (Barney 1991; Tyrell 2002). To explore issues that are inextricably connected to a specific context, a richer result is achieved by studying hospitals located in different and distinct healthcare systems. In this way we gained insights pertaining to improvisation, irrespective of style of healthcare system, size, and (or) expenditure.

Based on our research questions, two conditions emerged to form the basis for case study selection. First, the case study hospitals must aim to improve workflows and HIS through the adoption of the Kaizen philosophy of providing incremental and continual improvement. Second, both the case study hospitals improvise their HIS designs with a common aim that is to deliver superior healthcare-value.

Research access for the Singapore hospital (SH) was provided over a period of six months, with a total of 19 face-to-face interviews with individuals recommended by the Director of Operations. Most interviews were recorded and transcribed, with photos and additional notes taken.. Each interview session lasted between one and a half and 3 hours. Informants included nurses, IT specialists, doctors and senior management personnel with an average working experience of three years in SH. Similarly in the US case study, face-to-face interviews were conducted, but

Table 3.1 Summary of key indicators for healthcare systems

Location	Singapore	USA
Healthcare expenditure	3.4% of GDP	16.2% of GDP
	(Straits Times 2009)	(CMS 2008)
Total population	4,615,000	311,666,000
	(WHO 2008a)	(WHO 2008b)
Gross national income per capita (PPP international $)	USD$47, 940	USD$48,430
	(World Bank 2010a)	(World Bank 2010b)
Life expectancy at birth m/f (years)	79/85	76/81
	(Index Mundi 2010a)	(Index Mundi 2010b)

[1] www.healthreform.gov

over a longer time period. A total of 50 informants were interviewed including medical professionals, IT professionals and members of the senior management team.

All case study interviewees were provided with assurance of confidentiality and anonymity, especially when potentially sensitive information was sought (Walsham 2005). The questions asked were exploratory in nature, open-ended, and tailored to the interviewees' roles.

Data analysis is 'the heart of theory-building process' in case studies (Eisenhardt 1989, p. 539). In view of this, data analysis was performed in conjunction with data collection in an iterative process that involved cycling between the empirical data, the theoretical lens, and the relevant literature (Eisenhardt 1989). Based on the collected data, we identified the initial set of themes that was pertinent to construct improvisation as stated in the literature. Each new finding was then verified to ensure that it was supported by at least two sources of data (Klein and Myers 1999).

In turn, this set of themes (for example time, cost, and effort) was used to form our improvisation theoretical lens. In order to ensure that the chain of evidence was at all times clear, we provide narratives by adding specific quotes from informants on the identified themes (Pratt 2009). In this way we establish a visual mapping strategy to organize the empirical data (Langley 1999). Narratives and visual maps were then compared with the theoretical lens and the relevant literature to shape our emerging theoretical ideas. This data analysis process was continued until the state of theoretical saturation was reached; namely, when it became possible to explain the findings of the case studies comprehensively (Eisenhardt 1989).

3.4 Case Studies

3.4.1 Singapore Hospital (SH)

To support the government's newly declared healthcare delivery standard, the Minister for Health challenged a Singapore hospital (SH) (anonymous) that was performing below par to improve its service and performance by transforming itself into a state-of-the-art hospital. Faced with being one of the smallest hospitals and troubled with resource constraints, SH engaged in an uphill battle to improve. However, after 2 years of intense improvement, SH was transformed and rejuvenated into an iconic hospital. The Singapore healthcare industry expressed its awe by voting it the best patient service hospital each year from 2004 to 2008. Table 3.2 serves to summarize the key issues for SH in making the changes.

3.4.1.1 Phase I: Initiating Improvisation

This project began with a self-motivated group consisting of the Operations Manager, nurses, and doctors. After a week of serious discussions and in-depth study, they proposed to the hospital senior management that the change should target the two

Table 3.2 Summary of key criteria for case study comparison

Location	Singapore hospital (SH)	US hospital (USH)
Type of hospital	Public hospital	HMO
Type of HIS	Clinical Digital Dashboard (CDD) and Bed Management System (BMS)	Automated medical record system
Aim of HIS implementation	Reduce errors and improve efficiency and effectiveness	Reduce errors and improve efficiency and effectiveness
HIS design concept	Kaizen concept	Kaizen concept
Unit of analysis	Project level	Project level
Business strategy	Improvise and innovate	Improvise and innovate

problematic departments: the department of emergency (DE) and the bed management unit (BMU). Under the supervision of the Director of Operations, a team in DE was tasked to map out a typical patient workflow by physically tracing the patients' flow from one 'station' to the next. The rationale for this was guided by the Kaizen concept of identifying possible 'waste' in the procedures that could be streamlined for improvement.

The proposed outcome of studying the workflow was to assign a senior doctor (rather than a junior) to assess patient treatment and rank cases according to their priorities. Additionally, feedback from stakeholders mooted a new concept of a 'just-in-time' bed management system.. This improvised concept allows wards to 'pull' patients to the newly-available beds as against to the traditional 'push' system of emergency departments.

To overcome the constraint of a shortage of human resources, SH used volunteers from the existing medical staff, in particular junior doctors and nurses from the Ward 13. Within a month, as one difficulty after another was handled, they managed to iron out all discrepancies successfully and finalize the key concept of their ideal hassle-free and patient-centric systems. However, to implement this system the hospital was challenged for the second time, now with the lack of IT experts and funds. The creative solution SH management proposed tapped into the brainpower of polytechnic students who were offered the proposed concept as a business case, a prototype study for them to attempt to solve. In parallel, SH advertised the hospital project through the mass media, as a bait to attract IT solutions providers to prescribe the relevant panacea.

Figure 3.2 summarizes the SH effort, and the time spent in improvising with its limited resources, in its initiatives for HIS transformation with a strong complement from network bricolage.

3.4.1.2 Phase II: Deploying the Healthcare Information Systems Improvisation

A golden opportunity arose when Fujitsu and Cisco came forward and formed a strategic partnership with SH. Pulling together their resources and expertise, Fujitsu

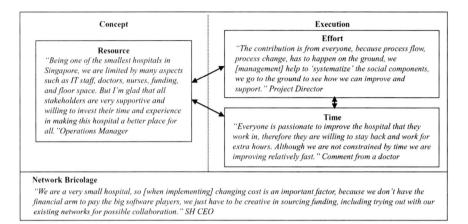

Fig. 3.2 Conceptualization of IS system improvisation in SH: Phase I

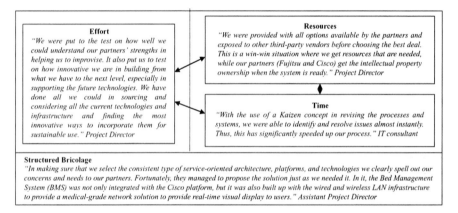

Fig. 3.3 Conceptualization of IS system improvisation in SH: Phase II

fine-tuned the prototype which had been created by the polytechnic students and worked closely with the enthusiastic group of DE and Ward 13 staff to identify more substantial user requirements. With feedback from staff users, and wish-lists from patients, a CDD prototype was finally deployed.

Contemporaneously Cisco was exploring ways their service-oriented architecture and platforms could complement with the hospital's existing infrastructure. Working closely with Cisco, SH was challenged to improvise their existing infrastructures to support future technologies, at minimal cost. After a feasibility study, SH eventually agreed to adopt the Cisco platform, integrating it with the existing bed-management and nurse-call systems.

The SH endeavour in improvising the HIS deployment was made possible by strong resource support. The timely system requirement revision analysis, with the complement of structured bricolage that provided fundamental guidance to unify all stakeholders in this phase, is summarized in Fig. 3.3.

3.4.1.3 Phase III: Embracing the Improvised HIS

A user training session of less than an hour was given prior to the deployment of the new CDD and BMS systems. This was to the satisfaction of senior doctors and nurses because they had been previously involved, in phase II, with the design of the systems, via Kaizen activities with the Fujitsu and Cisco IT consultants.

The CDD (all-in-one) database helped medical staff to handle patient priorities and allowed doctors to follow through cases that were processed, screened and categorized by senior doctors at the triage post. It also allowed doctors to attend to patients and prescribe medications on the spot, shortening the waiting and turn-around time for patients in DE. After the system was fully integrated there was no longer a need to provide the same basic information at every contact point, since patient information was online and computerized. Not only was much effort saved from both the medical professionals' and patients' points of view, this transformation also successfully halved the average DE waiting time per patient from 40 to 20 minutes.

Nurses at Ward 13 also displayed a strong willingness and commitment to adapt to the newly transformed ways of working. Of particular benefit to them was the BMS system, that provides a real-time online visual display of available beds, facilitating the process of allocating patients to beds, significantly reducing the communication hassles between nurses from BMU and Ward 13. Additionally the new system also triggers an alert for real-time housekeeping whenever there is an available bed ready for use. Hence, nurses could spend their time servicing patients rather than searching for a housekeeper, updating the paperwork and phoning the other DE whenever a bed was ready. This 'just-in-time' approach significantly reduced (by 30%) the patient waiting time for beds.

The implementation of these two systems successfully transformed the hospital, providing hassle-free solutions to patients and medical staff. The incorporation in the use of resources, effort and time successfully improvised the SH system performance improvement. The institutional bricolage enabled collective consensus to evolve from doctors and nurses in the process of transformation, which is summarized in Fig. 3.4.

3.4.2 US Hospital (USH)

The USH has national coverage in various parts of the United States. Its non-profit, group-practice pre-payment plan provides comprehensive medical and hospital services to more than 6.6 million enrolled members in 11 geographic regions and 16 states. One of the first HMOs (health maintenance organizations) in the United States, this USH began in the west and was opened to public enrolment in 1945. Today, nationally the USH has about 9,000 full-time physicians representing all specialties; 57% of these are primary care physicians (PCPs). In addition, UHS employs about 75,000 non-physician health care professionals and administrative,

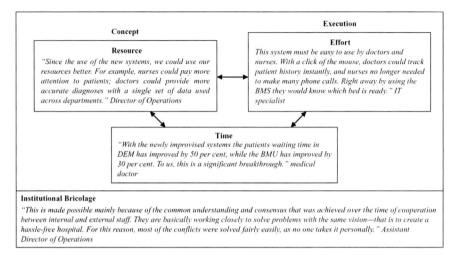

Fig. 3.4 Conceptualization of IS system improvisation in SH: Phase III

clerical, and technical employees. Nationally USH has 28 medical centres with approximately 7,400 licensed hospital beds and 255 medical office locations for outpatient services. The last column of Table 3.2 serves to summarize the pertinent details for USH.

The several systems that are prevalent in this environment fall into the following two main categories: Clinical systems and Business systems. The former includes systems that handle appointment scheduling, laboratory and radiology, document management (concerned with images), internal referral and messaging. Business systems includes those that handle membership and (or) benefits, claims, referrals and patient accounting.

The most important system for USH – the Automated Medical Record System, the newest and most significant information system in this organization – is the product of several integrated systems running in two distinct operating environments. The various application systems that comprise this Automated Medical Record System include: the Encounter System, the results component of the Laboratory Information System, the results component of the Radiology Information System, ACUMEN (a PC graphic user interface integration tool), MedSTAR (a document-management application), the Order Entry/Results Processing System and ACUXFER (a PC graphic user interface data transmission tool).

The project began with a clear need, expressed by the Medical Director, to provide more effective and efficient healthcare delivery. The Medical Director and several other medical personnel within this system were extremely IT savvy and thus an in-house system, or set of systems, was designed and developed. Given the innovative nature of the exercise, improvisation was a central focus and although specific management techniques such as Kaizen were not explicitly stated, it is still possible to map the dynamics of this project into our suggested improvisation framework, as seen in Fig. 3.5.

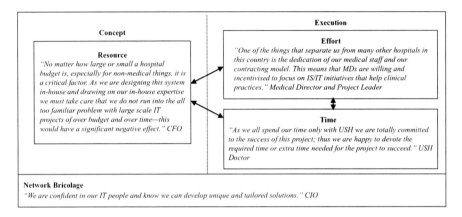

Fig. 3.5 Conceptualization of IS system improvisation in USH: Phase I

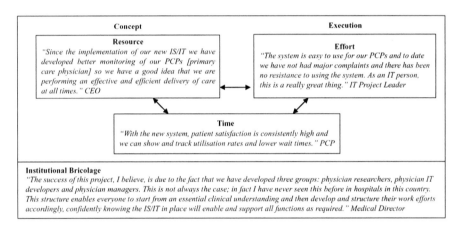

Fig. 3.6 Conceptualization of IS system improvisation end of UHS project

Figure 3.5 summarizes USH effort and time spent in improvisation regarding its HIS initiative.

At the end of data observation, in January 2007, it was possible to identify both the dynamic that occurred between developing clinical practice guidelines to work with the IS/IT designed and implemented, and the final steady state of the IS system improvisation (see Fig. 3.6). In particular, what Fig. 3.6 depicts is that equilibrium between resource–effort–time was established at the end of the data observation in January 2007, to that in the Singapore case study. In attaining this new state, variations to work roles had emerged; physicians tended to fall into one of three groups: those interested in research, those interested in IS/IT development, and those interested in management. This rationalization of effort, while not explicitly stipulated, appeared to be key in enabling a state of equilibrium to be reached.

3.5   Discussion

A conceptualization model of improvisation was inductively derived from the HIS design case studies conducted in Singapore and the United States. This conceptualization model suggests the shift in the emphasis of resource–time–effort occurring between conception and execution of ideas (Cunha et al. 1999) according to the different contexts (Burner 1993). Given that the model is inductively derived from empirical data, the following discussion provides an explanation of how the existing literature corroborates our model and how the model enriches the existing conceptualization of improvisation for HIS design.

3.5.1   Singapore Hospital

Prior literature has suggested that the nature of improvisation is helping to develop a more appropriate view of the patient recovery process (Cunha et al. 2009), and to improve service quality. As evident in the case, in order to overcome the lack of resources, the Singapore Hospital (SH) management initiated this project by using network bricolage for the purposes of HIS design improvisation – the collective creativity initiating from volunteer networks (Baker et al. 2003) to improvise the conceptual ideas and to execute them with the support of the self-motivated team's time-effort approach.

Together with resources from strategic partnerships, this has enabled the deployment of HIS design improvisation in the second phase. In this phase, the main challenge was the effort expended to understand and match multiple stakeholders' resources in conceptualizing the improvisation idea. Thus, SH management initiated structured bricolage as a guide to clarifying the hospital aims and goals for internal and external stakeholders. By doing so, it simplified stakeholder efforts in conceptualizing the improvisation ideas through the mix-and-match technique, with the available resources, to supplement the HIS design deployment phase.

The HIS design improvisation was formulated, in the last phase, with an equal emphasis on resource–time–effort principles. This final stage of improvisation was supplemented with institutional bricolage where different groups eventually formed a close bond, fostering cooperation to achieve what the institution needed (Cleaver 2003) to improvise. In the Singapore case study the application of the DSS and BMS systems not only improved patient waiting time, but also better allocated resources (medical staff) to provide better quality service to patients.

3.5.2   US Hospital

The development and deployment of an automated medical record system in the US hospital (USH) was a large and ambitious project. The system was unique and ahead of its time (as noted by many of the key informants). One key aspect that became apparent was the importance of institutional bricolage to enable and facilitate key medical staff, management and IT staff to work together in designing and developing an appropriate system. The other was that is took an equilibrium between resources, effort and time to be reached for the HIS project to be identified as successful; meeting not only all user needs and requirements, but also achieving improved patient waiting times and patient satisfaction.

As with the Singapore hospital, it appears that equal emphasis on resources–time–effort principles is the key to reaching a successful outcome, which in turn leads to the attainment of the healthcare-value proposition.

As with all case study research, in addition to uncovering data to support and (or) refute specific themes one also discovers unexpected findings. In regard to the USH case, these included the finding that three groups began to develop: physician researchers, physician IS/IT enthusiasts, and physicians as managers. As noted earlier, this appeared to develop organically and when asked the physicians all noted that this was the area in which they had the most interest. Moreover, structuring the physicians' efforts into different areas led to boundary-spanning behaviour, since the physicians in the respective areas started to take a strong position in ensuring that tasks under their area (research, IS/IT, or management) were being performed well. They were also interested to see their area fitted within the overall healthcare-value proposition. In this way, the development of self-monitoring to ensure that appropriate utilization targets and other medical metrics were being met contributed to successful project outcomes. Thus, what can be seen is that institutional bricolage can enable and facilitate changes in structures and roles of key players within an organization. Changes needed to reach the state of equilibrium between resources–effort–time and facilitate the attainment of key goals.

3.6 Conclusion

The purpose of this chapter is to enhance current understanding of HIS design by the conceptualization, through improvisation, of an HIS process model, a resource-based view and the bricolage literature. Through our Singapore and US case studies we discovered some interesting findings. Notably, that HIS design improvisation, coupled with network, structure, and institutional bricolage was formulated to source, manoeuvre and complement resources with collective creativity in achieving design improvisation – the equilibrium stage between resource–time–effort in IS system improvisation (refer to Fig. 3.7).

Theoretically, this study proposes and clarifies a series of structured activities and systematic processes through improvising the HIS model. The outcome of HIS improvisation seen through the two case studies further validates the claim in previous literature of the shift in emphasis of resource–time–effort occurring between conception and execution of ideas (Cunha et al. 1999), as being strongly dependent on the context (Burner 1993). In addition, this study advances the state of existing literature and knowledge by providing specific and testable propositions about attaining IS system improvisation that are grounded in the empirical reality of real-world organizations.

Fig. 3.7 Conceptualization of IS system improvisation

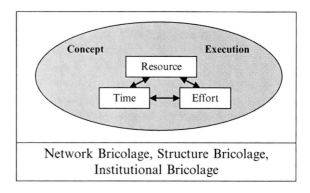

For professionals, this study contributes three key insights for IS system improvisation in the healthcare industry. First, practitioners need to be open-minded and creative in achieving a network bricolage strategy for sourcing, manoeuvring, and complementing available resources. Second, it is important to obtain a structure bricolage strategy appropriately for project governance. Last, it is critical to introduce an institutional bricolage strategy to harmonize working relationships, and thus balance the use of resources to achieve creative improvisation.

The major limitation of this study is that only two case studies were examined. Even though we were only able to examine these two, we believe our study provides strong directional data to suggest that more empirical work is necessary to theorize and refine this IS system improvisation model. In addition, we note that more confirmatory research is needed to support these initial findings. We believe that with such studies would come an ability to develop a taxonomy for appropriate steps to be taken with regard to HIS improvisation.

HIS is in its infancy. Countries are beginning to focus on attempts to make their healthcare system effective and efficient through the adoption of IS/IT, especially embarking on a plethora of e-health initiatives. We contend that IS/IT is, and will become, an even more integral part of achieving the healthcare-value proposition. This makes prudent design and implementation of HIS critical. Our case study data indicates that HIS improvisation is an approach in the right direction to facilitate optimal design and implementation of HIS in a healthcare context. We plead for more research in this and related areas to encourage the design of e-health, in particular and HIS in general, to embrace the techniques of improvisation.

References

Aktas, E., Ulengin, F., & Sahin, S. O. (2007). A decision support system to improve the efficiency of resource allocation in healthcare management. *Socio-Economic Planning Sciences, 41,* 130–146.

Ash, J. S., Berg, M., & Coiera, E. (2004). Some unintended consequences of information technology in health care: The nature of patient care information system-related errors. *Journal of the American Medical Informatics Association, 11,* 104–112.

Baker, T., Miner, A. S., & Eesley, D. T. (2003). Improvising firms: Bricolage, account giving and improvisational competencies in the founding process. *Research Policy, 32*, 255–276.

Barney, J. (1991). Firm resources and sustained competitive advantage. *Journal of Management, 17*(1), 99–120.

Burner, E. (1993). Epilogue: Creative persona and the problem of authenticity. In S. Lavie, K. Narayan, & R. Rosaldo (Eds.), *Creativity/Anthropology*. Ithaca: Cornell University Press.

CMS (Center for Medicare and Mediade), (2008). https://www.cms.gov/NationalHealthExpend Data/25_NHE_Fact_Sheet.asp. Cited 13 Nov 2010.

Ciborra, C. (1999). Notes on improvisations and time in organizations. *Accounting, Management and Information Technologies, 9*, 77–94.

Cleaver, F. (2003). Reinventing institutions: Bricolage and the social embeddedness of natural resource management. In T. A. Benjaminsen & C. Lund (Eds.), *Securing land rights in Africa*. London: Frank Cass.

Cunha, M. P., Cunha, J. V., & Kamoche, K. (1999). Organizational improvisation: What, when, how and why. *International Journal of Management Reviews, 1*, 299–341.

Cunha, M. P., Cunha, J. V. D., & Clegg, S. R. (2009). Improvisation bricolage: A practice-based approach to strategy and foresight. In L. A. Costanzo & R. B. MacKay (Eds.), *Handbook of research on strategy and foresight*. USA: Edward Elgar Publishing.

Eisenhardt, K. M. (1989). Building theories from case study research. *Academy of Management Review, 14*, 534–550.

Ferneley, E., & Bell, F. (2006). Using bricolage to integrate business and information technology innovation in SMEs. *Technovation, 26*(2), 232–241.

Garud, R., & Karnoe, P. (2003). Bricolage versus breakthrough: Distributed and embedded agency in technology entrepreneurship. *Research Policy, 32*, 277–299.

Heeks, R. (2006). Health information systems: Failure, success and improvisation. *International Journal of Medical Informatics, 75*, 125–137.

Index Mundi. (2010a). Singapore Demographic Profile, http://www.indexmundi.com/singapore/demographics_profile.html. Cited 14 Nov 2010.

Index Mundi. (2010b). United State Demographic Profile, http://www.indexmundi.com/united_states/demographics_profile.html. Cited 14 Nov 2010.

Innes, J. E., & Booher, D. E. (1999). Consensus building as role playing and bricolage: Toward a theory of collaborative planning. *Journal of the American Planning Association, 65*, 9–26.

Klein, H., & Myers, M. (1999). A set of principles for conducting and evaluating interpretive field studies in information systems. *MIS Quarterly, 23*, 67–94.

Langley, A. (1999). Strategies for theorizing from process data. *Academy of Management Review, 24*, 691–710.

Levi-Strauss, C. (1966). *The savage mind*. Oxford: Oxford University Press.

Mintzberg, H. (1994). *The rise and fall of strategic planning*. New York: Free Press.

National Center for Policy Analysis. (2004). Singapore's health care ranked first in an international comparison, http://www.ncpa.org/sub/dpd/index.php?Article_ID=7923. Cited 17 April 2010.

Oliver, J. (2009). Creativity as openness: Improvising health and care 'situations'. *Health Care Analysis, 17*, 318–330.

Pentland, B. T. (1999). Building process theory with narrative: From description to explanation. *Academy of Management Review, 24*(4), 711–724.

Pratt, M. G. (2009). From the editors: For the lack of a boilerplate: Tips on writing up (and reviewing) qualitative research. *Academy of Management Journal, 52*, 856–862.

Sirmon, D. G., Hitt, M. A., & Ireland, R. D. (2007). Managing firm resources in dynamic environments to create value: Looking inside the black box. *Academy of Management Review, 32*(1), 273–292.

Straits Times. (2009). Singapore healthcare spending compared with other countries. Available via http://www.pressrun.net/weblog/2009/05/singapore-healthcare-spending-compared-with-other-countries.html. Cited 17 Feb 2010.

Tyrell, S. (2002). *Using information and communication technology in healthcare*. Oxford: Radcliffe Medical Press.

Vendelo, M. T. (2009). Improvisation and learning in organizations – An opportunity for future empirical research. *Management Learning, 40*, 449–456.

Von Lubitz, D., & Wickramasinghe, N. (2006). Healthcare and technology: The doctrine of network centric healthcare. *International Journal of Electronic Healthcare, 4*, 322–344.

Walsham, G. (1995). Interpretive case studies in IS research: Nature and method. *European Journal of Information Systems, 4*, 74–81.

Walsham, G. (2005). "Doing Interpretive Research", European Journal of Information Systems, *15*, pp. 320–330.

Weick, K. E. (1993). Collective mind in organizations: Heedful interrelating on flight decks. *Administrative Science Quarterly, 38*, 357–381.

Weick, K. E. (1998). Improvisation as a mindset for organizational analysis. *Organization Science, 9*(5), 357–381.

WHO. (2000). The World Health Organization's ranking of the world's health systems. http://www.photius.com/rankings/healthranks.html. Cited 17 April 2010.

Wickramasinghe, N., & Silvers, J. B. (2003). IS/IT the prescription to enable medical group practices to manage managed care. *Health Care Management Science, 6*, 75–86.

Wickramasinghe, N., Bali, R. K., & Geisler, E. (2007). The major barriers and facilitators for the adoption and implementation of knowledge management in healthcare operations. *International Journal of Electronic Healthcare, 3*, 367–381.

Wickramasinghe, N., Bali, R. K., Gibbons, M. C., et al. (2009). A systematic approach: Optimization of healthcare operations with knowledge management. *Journal of Healthcare Information Management, 23*, 44–50.

World Bank. (2010a). World Development Indicators. http://www.google.com/publicdata?ds=wb-wdi&met=ny_gnp_pcap_pp_cd&idim=country:USA&dl=en&hl=en&q=gni+per+capita+in+ppp+dollars,+united+states#met=ny_gnp_pcap_pp_cd&idim=country:SGP. Cited 13 Nov 2010.

World Bank. (2010b). World Development Indicators. http://www.google.com/publicdata?ds=wb-wdi&met=ny_gnp_pcap_pp_cd&idim=country:USA&dl=en&hl=en&q=gni+per+capita+in+ppp+dollars,+united+states. Cited 13 Nov 2010.

World Health Organization. (2006). Regional Office for the Western Pacific: Singapore, http://www.wpro.who.int/countries/sin/national_health_priorities.htm. Cited 13 April 2008.

World Health Organization. (2008a). Singapore Statistics. http://apps.who.int/ghodata/?vid=20800. Cited 17 Nov 2010.

World Health Organization. (2008b). United Nation of America Statistics. http://apps.who.int/ghodata/?vid=20800. Cited 17 Nov 2010.

Chapter 4
Assimilation of Healthcare Information Systems (HIS): An Analysis and Critique*

Hidayah Sulaiman and Nilmini Wickramasinghe

Abstract The assimilation of information systems throughout the healthcare industry has increased dramatically since it is now perceived that Information Systems/ Information Technology (IS/IT) will be able to bring about immense benefit to medical personnel in delivering better services. However, the enthusiasm of having new information systems implemented usually deteriorates dramatically once the system is acquired. This causes a major issue in the assimilation of the newly implemented technology which could provide a negative impact on the successful use of the information system. This study describes the design and preliminary analysis on the technology innovation assimilation issues in a healthcare setting with the aim of developing a technology innovation assimilation model for hospitals to successfully assimilate and sustain the use of the healthcare information systems. Findings indicate that there are various technology, organization and environment elements that should be considered and also barriers that relevant healthcare factions need to overcome in order to successfully assimilate the healthcare information systems.

Keywords Assimilation • Technology innovation • Technology-organization-environment • Healthcare information system • Healthcare

4.1 Introduction

The healthcare industry has been criticized for being slow in the adoption of technology to support delivery of care (Barnes 2001; Spil and Stegwee 2001; Suomi 2001; Wager et al. 2005; Wickramasinghe 2000). Nevertheless, various innovative

---

*An earlier version of this material was presented at PACIS (Pacific Asia Conference on Information Systems) in Taiwan July 9–12, 2010

H. Sulaiman • N. Wickramasinghe (✉)
School of Business IT and Logistics, RMIT University, Melbourne, VIC, Australia
e-mail: nilmini.wickramasinghe@rmit.edu.au

technologies have successfully been introduced with the aim of improving hospital's performance and providing better healthcare services. However, the delivery of these technologies is perceived to be less than appropriate or adequate for the medical staff (Wager et al. 2005). The introduction of new technology begins with great enthusiasm and extensive spread of initial acquisition, however the new technology fails to be deployed and sustained in many acquiring firms (Fichman and Kemerer 1999). This causes the existence of an assimilation gap for a technology innovation as the initial acquisition of the technology does not always lead to sustainability of the technology usage.

The purpose of this chapter is to discuss a current research study that focuses on the issues that too many hospitals are facing in the implementation or acquisition of a healthcare information system. Specifically, this study will explore the technology innovation assimilation issues and contribute to the current body of literature of information technology innovation assimilation. Through the development of a focused theory tailored specifically to the technology implemented in the healthcare setting, it is hoped that this research will provide a technology assimilation process model for IS/IT managers, hospital chief information officers and IS/IT executives in implementing or adopting healthcare information technology applications with the aim of delivering better healthcare services that can be fully utilized by medical personnel.

4.2 The Malaysian Hospital Context

The context of this research is the implementation of HIS in a Malaysian public hospital which covers both clinical information systems and non-clinical systems. There have been various definitions for hospital information systems which mainly covers the clinical side of the healthcare information systems. Thus in this research, a specific focus is given to Total Hospital Information Systems (THIS) which covers all aspects of the hospital workflow from patient registration, diagnostics, wards, outpatient clinics to billing. Hence the context of a Healthcare Information Systems (HIS) is best suited to this information system which was implemented at a Malaysian public hospital in 1999. The hospital is taken as a case study since it complies with the definition of being a hospital that has gone through the series of assimilation stages from initiation to adoption and routinization. This hospital was uniquely designed to have a hospital wide use of IS/IT and was only opened to public after thorough testing was done by medical and non-medical personnel for a period of 2 years. The hospital comprises of 19 medical departments, an IT department, administration and pharmacy. Since the hospital was built to have a hospital wide use of information systems, all hospital staffs are considered potential interview participants. The hospital staff are interviewed on their experiences of using the HIS highlighting its problems and issues with the implementation. Primary focus is given to the hospital staff that have been in the hospital throughout the planning and implementation stage in order to gauge their views and experiences in each of the assimilation stages.

The hospital operates with a total of 960 beds spread across 5 floors and a total of 19 clinical departments as listed in the hospital's organizational chart. The daily operations of the Alpha Hospital basically involve processing of patient admission and outpatient clinic. The outpatient clinic is on appointment basis where referred patients from other medical centers register themselves as a patient in the Alpha Hospital with their demographic data taken via the patient registration system and given the appropriate appointment to see the specialist based on the specialists' schedule. This could take between 1 week to 6 months. It is only after the appointment with the referred specialist that the patient is assessed if they are to become an inpatient of the Alpha Hospital. Otherwise they would either be treated during the appointment by prescription of medication or a follow up treatment on another day.

A typical government hospital patient usually comes in with a guarantee letter which states that the patient is either working for the government which is commonly referred to in Malaysia as a government servant or the spouse, dependent or parents of the government servant. This guarantee letter exempts the patient from paying hospital bills and acts as a hospital deposit. Government servants are entitled to free or heavily subsidized hospital care and privileged to different classes of services according to their ranks (Chee and Barraclough 2007). The general public without guarantee letter are considered full paying patient which could also seek free or heavily subsidized inpatient and outpatient care or choose to pay more for higher class wards (Chee and Barraclough 2007; MOH-Malaysia 2010).

The inpatient has to go through a process of admission registration where it involves bed allocation and clerking of demographic data. Patients requiring inpatient care in the Alpha Hospital needs to be registered for the visit through inpatient admission process. Once registered the patient can be admitted to an inpatient facility and allocated a bed. During the stay, patient may be moved or transferred from one room to another or one ward or unit to another. At the end of the stay the visit is terminated or in other words the patient is discharged.

An inpatient is given a standard name according to the type of service provided and a unique identifier known as the Medical Record Number (MRN) to enable the accounting of all services and products provided to the patient. The registration process is done via counter in the lobby of the hospital by an administrative clerk through the Patient Registration System. The information is then made accessible to the ward expecting to receive the inpatient. Bed allocation is done manually by the ward nurses and clerks. Depending on the ward availability the patient or patient care taker may choose to be assigned to different classes of wards either through the assigned class ranking from the guarantee letter or choose to pay a higher amount for higher class. A typical third class ward in the Alpha Hospital consists of four to eight beds in an area, whereas class two wards are a two bedded sharing room and first class is a single room. Once patient is safely assigned to the respective ward the investigation and diagnosis begins.

During investigation, tasks or procedures are performed and goods such as drugs or prosthesis are provided. For financial accounting and statistical calculation, all these encounters, tasks, procedures and events need to be named and listed using standard nomenclature usually using codes. Various responsibilities are involved in the care of a patient. A team of doctors, nurses and medical assistants in some instances are responsible for overall planning and care of the patient. A doctor usually the specialist leads the team and is said to be the doctor-in-charge of the patient. The doctor in-charge or attending physician has the prerogative of inviting other clinicians or other categories of caregivers to be involved in the care of the patient by requesting for their services or referring the patient to them in request for their consultation. The procedures involved in the investigation are fairly standard for all clinical units and cover a range of processes that includes:

1. Clinical data gathering: Interviewing and examining the patient
2. Carry out further investigations
3. Making diagnosis: Identifying problems and needs
4. Planning for treatment or surgery
5. Carrying out treatment or surgery
6. Review of progress of disease or performing post operative care
7. Monitoring of effects of treatment
8. Review of diagnosis
9. Review of treatment including determination of outcome
10. Final disposal of the case

The information gathered throughout the investigation is crucial to be stored for real time accessibility of data and future references. The data gathered and stored are records of clinical processes performed during the care of the patient, the results of these processes and any other events occurred on the patient.

The patient data in digital format are sent to the electronic medical record and billing application to calculate the services and procedures involved during the stay. The charts or scribbling done manually will be hand delivered to the Medical Record Office to be physically stored inside large filing cabinets in the medical record office's storage room. Inpatients that are discharged from wards are also given a single prescription for supply of medication for a fixed duration. The doctor in charge in the ward places the order in the EMR as well as prints the prescription to the patient. The patient may obtain the drug from the dispensary counter or in exceptional cases the drugs may be delivered to the patient.

4.3   Theoretical Background

Based on the innovation diffusion literature, assimilation can be defined as a series of stages beginning from the organization's initial evaluation of the potential system to be used to its formal adoption and finally to a well accepted deployment of the system to a point where it becomes an important part of the value chain activities (Fichman 2000). The final stage where the system becomes part of the value chain activities is called routinization (Zhu et al. 2006). Previous literature on technology innovation and diffusion was mostly based on the work of Everett Rogers through his diffusion of innovation (DOI) theory (Agarwal et al. 1997; Ahmed et al. 2007; Burke et al. 2002; Gallivan 2001; Greenhalgh et al. 2004). Although this model has been extended in some other researcher's work (Moore and Benbasat 1991) and has created an insightful role in moulding the basic idea, terminologies and scope of the field, nevertheless this model does not "apply equally well to all kinds of innovation in all adoption context" (Fichman 2000). In this case, Rogers also suggested that innovations in a non-profit sector often encounter a huge diffusion difficulty, hence a study on healthcare innovations which can bring about good to the public but has diffusion and other related innovation issues is worth of a study (Mcgrath and Zell 2001). Therefore, a study that looks into the organization, individual and technological level focusing on how a technology can be sustained throughout the innovation assimilation stages and why the assimilation gap exists is also worth looking into. Moreover, how and why do people in the organization reject or refuse to make use of the innovation after the acquisition process which can cause discontinuance of the innovation is also crucial in understanding this scenario (Greenhalgh et al. 2004). Further, there are also lack of theories being developed to a specific type of technology and to a particular adoption context due to the lack of generic theory of technology innovation (Fichman 2000). Therefore, this provides a motivation to this research in developing a technology innovation assimilation model for hospitals to successfully assimilate thus sustain the use of healthcare information systems.

4.3.1 Diffusion Innovation Theory

The diffusion of an innovation can be described as the process in which knowledge of an innovation spreads across a population, and through the decision made by a unit in the organization the innovation is eventually adopted or rejected (Carter et al. 2001; Rogers 2003a). Studies on the diffusion of innovation research began with Rogers' work on the diffusion of agricultural innovation through the observation of the state of Iowa farmers in America who delayed the adoption of new innovation that is known to be beneficial for them (Rogers 2003b). Findings indicate that adopters of any new innovation or idea can be categorized as innovators, early adopters, early majority, late majority and laggards, based on the mathematically-based Bell curve. However, adoption over time will indicate an "s-shaped curve" or better known as an "S curve" to show that the technology adopters may be slow at start, more rapid as adoption increases, then taking off at a more level state (Rogers 2003a). This is more widely known as the diffusion of innovation model (Rogers 2003b). While Rogers' model was considered the first process model of innovation adoption and implementation, over the years there have been many other models proposed namely in the area of management (Meyer and Goes 1988) as well as information technology (Cooper and Zmud 1990; Kwon and Zmud 1987; Saga and Zmud 1994). Based on the diffusion of innovation literature, a summary of studies relevant to this research has been identified and categorized into organizational issues, innovation assimilation and usage of traditional DOI.

Based on the selected literature identified in the table above, there is a need for more research to be done on the IT innovation assimilation area grounded through the diffusion of innovation literature in finding out reasons behind the failure or rejection of innovation usage amongst a population of a particular context. The review of relevant theoretical work carried out in the area of IS/IT innovation assimilation based on the diffusion of innovation literature and specifically focused on the healthcare industry is discussed in the next section.

4.3.1.1 Theory of Innovation Assimilation

Innovation can be defined as an idea, practice, technology or entity that is considered to be new by an individual, a group or any other units of adoption (Rogers 2003b). The need for an innovation assimilation process can be seen in many of the healthcare information system implementation literature (Heeks 2002; Jayasuriya and Anandaciva 1995; Littlejohns et al. 2003). In a study of the implementation of healthcare information systems in developing countries such as South Africa and Philippines, when the HIS are being evaluated, three quarters are found to have failed with no evidence that the system have actually improved healthcare professional's productivity (Littlejohns et al. 2003; Willcocks and Lester 1996). These hospitals undoubtedly suffered from a severe assimilation gap during its implementation and operation (Heeks 2002). The systems did not meet healthcare personnel's requirements and was abandoned within less than a year (Heeks 2002). Millions have been spent in the entire process of implementing the information system however due to mismanagement of assimilating the new technology to the healthcare personnel, the information system failed to proclaim its benefits (Littlejohns et al. 2003). Therefore, a study on the processes of innovation assimilation is worth looking into based on the issues identified in the healthcare information systems implementation.

4.3.2 Technology-Organization-Environment Framework

In finding out how to address assimilation gaps, there is a need to consider elements that influence the innovation assimilation process. Based on the reviewed literature, the technology-organization-environment (TOE) framework (Tornatzky and Fleischer 1990) provides aspects that firms should consider when studying influences to assimilation of technological innovation. These concepts are grouped in three firm's aspects: technological context, organizational context and environmental context (Tornatzky and Fleischer 1990; Zhu et al. 2006).

Technology context: Comprises of the internal and external technologies pertaining to the firm involved that includes both equipment and processes (Tornatzky and Fleischer 1990).

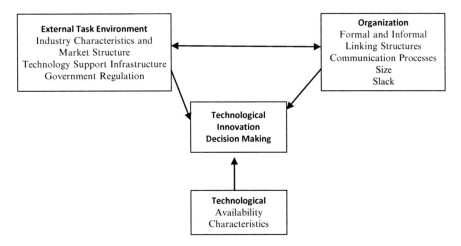

Fig. 4.1 TOE model: The original TOE model (Tornatzky and Fleischer 1990)

Organizational context: This involves the characteristics and resources of the firms such as firm size, managerial structure, human resources, amount of slack resources and linkages among employees (Tornatzky and Fleischer 1990).

Environmental context: This includes structure of the industry, the firm's competitors, the macroeconomic concept and the regulatory environment (Tornatzky and Fleischer 1990).

These elements has been argued as being both the constraints and opportunities for technological innovation, thus it is also considered as elements that influences the way a firm sees the need, the search and the way to adopt new technology (Tornatzky and Fleischer 1990).

A version of this framework is also applied in the work of Zhu et al. (2006) studying factors that influence e-business assimilation stages in both developed and developing countries (Fig. 4.1).

From this study, the germane findings included that factors such as technological readiness and regulatory environment are significant in innovation assimilation process. In addition, it was shown that the organizational context factors such as firm size and managerial obstacle which has been verified in the IS literature impacts IS/IT adoption and usage (Gurbaxani and Whang 1991; Zhu 2004). Firm size is seen as an important organizational attribute for innovation diffusion (Rogers 2003a). With regard to the assimilation stages, Damanpour (1996) argued that the relation between firm size and assimilation stages may differ due to differences in activities carried out in each of the assimilation stages. Further, larger firms usually initiate and adopt innovations due to their resource advantages in terms of financial, managerial and technical resources (Zhu et al. 2006).

The managerial obstacle element is referred to as the organization's lack of managerial skills and efficiency in handling change management, thus causes the

Table 4.1 IS/IT resource elements (Ross et al. 1996)

Resource	Elements
IS/IT human resources	Strong competent technical skills
	Excellent understanding of the business
	Empowered IS/IT teams to work closely with clients in addressing business needs
Technology	Sharable technical platform and databases
	Well defined technology architecture data and platform standards
Relationship	Ownership and accountability of IS/IT projects from both IS/IT and client
	Top management leadership in establishing IS/IT priorities

ineffectiveness of managing technology adoption and adaptation (Roberts et al. 2003). This is inline with Mata's et al. (1995) view that the ability to merge managerial and IT skills highly depends on the firms' ability to assimilate information technology. Hence this requires firms to possess relevant managerial skills and overcome barriers in adopting and assimilating new technology. In line with the health-care information systems assimilation study, this research will adapt some of the influencing elements in the TOE framework such as hospital size and managerial obstacles as an influence to the HIS assimilation process.

4.3.3   IS/IT Resources in Resource Based View

The resource based view literature on IS/IT resources classification begins with Grant's (1995) classification of key IS/IT-based resources, and was categorized into:

IS/IT infrastructure: The tangible resource which includes IS/IT infrastructure components

IS/IT expertise: The human IS/IT resources which is divided into technical and managerial IS/IT skills

IS/IT enabled intangibles: The intangible IS/IT enabled resources such as knowledge assets, and customer focus

Ross et al. (1996) further extended the study by suggesting that the relationship and use of resources such as IS/IT human resources, reusable technology infrastructure and strong IS/IT-business partner relationship together would result to a faster strategic business needs in terms of cost effectiveness as compared to the organization's competitors. Elements of these resources as defined by Ross et al. (1996) are listed in Table 4.1.

Merging the studies of both Ross et al. (1996) and Grant (1995), Bharadwaj (2000) extended these concepts of IS/IT resources through an empirical study of the relationship between the IS/IT resources to organization's superior performance. Bharadwaj (2000) defines all three resources according to Grant's classification and

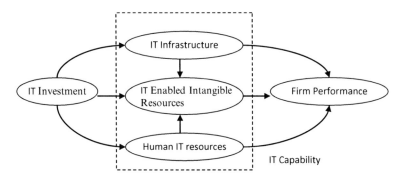

Fig. 4.2 IS/IT resources framework: Research framework in the study of Huang et al. (2006)

Table 4.2 Glaser's (2002) definition of the organization IS/IT resources

Resource	Description
Technical architecture	Basic infrastructure comprising of networks, programming languages, operating systems, workstations and other basic technologies that form the foundation for the applications
IS/IT staff	Analyst, programmers, computer operators who manages IS/IT in the organization
IS/IT governance	Organization mechanisms which include committees, policies, procedures, and best practices by which IS/IT strategies are formed, priorities are set, standards are developed and projects are managed

refers to them as IS/IT capabilities. Huang et al. (2006) then further explored the study by Bharadwaj (2000), through the similar usage of IS/IT resource based-view and concentrated on the same three resources. Their study however is focused on the use of the IS/IT resources in relation to IS/IT investment. An interesting outcome from this study is the revelation that the IS/IT infrastructure and human IS/IT resources cannot directly influence firm's performance. However, the two resources provide an influence to intangible resources such as knowledge assets, improved customer service through IS/IT, management of organizational knowledge, better synergy, improved coordination and sharing of resources across organizational divisions (Bharadwaj 2000; Huang et al. 2006). Hence, these intangibles are grouped as IS/IT enabled intangibles (Bharadwaj 2000) which will directly influence the firm's performance. Figure 4.2 denotes the original conceptual diagram used in Huang et al.'s (2006) research.

A study by Glaser (2002) on the strategic applications of IS/IT in healthcare organization has brought about the identification of healthcare organizational IS/IT resources that was aimed towards "furthering organizational strategies and advancing the organization's abilities to achieve its goals". The resources identified relevant to this study are listed in Table 4.2.

Another study on the identification of IS/IT resources in healthcare is a conceptual study done by Khatri (2006) which has identified important resources for healthcare organizations through literatures of resource based view. It is interesting to note that the identified resources are similar to the resources identified by Grant (1995) as well as the ones tested by Bharadwaj (2000) and Huang et al. (2006). Furthermore Khatri (2006) also feels that it is worth examining the relationship between these resources and clinical outcomes through mediating variables such as organizational processes. Therefore, this study identifies the influence of these resources to the innovation assimilation of healthcare information systems within a healthcare organization.

4.4 Development of the Conceptual Framework

Integral to the design and development of the proposed research model is the need to present the theoretical basis to answer the research question of how systematic focuses on assimilation can facilitate sustained use of healthcare information systems (HIS)? It also identifies the assimilation gaps and different components of technology, organization and environment which acts as an influence to the success of the HIS innovation assimilation. This model is derived from a combination of previous work done by Huang et al. (2006) and Zhu et al. (2006), in consistent with the classic conceptual work of Tornatzky and Fleischer (1990), Rogers (1995), Thompson (1965), Zmud (1982) and Grover and Goslar (1993). With the proposed model, this research will explore the interrelationship between innovation assimilation stages and contributing concepts that consist of technology, environment and organizational context to address the assimilation gaps. In line with the main aim of this research, this model deals with developing a healthcare information systems assimilation model for hospitals to successfully implement and utilize the healthcare information systems (Fig. 4.3).

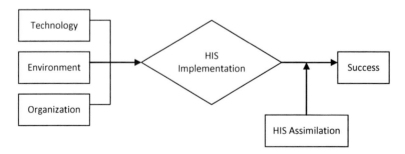

Fig. 4.3 Conceptual model of the research: HIS assimilation model

Fig. 4.4 HIS assimilation stages

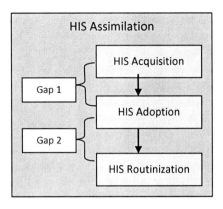

4.4.1 The HIS Assimilation Stages

Applying the innovation assimilation concept to the healthcare setting, this study will adopt the view of Zhu et al. (2006) and Ammenwerth et al. (2005), in classifying both awareness and evaluation in the initiation stage. This is inline with the conceptual framework of Thompson (1965) and many other empirical research (Agarwal et al. 1997; Chengalur-Smith and Duchessi 1999; Cooper and Zmud 1990; Gallivan 2001; Grover and Goslar 1993; Pierce and Delbecq 1977; Zhu et al. 2006; Zmud 1982) which considers "initiation" to be the first stage in assimilation.

Subsequent to initiation is the adoption stage, where this involves the successful usage of the technology acquired (Agarwal et al. 1997). A gap is identified between the stages of acquisition and adoption as there is usually the enthusiasm of acquiring new technology however once it has been adopted, many failed to meet its purpose and was not able to sustain its use (Fichman and Kemerer 1999).

Hence, adoption does not always indicate that the technology has been widely used in the organization, therefore this has to be followed by the utilization and institutionalization of the technology throughout the organization to a point where the technology adopted is becoming part of the organization's value chain (DeLone and McLean 1992; Devaraj and Kohli 2003; Sethi and King 1994; Zhu et al. 2006). This stage is then known as routinization. However, there exist another gap between adoption and routinization as it is also highlighted that after a new information technology or systems are being adopted, the organization and its members usually lack sufficient knowledge to gain control and manage the system thus causes an issue with the fit between the technology implemented and the end user's work context (Fichman and Kemerer 1999; Zhu et al. 2006), leading the system to be abandoned. The HIS assimilation stages for this research is depicted in Fig. 4.4.

The research model will also include several concepts identified from the TOE framework namely those which have been identified to be relevant with this research. Among the selected concepts are regulatory environment, technology readiness context, firm size and managerial obstacle as shown in Fig. 4.6.

Regulatory environment is an important concept to consider in this research as this study involves a government owned healthcare setting which centralizes control over the country's health policy through its constitutional powers. Hence the healthcare organizations are abide to any regulatory changes and implementation (Chee and Barraclough 2007) as the government's regulatory influences would have an impact on the HIS assimilation in a hospital. Technological readiness involves infrastructure, relevant systems and technical expertise which is considered important influences to the success of IS adoption (Armstrong and Sambamurthy 1999; Kwon and Zmud 1987). This concept is similar to the concept of IS/IT resources in the resource based view theory. Hence this research will merge the TOE technology readiness concept with the IS/IT resources concept identified from a combination of resource based view literature that relates to the influence of resources to organization's sustainability and performance (Bharadwaj 2000; Grant 1991, 1995; Huang et al. 2006; Khatri 2006; Ross et al. 1996).

Based on the studies done by Grant (1995), Ross et al. (1996), Bharadwaj (2000) and Huang et al. (2006) the identification of resources for this research shall include all of the three common resources (IS/IT Infrastructure, human IS/IT resources, IS/IT enabled intangibles) in the conceptual framework. These resources are deemed significant in finding out the influence that the IS/IT resources could provide to the HIS innovation assimilation. Hence, exploring how they are being utilized, and how they can be leveraged in sustaining the use of HIS is relevant to this study.

Apart from that, IT governance is also included as an influencing resource as many organisations including the healthcare industry adopted IT governance to ensure that IS/IT is aligned with organization goals and objectives (Cater-Steel and Tan 2005). In order to sustain the use of technology, there is a necessity in establishing some order and control in the management of IS/IT resources (Zachman 1987). Hence, in managing IS/IT resources, effective IT governance is required.

The firm size concept is incorporated in this framework due to its importance for innovation diffusion (Rogers 2003b) and to distinguish between activities that are carried out between large and small firms in each of the assimilation stages according to their resource advantages (Zhu et al. 2006). The managerial obstacles under the organizational context are also considered an important concept as the success of technology innovation will not only rely on the innovation itself and the behaviour of the adopters but also the strength and support provided by the management (Attewell 1992; Greenhalgh et al. 2008; Yetton et al. 1999; Zmud 1984). Considering the theoretical aspect and literature above, the research model will portray the three innovation assimilation stages: initiation, adoption, routinization, the relevant TOE concepts and the gaps which will be explored in the healthcare setting as depicted in Fig. 4.5.

Fig. 4.5 HIS assimilation stages

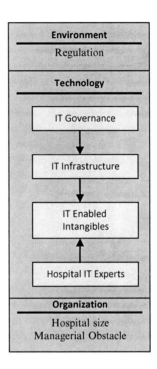

4.5   Methodology

This research examines the issue of IS/IT assimilation in healthcare and thus necessitates much investigation on the innovation assimilation with the influence of organizational, environment and technology resources. This in turn requires the adoption of qualitative research methods to be employed as it supports the investigation of "little known phenomena and complex processes in their natural setting" (Mantzana et al. 2007) and it is also crucial to answer the research questions by obtaining the point of view of the participants using the healthcare information systems in their hospital addressing their issues and problems explicitly. The use of interpretive case study research was adopted to enable an extensive understanding of the healthcare information systems assimilation process and enable a better understanding of the current organizational status directly from informants within the organization (Yin 2003). This study was guided through diffusion innovation and TOE theoretical concept with identified resources from the resource based view perspective. This provides a more detailed and insightful explanation of the study, hence the use of these theories acted as an initial guide to design and data collection (Walsham 1993, 1995). However, the theories were used in a very cautious manner, in order not to allow the research to be too rigid in only seeing what the theories suggest (Walsham 1995). An open mind was kept in order to discover new issues and areas for exploration leading to any modification of initial assumption and theories (Walsham 1995).

For this study an embedded single case design was used as the case selected is considered a critical case in testing well formulated theories. In the area of health-care information systems research, a case where the healthcare organization has undergone a series of healthcare information systems assimilation stages for a significant number of years up to a routinization point is considered as a critical case. In this manner, the choice of the single case with combination of the three chosen theories would represent a significant contribution to knowledge and information systems assimilation theory building. Adopting the critical case would also result to refocus future investigations in an entire field of healthcare information systems in other context (Yin 2003).

This research adopts a single case study approach with multiple units of analysis embedded within the case. One of Malaysia'a public hospital which has had a significant number of years assimilating healthcare information systems was selected as a case which provides the setting but within the hospital several instances of the phenomena is present. This supports Yin (1981) and Eisendhart's (1991) argument that contrasting observations from several units of analysis within one case can create and highlight theoretical constructs. A major reason for the choice of this hospital as a single case study was that in studying assimilation of information system, this involves a number stages from initiation, to adoption and finally to routinization. Hence, looking for a hospital equipped with end-to-end IS/IT utilization and adhering to the specific timeframe is crucial. A Malaysian public hospital which will be known as Alpha Hospital in this study was designed constructed and equipped for total hospital wide information systems environment with the ultimate aim of paperless and filmless hospital operation. This hospital is seen as the best choice as it was the first hospital in Malaysia that was build to operate with an end-to-end hospital wide computerization covering all aspects of its operation. It is anticipated that a number of implications would be derived from an in-depth case study of the assimilation of HIS in this public hospital which has gone through the assimilation stages by having IS/IT as its main hospital wide facilities for the last 11 years.

The common question when adopting a single case study approach would be "How can you generalize from a single case study?", with this a short answer from Yin (1981) states that case studies are generalizable to theoretical proposition. However, since this research takes on the interpretivist view, Walsham (1995) further extends this answer by claiming that interpretive case studies can be generalized through the development of concepts, generation of theory, drawing of specific implications and contribution of rich insights. To further strengthen the stand on adopting a single case study, this research also supports the argument of Markus (1989) where single cases may also be used for theory testing and disconfirming theory.

A variety of data collection methods were employed in getting a better depth of the study. The methods included interviews, researcher observation and document analysis. There were 31 participants for the main interview at the Malaysian public hospital and 2 participants were recruited for the pilot study. The participants for the pilot study were a medical specialist from the targeted Malaysian hospital and a

Table 4.3 Data collection details

Type of study	Number of interviewee	Positions	Department
Pilot	2	Medical personnel Subject matter expert	Departments chosen based on informant suggestion.
Main	31	Medical personnel, administrators, clerks and IT executives	1. Director's office 2. Hand and micro surgery 3. Pharmacy 4. Emergency 5. E & T 6. Gynaecology 7. Laboratory services 8. Admissions 9. Paediatrics 10. Information technology department 11. Emergency

subject matter expert on information systems in healthcare. The participants for the main interview were recruited across multiple departments in the hospital ranging from the pioneering group that was setting up the hospital to the very junior medical team. The participants were approached after permission was sought through the hospital's Deputy Director of Medical with some names being suggested as the point of contact for the relevant department. Participants were mostly contacted via email and appointment was scheduled according to the participant's availability. Table 4.3 summarizes the pilot and main data collection details.

This research adopts a semistructured interview method where the interviews were conducted on the basis of a loose structure consisting of open ended questions. These questions are there to provide a guide to the area to be explored initially however as the interviews progresses, the interviewer or interviewees may diverge in order to produce a more detailed description to the issues being discussed (Britten 1995).

Based on the experience of the researcher the semistructured interview was chosen in order to have a better guide and produce a more informative interview session. The questions in the semistructured interview was designed adapting the suggested list by Patton (1980) which starts by asking the interviewees background and demographic, followed by their opinion, experience, feelings and knowledge. The semistructured interview consists of 11 questions where some questions were merged and devised by the researcher during the interviews in order to provide better explanation and understanding especially to clinical staffs who are not quite well versed with IS/IT technological terms. All interviewees were given explanation on the research question, definition of assimilation and details on the assimilation stages to obtain more insight and in-depth responses. The interviews were digitally recorded upon approval of the interviewees and notes were taken where necessary.

4.6   Prelimenary Findings

The analysis was carried out with the initial conceptual framework in mind and emerging data from the interview translation. The interviews were transcribed and themes were identified from the transcription. The use of thematic analysis was applied in the analysis of data in this study as it provides a structured way of understanding how to develop thematic codes and sense themes. There were 3 stages involving the use of thematic analysis; Stage 1 involves deciding on sampling and design issues; Stage 2 involves developing themes and codes; stage 3 involves validating and using the codes (Boyatzis 1998). There are various ways of conducting the second stage either through theory driven, prior research or prior data driven and inductive. This study undertakes the theory and prior research driven approach to develop the themes and codes. The themes were first identified from the initial conceptual model, followed by some occurring themes identified through interview transcriptions. Any concepts that were not suitable to be categorized in any of the themes were placed in the "others" category. Figure 4.6 describes the themes identified with the issues discovered through the interviews.

The responses from the medical personnel were methodically and carefully scrutinized to be categorized into the identified themes. These themes are defined and described in the next section.

4.6.1   Organization

The organization theme refers to the characteristics and resources of the firms such as firm size, managerial structure, human resources, amount of slack resources and linkages among employees (Tornatzky and Fleischer 1990). This research has identified several sub-themes which are coded into financial, people and process.

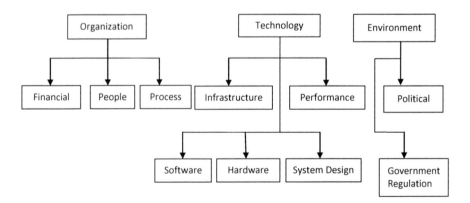

Fig. 4.6 Identified themes

Financial capacity has been argued as one of the most salient characteristics of having HIS innovation in a hospital setting (Jaana et al. 2006; Paré et al. 2009). A number of research in the technology innovation adoption in healthcare have also claimed that adequate financial resources, high costs, and calculating return on investment are among the top challenges and significant contribution to HIS technology adoption (Chang et al. 2007; Radhakrishnan et al. 2008; Yasunaga et al. 2008). Hence this research would like identify whether these issues are commonly described as a barrier towards HIS assimilation.

People or human resources are a crucial element to the success of assimilation. The IS/IT resources have been argued to require strong IS/IT competencies and skills in order to be able to solve business problems and handle business opportunities through the use of information technology (Ross et al. 1996). This research would like to identify if the IS/IT resources are seen as crucial to HIS assimilation or it requires more than just the skills of the IS/IT personnel.

Organization process is crucial in order to ensure the organisation's use of IS/IT sustains and planning of the organisation's strategy would be able to extend further in meeting newer requirements and needs (Sallé 2004). How does the process influence the HIS assimilation and what are the issues with the current process will be identified through further analysis of the data.

4.6.2 Technology

Technology refers to the readiness of the organization in providing the right infrastructure, relevant systems, technical expertise and other intangible IS/IT related matters concerning the proper assimilation of HIS. The sub-themes identified for this research has the technology characteristics divided into infrastructure (software and hardware), performance and system design.

Technology infrastructure refers to the physical IS/IT assets that forms the IS/IT backbone of the organization including the communication technologies, shareable technical platforms and databases (Bharadwaj 2000; Ross et al. 1996). Hence, this research identifies if the hospital's infrastructure has been expanded to the entire hospital, allowing them to evolve in taking care of the distribution and management of hardware, software, and other support services.

4.6.3 Environment

Environment refers to the higher level issues that surround the hospital administration namely in assimilating HIS. Political characteristics refer to any decisions or behaviour of any relevant parties within and outside the hospital which causes an impact towards the assimilation of HIS in the hospital. Since the setting of this research is in a public hospital, therefore government regulation is inevitable to be included and analysed on how the policies and regulations has provided a direct or indirect influence to the assimilation of HIS.

4.7   Discussion

The benefits of assimilating HIS in a public hospital is seen to provide great benefits in terms of data and information sharing amongst clinicians, availability of current and historical data, automated transactions and data analysis for audit and planning purposes. Unfortunately, with some inevitable barriers such as the lack of information and knowledge management planning, the misalignment of goals between the hospital and vendors and the lack of clinical IS/IT knowledge in the organization will not enable the benefits to be fully realized. Knowledge and information management was found to be one of the most critical barriers to the assimilation of HIS in the Malaysian public hospital. The initiation stage of the HIS assimilation of Alpha Hospital was done through various uncertainties and many unfamiliar territories. The inexistence of ready made documented policies, procedures, roles and responsibilities for information management in the hospital caused a major issue that was carried on until the routinization phase. Although the operations data were stored in a database, however with an unplanned and unstructured process of handling the data, accessing, extracting, aggregating and statistically analysing data to generate information on a single patient or a population of patients is seen as a constant failure. The root cause of this issue is due to the current business process of a public hospital which had too much dependency on contractors and vendors especially during the initiation stage which causes the management to loose control over various aspects of the HIS assimilation especially on knowledge and information management planning.

Due to obtaining the HIS through an off the shelf software and the lack of technical expertise in the hospital, there is the existence of one or more development and maintenance vendor. The hospital has an ultimate goal of having an efficient and effective HIS to be successfully assimilated across the entire hospital in assisting their daily clinical activities. This goal has to be aligned with any vendor that has the responsibility of deploying HIS to the entire hospital. Nevertheless, there were cases where unethical and incompetent vendors who managed to secure projects on the HIS development and maintenance through political influences, hence resulted to serious failure of providing a usable and workable HIS. This indicates a huge inter-organization misalignment of goals as on one hand we have an organization that wants to improve their work practices with the assistance of an information systems but on the other hand we have the supplier who were just there for their own benefits and personal agenda. The prolong practice of this situation is very damaging for the entire healthcare system. The way forward in achieving common goals will never be sought unless there is an intervention from the highest healthcare and country leadership in providing intelligent, fair and transparent affirmative policies instead of the current arbitrary and patronage-driven government policies relating to project procurement process. Dealing with human lives is an upmost priority that the relevant parties involved have to understand. If HIS were assimilated in hospitals, it should be seen as an enabler to expedite an existing service or enhance new services which would bring about immense benefit to the nation's healthcare and wellbeing. This can only be realized through a common understanding of the healthcare information systems' potential, capabilities, limitations and pre-requisites by the relevant parties involved such as the government, the hospital and vendors.

The lack of clinical IS/IT knowledge involves both the clinicians and IS/IT department. Whilst traditionally you have a common practice of users logging calls via helpdesk and troubleshooting of problems carried out by the IS/IT department, this creates a "language" barrier in a hospital with HIS. In order succeed in assimilation of HIS, the clinicians involved should somehow be able to have basic IS/IT knowledge such assessing system functionalities, identification and prevention of potential problems with the applications being used, and relaying these issues with their needs to the systems manager. It takes the champion to make the initiation and adoption stage a success, however to fully succeed in assimilating the information systems right to the routinized stage, the clinicians and IS/IT department needs to "speak" the same "language".

4.8 Conclusion

In summary, this study provides an overview of the issues which surrounds the design and preliminary findings of technology innovation assimilation in a healthcare environment. Aspects of technology innovation assimilation stages, the roles of the technology-organization-environment context have been explained to articulate the complex requirements of the HIS innovation assimilation. Further, it is necessary to address the assimilation gaps and this also foresees the important role of the contributing elements identified through the case study in successfully assimilating the HIS. Thus, this study addresses the gaps and challenges by merging different or commonly disparate theoretical frameworks to explore the technology assimilation stages, contributing elements and barriers to successfully assimilate the HIS. Given the huge reliance today on HIS by healthcare organisations globally this research will serve to facilitate better, more effective and efficient use of HIS and thereby support superior value driven healthcare delivery.

References

Agarwal, R., Tanniru, M., & Wilemon, D. (1997). Assimilating information technology innovations: Strategies and moderating influences. *IEEE Transactions on Engineering Management, 44*(4), 347–58.

Ahmed, H., Daim, T., & Basoglu, N. (2007). Information technology diffusion in higher education. *Technology in Society, 29*(4), 469–82.

Ammenwerth, E., Gräber, S., Bürkle, T., & Iller, C. (2005). Evaluation of health information systems: Challenges and approaches. In T. A. M. Spil & R. W. Schuring (Eds.), *E-health systems diffusion and use: The innovation, the user and the USE IT model*. Hershey, PA: Idea Group Publishing.

Armstrong, C. P., & Sambamurthy, V. (1999). Information technology assimilation in firms: The influence of senior leadership and IT infrastructures. *Information Systems Research, 10*(4), 304–27.

Attewell, P. (1992). Technology diffusion and organizational learning: The case of business computing. *Organization Science, 3*(1), 1–19.

Barnes, S. J. (2001). Experiences in strategic information systems implementation in UK healthcare. In R. Stegwee & T. A. M. Spil (Eds.), *Trategies for healthcare information systems* (pp. 11–30). Hershey, PA: Idea Group Publishing.

Bharadwaj, A. S. (2000). A resource-based perspective on information technology capability and firm performance: An empirical investigation. *MIS Quarterly, 24*(1), 169–96.

Boyatzis, R. E. (1998). *Transforming qualitative information: Thematic analysis and code development*. California: SAGE Publications.

Britten, N. (1995). Qualitative research: Qualitative interviews in medical research. *British Medical Journal, 311*, 251–3.

Burke, D. E., Wang, B. B. L., Wan, T. T. H., & Diana, M. L. (2002). Exploring Hospitals' adoption of information technology. *Journal of Medical Systems, 26*(4), 349–55.

Carter, F. J., Jambulingam, T., Gupta, V. K., & Melone, N. (2001). Technological innovations: A framework for communicating diffusion effects. *Information Management, 38*(5), 277–87.

Cater-Steel, A., & Tan, W. G. (2005). Implementation of IT infrastructure library (ITIL) in Australia: Progress and success factors. *Paper presented to IT governance international conference*, Auckland, New Zealand, pp. 14–16.

Chang, I. C., Hwang, H. G., Hung, M. C., Lin, M. H., & Yen, D. C. (2007). Factors affecting the adoption of perspective of hospital electronic signature: Executives' information department. *Decision Support Systems, 44*(1), 350–9.

Chee, H., & Barraclough, S. (2007). *Health care in Malaysia: The dynamics of provision*. Routledge, Hoboken: Financing and Access.

Chengalur-Smith, I., & Duchessi, P. (1999). The initiation and adoption of client–server technology in organizations. *Information Management, 35*(2), 77–88.

Cooper, R. B., & Zmud, R. W. (1990). Information technology implementation research: A technological diffusion approach. *Management Science, 36*(2), 123–39.

DeLone, W. H., & McLean, E. R. (1992). Information systems success: The quest for dependent variable. *Information Systems Research, 3*(1), 60–95.

Devaraj, S., & Kohli, R. (2003). Performance impacts of information technology: Is actual usage the missing link? *Management Science, 49*(3), 273–89.

Eisenhardt, K. M. (1991). Better stories and better constructs: The case for rigor and comparative logic. *Academy of Management Review, 16*(3), 620–7.

Fichman, R. G. (2000). *The diffusion and assimilation of information technology innovations*. Pinnaflex Publishing.

Fichman, R. G., & Kemerer, C. F. (1999). The illusory diffusion of innovation: An examination of assimilation gaps. *Information Systems Research, 10*(3), 255–75.

Gallivan, M. J. (2001). Organizational adoption and assimilation of complex technological innovations: Development and application of a new framework. *SIGMIS Database, 32*(3), 51–85.

Glaser, J. P. (2002). *The strategic application of information technology in health care organizations*. San Francisco: Jossey-Bass.

Grant, R. M. (1991). The resource-based theory of competitive advantage – Implications for strategy formulation. *California Management Review, 33*(3), 114–35.

Grant, R. M. (1995). *Contemporary strategy analysis*. Oxford, UK: Balckwell Publishers.

Greenhalgh, T., Robert, G., & Bate, P. (2008). *Diffusion of innovations in service organizations: A systematic literature review*. Wiley Blackwell.

Greenhalgh, T., Robert, G., MacFarlane, F., Bate, P., & Kyriakidou, O. (2004). Diffusion of innovations in service organizations: Systematic review and recommendations. *The Milbank Quarterly, 82*(4), 581–629.

Grover, V., & Goslar, M. D. (1993). The initiation, adoption, and implementation of telecommunications technologies in U.S. organizations. *Journal of Management Information System, 10*(1), 141–63.

Gurbaxani, V., & Whang, S. (1991). The impact of information systems on organizations and markets. *Communications of the ACM, 34*(1), 59–73.

Heeks, R. (2002). Information systems and developing countries: Failure success, and local Improvisations. *The Information Society, 18*, 101–12.

Huang, S.-M., Ou, C.-S., Chen, C.-M., & Lin, B. (2006). An empirical study of relationship between IT investment and firm performance: A resource-based perspective. *European Journal of Operational Research, 173*(3), 984–99.

Jaana, M., Ward, M. M., Paré, G., & Sicotte, C. (2006). Antecedents of clinical information technology sophistication in hospitals. *Health Care Management Review, 31*(4), 289–99.

Jayasuriya, J., & Anandaciva. (1995). Compliance with an incident report scheme in anaesthesia. *Anaesthesia, 50*(10), 846–9.

Khatri, N. (2006). Building IT capability in health-care organizations. *Health Services Management Research, 19*(2), 73.

Kwon, T. H., & Zmud, R. W. (1987). Unifying the fragmented models of information systems implementation. In *Critical issues in information systems research*. John Wiley & Sons, Inc. pp. 227–251.

Littlejohns, P., Wyatt, J. C., & Garvican, L. (2003). Evaluating computerised health information systems: Hard lessons still to be learnt. *British Medical Journal, 326*(7394), 860–3.

Mantzana, V., Themistocleous, M., Irani, Z., & Morabito, V. (2007). Identifying healthcare actors involved in the adoption of information systems. *European Journal of Information Systems: Including a Special Section on Healthcare Information, 16*, 91–102.

Markus, M. L. (1989). Case selection in a disconfirmatory case study. In *The information systems research challenge* (pp. 20–26). Boston, MA: Harvard Business School Press.

Mata, F. J., Fuerst, W. L., & Barney, J. B. (1995). Information technology and sustained competitive advantage: A resource-based Analysis. *MIS Quarterly, 19*(4), 421.

Mcgrath, C., & Zell, D. (2001). The future of innovation diffusion research and its implications for management: A conversation with Everett Rogers. *Journal of Management Inquiry, 10*(4), 386–91.

Meyer, A. D., & Goes, J. B. (1988). Organizational assimilation of innovations: A multilevel contextual analysis. *Academy of Management Journal, 31*(4), 897–923.

MOH-Malaysia (2010). *Ministry of Health Official Website*, viewed 05 April 2010, <http://www.moh.gov.my/>

Moore, G. C., & Benbasat, I. (1991). Development of an instrument to measure the perceptions of adopting an information technology innovation. *Information Systems Research, 2*(3), 192–222.

Paré, G., Jaana, M., & Sicotte, C. (2009). Exploring health information technology innovativeness and its antecedents in Canadian hospitals. *Methods of Information in Medicine, 49*(1), 28–36.

Patton, M. Q. (1980). *Qualitative evaluation methods*. CA: Sage Publications.

Pierce, J. L., & Delbecq, A. L. (1977). Organization structure, individual attitudes and innovation. *Academy of Management Review, 2*(1), 27–37.

Radhakrishnan, A., David, D., & Zaveri, J. (2008). *Challenges with adoption of electronic medical record systems*. Hershey, PA: IGI Global.

Rogers, E. (1995). *Diffusion of innovations*. New York: Free Press.

Rogers, E. (2003a). *Diffusion of innnovations* (5th ed.). New York: Free Press.

Rogers, E. (2003b). *Diffusion of innovations*. New York: Free Press.

Ross, J. W., Beath, C. M., & Goodhue, D. L. (1996). Develop long-term competitiveness through IT assets. *Sloan Management Review, 38*(1), 31–42.

Saga, V. L., & Zmud, R. W. (1994). The nature and determinants of IT acceptance, routinization, and infusion. Paper *presented to Proceedings of the IFIP TC8 working conference on diffusion, transfer and implementation of information technology.*

Sallé, M. (2004). *IT service management and IT governance: Review comparative analysis and their impact on utility computing.* Palo Alto: HP Laboratories.

Sethi, V., & King, W. R. (1994). Development of measures to assess the extent to which an information technology application provides competitive advantage. *Management Science, 40*(12), 1601–27.

Spil, T. A. M., & Stegwee, R. A. (2001). Strategies for healthcare information systems. In R. Stegwee & T. A. M. Spil (Eds.), *Trategies for healthcare information systems* (pp. 1–10). Hershey, PA: Idea Group Publishing.

Suomi, R. (2001). Streamlining operations in healthcare with ICT. In R. Stegwee & T. A. M. Spil (Eds.), *Strategies for healthcare information systems* (pp. 31–44). Hershey, PA: Idea Group Publishing.

Thompson, V. A. (1965). Bureaucracy and innovation. *Administrative Science Quarterly, 10*(1), 1–20.

Tornatzky, L. M., & Fleischer, M. (1990). *The process of technological innovation.* Lexington, MA: Lexington Books.

Wager, K. A., Lee, F. W., & Glaser, J. P. (2005). *Managing health care information systems: A practical approach for health care executives.* San Francisco: John Wiley.

Walsham, G. (1993). *Interpreting information systems in organizations.* Chichester: Wiley & Sons.

Walsham, G. (1995). Interpretive case studies in IS research: Nature and method. *European Journal of Information Systems, 4,* 74–81.

Wickramasinghe, N. (2000). IS/IT as a tool to achieve goal alignment. *International Journal of Healthcare Technology and Management, 2*(1), 163–80.

Willcocks, L., & Lester, S. (1996). Beyond the IT productivity paradox. *European Management Journal, 14*(3), 279–90.

Yasunaga, H., Imamura, T., Yamaki, S., & Endo, H. (2008). Computerizing medical records in Japan. *International Journal of Medical Informatics, 77*(10), 708–13.

Yetton, P., Sharma, R., & Southon, G. (1999). Successful IS innovation: The contingent contributions of innovation characteristics and implementation process. *Journal of Information Technology, 14*(1), 53–68.

Yin, R. K. (1981). The case study crisis: Some answers. *Administrative Science Quarterly, 26*(1), 58–65.

Yin. (2003). *Case study research: Design and methods* (3rd ed.). Newbury Park: Sage Publications.

Zachman, J. (1987). Framework for information systems architecture. *IBM Systems Journal, 26*(3), 276.

Zhu, K. (2004). The complementarity of information technology infrastructure and E-commerce capability: A resource-based assessment of their business value. *Journal of Management Information System, 21*(1), 167–202.

Zhu, K., Kraemer, K. L., & Xu, S. (2006). The process of innovation assimilation by firms in different countries: A technology diffusion perspective on E-business. *Management Science, 52*(10), 1557–76.

Zmud, R. W. (1982). Diffusion of modern software practices: Influence of centralization and formalization. *Management Science, 28*(12), 1421–31.

Zmud, R. W. (1984). An examination of 'Push-Pull' theory applied to process innovation in knowledge work. *Management Science, 30*(6), 727–38.

Chapter 5
e-Health in China: An evaluation*

Yu Yun, Wilfred Huang, Juergen Seitz, and Nilmini Wickramasinghe

Abstract China welcomes e-health service as it is developing globally, but like many other nations it encounters both opportunities and challenges. The rapid development of e-commerce and the wide application of ICT have accelerated their uses in healthcare service. Therefore, the assessment of e-health is becoming more important. We analyze the current situation in China and assess its goals of realizing e-health and the challenges of developing e-health.

Keywords e-health • ICT infrastructure • Electronic health record (EHR) • China • e-commerce

---

*An earlier version of this material was presented at the 23rd Bled eConference, Slovenia, June 20–23, 2010.

Y. Yun
School of Business, China University of Geosciences (Wuhan),
Wuhan, China
e-mail: yuyun.huihui@163.com

W. Huang
School of Business, Alfred University, New York, USA
e-mail: fhuang@alfred.edu

J. Seitz
Business Information Systems, DHBW Heidenheim,
Heidenheim, Germany
e-mail: seitz@dhbw-heidenheim.de

N. Wickramasinghe (✉)
School of Business IT and Logistics, RMIT University,
Melbourne, Victoria, Australia
e-mail: nilmini.wickramasinghe@rmit.edu.au

N. Wickramasinghe et al. (ed.), *Critical Issues for the Development
of Sustainable E-health Solutions*, Healthcare Delivery in the Information Age,
DOI 10.1007/978-1-4614-1536-7_5, © Springer Science+Business Media, LLC 2012

5.1 Introduction

The World Health Organization (2003) defines e-health as "being the leveraging of the information and communication technology (ICT) to connect providers and patients and governments; to educate and inform healthcare professionals, managers and consumers; to stimulate innovation in care delivery and health system management; and, to improve our healthcare system" (Wickramasinghe et al. 2004). Hence, e-health is a very broad term encompassing various activities in a developing field. As such, for practical reasons, in this paper we accept the assertion that e-health is basically enabled and driven by the use of ICT in healthcare with the potential to change the healthcare industry worldwide in terms of infrastructures as well as the costs and quality of services (Wickramasinghe and Goldberg 2004; Wickramasinghe and Misra 2004).

According to the World Health Organization, e-health evaluation may be carried out during planning, development, or operation of an e-health system (Brender 2006). The purpose is to provide the basis for the decisions about an e-health system under investigation or its implementation context. This paper will assess e-health in China to evaluate the risks and benefits for government, medical institutions and patients.

5.2 e-Health in China

Globally healthcare services are considered to be the biggest service industry, and they are taking top priority, receiving enormous investments, and are growing at a rapid pace in most developed countries (Mitchell 2000; Pan American Health Organization 1999). In China, the current focal point is the basic healthcare services in the rural areas. In 2008, the government focused its effort to expand domestic demand and promote economic growth in 10 measures, including Article IV stating the importance of "strengthening basic healthcare service system". According to the China Development and Reform Commission statistics, at the end of 2007, the central public finances have invested 9.4 billion RMB special funds to transform and build needed healthcare infrastructure. The positive attitude of the healthcare services reflects the e-health development potential in China.

Since the emergence and the growth of ICT it has brought opportunities and challenges to China. China has what is likely the world's largest untapped pool of ICT skills. One of the more impressive forecasts is that the number of Internet users in China is expected to exceed 360 million by the end of 2009 (National Bureau of Statistics of China, 2009). Table 5.1 provides the number of Internet users and highlights China's role in e-commerce and ICT development. Both, the central and regional governments, are strongly committed to provide the incentives and public goods needed to support e-commerce development in China. Consequently, the e-commerce sector grows at an unprecedented rate and exerts major impact on the economy in China.

Table 5.1 1997–2009 the number of Internet users in China (million) (Source: CNNIC)

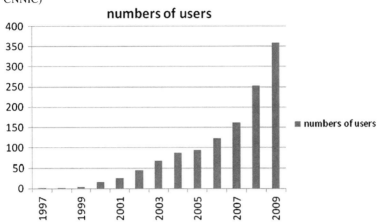

Each country is positioned differently and has varying potential and preparedness regarding embracing e-commerce technologies generally and e-health in particular (Wickramasinghe 2005). China has steadily carried out the development of e-commerce, which yields the opportunity for the advance of e-health. While e-health is increasing its efficiency in the healthcare services and ICT infrastructures, it may also bring risks. For example, information technology may be applied improperly, occurrence of errors, collapse of the information systems, etc. e-Health can bring serious consequences, so it is necessary to make an assessment. Given the macro level nature of issues pertaining to the development of e-health (Alvarez 2002) and to be more effective in their e-health initiatives, it is valuable to have an integrative framework that enables the assessment of e-health in China. A necessary first step is to identify the goals of e-health in China.

5.2.1 The Goals of e-Health

E-health in China aims to improve the traditional healthcare services. So, the goals are to remove the inequities, inefficiencies, poor quality, shortage of health resources, and improper distribution of health resources. They match the goals of e-health, which are efficiency, quality of care, evidence-based, empowerment of consumers and patients, education of physicians, widening the scope of healthcare, ethics and equity (Wickramasinghe et al. 2004).

The Ministry of Health in China has included e-health in the national long-term scientific and technological development plans, and is the main objective of the "The Eleventh Five-Year Plan "of China's health information (2005). In 2009, China published policy documents focusing the medical and health information technology on establishing a unified electronic health record (EHR) and national health information data dictionary. In summary, the following three goals for China's e-health include:

- Every citizen holds a safe and effective e-health record.

EHR is a necessary clinical information resource that modern medical institutions require to develop efficient, high-quality clinical practice and medical management. EHR can improve the quality and efficiency of medical and health services, prevent and reduce medical errors, control and reduce medical and health costs.

- Every citizen enjoys the disease prevention (immunization), healthcare and health counseling services, which can be multi-agency, cross-regional, inter-departmental and cross-ownership.

The development of health information technology development should support sharing of health information to improve healthcare efficiency and quality, to improve healthcare access, to reduce healthcare costs, and to reduce medical risks (Ma and Zhu 2005). Health information sharing depends on the computer and network technology in place (Nazi, 2002). Overall when compared to other industries the e-health is still fragile in this regard. E-health information is inevitably forming a large number of silos, which significantly slows down the information sharing process of the health sector. It is essential to improve healthcare structures so that they are multi-agency, cross-regional, inter-departmental and cross-ownership which will in turn enable health information to flow more seamlessly with the end result being that every citizen can enjoy the disease prevention (immunization), healthcare and health counseling services.

- Every citizen gains the corresponding food security and health insurance.

E-health must be connected to the national information database. It will become an efficient management and monitoring information platform in the market and knowledge-based economy.

5.2.2   Key Challenges of e-Health in China

To develop optimal partnerships between consumers and other groups of healthcare stakeholders, the key challenges in China include:

- Meaningful collaboration with healthcare recipients,
- Efficient strategies and techniques to monitor patterns of Internet use among consumers,
- Preparation for upcoming technological developments,
- Balancing between connectivity and privacy,
- Better understanding of the balance between face-to-face and virtual interactions,
- Equitable access to technology and information across the globe.

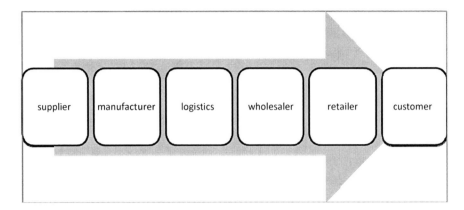

Fig. 5.1 Pharmaceutical supply chain in China

When we consider the domain of e-health at the macro level, three important issues must be carefully considered (Cyber Dialogue); namely procurement, connectivity and benefits.

5.2.2.1   E-Procurement

According to China's pharmaceutical supply chain model, the pharmaceutical manufacturers cannot directly sell drugs (Pharmaceutical Commerce, 2002). This is illustrated in Fig. 5.1. Pharmaceutical wholesale businesses are the intermediaries for the sales, especially for hospitals. Since the hospitals make up to 80% of the total drug sales in China, e-procurement mainly takes place between the wholesalers and the hospitals. In 2008, there were 19,712 general hospitals in China. There are a large number of pharmaceutical businesses and they are each of small scale. According to the National Bureau of Statistics of China, there are more than 25,000 wholesale enterprises. Less than 5% of these enterprises have annual sales of more than 20 million RMB, and the top 10 wholesale enterprises account for 20% of the total sales (Li and Duan 2003). This situation leads to drug operation disorder, bribery, kickbacks and other unethical practices, hence increasing the cost throughout the pharmaceutical supply chain.

Modern e-commerce tools enhance the transparence of the medical market and vigorously strengthen the information technology, thus allowing for better connection with government, market, and consumers. At the same time, under all levels of law enforcement supervision, the channels of all medicine selling and buying will be recorded by means and processes through the appropriate government agencies. Such market channels and the corresponding trading patterns will not only improve the efficiency of drug distribution, but reduce the costs of medicine in circulation.

Over the past decade, SeaRainbow Holding Corp, who had researched and developed SeaRainbow Medical E-commerce Solutions 2.0, had set up e-commerce business and quickly becomes the largest e-commerce platform in China. Its medical e-commerce revenue has reached $845.6 million in 2009. More and more pharmaceutical companies such as SeaRainbow Holdings Corp are actively operating on e-commerce of the medical market in China, who has accelerated the development of e-commerce of the medical market. However, most of these enterprises are also very conservative. Since the existing B-to-B e-commerce model has remained largely confined to providing medical information search and publishing platform, protecting trade secrets, and other considerations, the information released is limited to pharmaceutical companies on price and volume of transactions. So, the traditional procurement method is still preferred as the final means.

The current situation of B-to-C e-commerce in China is a stumbling block to the development of e-health. There are only 11 qualified online pharmacies and they are insignificant compared to China's vast pharmaceutical market. The primary reason for this is that the government strictly limits the online pharmaceutical market; i.e. the State Food and Drug Administration issues the "Certificate Internet Drug Information Service Qualification Certificate" and the "Internet Drug Transaction Services Qualification Certificate" which are very difficult to obtain. Drugstore chains are in fierce competition, yet the network monitoring is weak. Hence we contend that it will be a great challenge to establish e-procurement in China.

5.2.2.2   E-Connectivity

In 2009, the Ministry of Health of China issued the "Health Profile of Basic Architecture and Data Standards" (for trial implementation) (The Ministry of Health of China, 2009). The purpose of the implementation is to make personal health records more uniform and standardized. The provincial cities have been gradually implementing EHRs, and its footprint has gradually expanded to every province in 2009. However there are several difficulties in the rural areas. For example, the Hainan Health Department announced that in 2009 EHR coverage in the city had reached 30%, but in rural areas the archiving rate reached only 5%.

EHR informative sources can be found in: (1) the process of health services in a variety of services records; (2) the regular or irregular physical examination records; (3) thematic survey records of health or disease. Urban residents can go to a general hospital or the community hospital to establish their EHRs, but this is difficult in rural areas. The rural healthcare infrastructure is lagging behind and is burdened by obsolete infrastructure and medical equipment, which exacerbates the low utilization rate.

EHR requires a multitude of professionals, but according to a survey only 19.3% of the specialists in the rural hospitals have a technical secondary school diploma or above. Thus a substantial investment on the personnel training, a personnel training system and re-learning scheduling is vital as well as addressing the deficiencies with the current ICT infrastructure. The 2008 China Statistical Yearbook shows that there are 721 million in rural population; to develop an EHR for everyone will be difficult if not impossible given the current state.

5.2.2.3   E-Benefits

Since the launch of the new cooperative health cards and health insurance cards, e-commerce in healthcare service has been receiving much attention. The basic health insurance system uses the health insurance cards for every citizen. The health insurance card is identified by the ID card, which is issued by the government. It stores the name, gender, transferred account payment, consumption patterns, etc. The employer allocates money to employees' health insurance card through a bank. One can use the health insurance card in designated hospitals and drug stores. While visiting a doctor and buying medicine, the health insurance card can be used with authentication except to withdraw or transfer cash. Many cities in China have commenced providing social security cards and gradually replacing the health insurance card. It is not only for paying medical bills, but also for the retirement payment, job registration and unemployment registration.

If every Chinese has a health insurance card, it will greatly accelerate the development of e-health. However, China has a different development between urban and rural areas (Xiao, 2005). The Statistical Information Center of The Ministry of Health of China issued the "China's health development in 2008 Statistical Communiqués" which shows that in 2006 the nation's total health costs amounted to 984.3 billion RMB. Urban health costs accounted for 67% of total health costs and rural areas accounted for 33%. In the same year, the population was 1.314 billion, 44% were urban residents, and 56% were rural residents. Urban per capita health expenditures were 1,145 RMB; rural per capita health costs were 442 RMB. There has been a significant difference between urban and rural health and medical services. The main reasons are due to: (1) The urban-rural dual standards – Major investment of the government is focused on urban workers, along with individual investments to supplement the health insurance. Rural cooperative healthcare is primarily dependent on individual investments and small government support. (2) The government financial system – The financial resources of governments at all levels is uneven, the health investment cannot be guaranteed simply by transferring or sharing the resources. (3) Outdated market – Most of the peasants lack the purchasing capacity, causing the rural health service system to be deteriorated with poor regions being in a critical state.

5.3   Assessing e-Health Potential in China

We use the framework published in Wickramasinghe et al. (2004) to assess the e-health potential and preparedness of nations. The framework takes a macro perspective containing four main pre-requisites, four main impacts, and the implications of these pre-requisites and impacts to the goals of e-health. ICT infrastructure, standardization policies, user access infrastructure and governmental regulation make up the four essential prerequisites while the four key impacts are on IT education, morbidity rate, culture and economy. By examining both the pre-requisites and the impacts we can assess the potential of China and its preparedness for e-health as well as its ability to maximize the goals of e-health.

5.3.1 Prerequisites for e-Health

In sum, the four critical pre-requisites for any successful e-health initiative include ICT architecture/infrastructure, standardized policies, protocols and procedures, user access and accessibility policies and infrastructure, and finally government regulation and control.

5.3.1.1 ICT Architecture/Infrastructure

China's medical ICT has new applications, e.g. telemedicine, follow-up treatment, the patient data management, drug tracking, cell phone for help, the patient data collection, medical waste tracking and messaging communication. These new applications are supported by current ICT infrastructure.

By October 2009, the number of broadband Internet users exceeded 103 million. By December The Ministry of Industry and Information Technology of China 2009, the Chinese mobile phone users exceeded 747 million (date resource from Ministry of Industry and Information Technology of China). The 3G network has already been in full swing in China since 2009, the investment in wireless infrastructure rose 13.2% from 55 billion U.S. dollars in 2008 to 62 billion in 2009 (Kong 2009). In May 2008, the Chinese government has finally announced that it would issue three 3G licenses as part of its overall redevelopment plan. In the reconstruction program, the government plans to set up three telecommunication service providers – China Mobile, China Netcom (GSM) and China Unicom/Telecom. Each provider offers not only fixed-line but also mobile services. China Mobile has already built up TD-SCDMA trial network in some major cities. China Unicom and China Telecom gained the official 3G in the first quarter of 2009. China Unicom in 2009 has launched its W-CDMA and China Telecom is ready to expand its 3G CDMA2000-1x-EV DO network (Kong 2009).

In spite of this, the development of ICT infrastructure is still behind other nations. The mainland of China has only a 21% broadband penetration rate which ranks 43rd in the world. Chinese cable broadband (ADSL and cable modem) cannot keep pace with the demand for broadband access users. In 2007, the average network downlink transmission rate of major nations reached 17.4MB, while China had less than 4MB. So, transmission has become a bottleneck in the development of broadband. Currently, China's broadband development is mostly dependent on the market behavior of the telecom operators, less government involvement. Government's deployment of broadband will be a key step towards stimulating domestic demand by the state-led development strategy to promote broadband. The usage of Wi-Fi, CDMA, EV-DO, PHS and other wireless broadband technologies will lead to a better network coverage in China. The implementation in ICT infrastructures will gradually lead to the large-scale development of e-health.

5.3.1.2   Standardization Policies, Protocols and Procedures

To enable such a far-reaching coverage, significant amounts of document exchanges and information flows must be accommodated. Standardization is the key to this (Wickramasinghe 2005). In China, the medical reform proposed in 2009 was to establish the sharing medical and health information. The Ministry of Health also drafted a "Health Profile of Basic Architecture and Data Standards (for trial implementation)". The implementation of the program has three objectives: (1) establish a national unified, standardized health record of the population; (2) establish the basic framework for national EHRs and data standards; (3) establish the national health information data dictionary. The new standards require five types of EHRs to be standardized; they are the basic personal health information record, disease control record, maternal and child health record, medical services and community health record. Today, there are 35 cities, 2,406 community health service centers and 9,726 community health service stations in China who have established EHRs for a vast number of community residents. The content of EHRs and data structures strictly abides the uniform national norms and standards. The standardization of EHRs is to achieve integration of different sources of information, accessibility and sharing of mobile use, the necessary safeguards to eliminate information silos. It shows that the government strongly supports the development of China's EHRs.

However, there is a lack of the uniform "Community Health Service Information Management Systems" software. People rely on the hospital HIS system to establish EHR, therefore standardized health records do not exist since different software developers and software contractors create different hospital HIS systems. It is not the best choice for the community or general hospitals to establish EHR. Using Internet technology and the support from hospitals and community health service centers, a region which has independent financial support and a complete medical and health system of administration (The Ministry of Health of China 2009a–c) can establish a network information service center. The center can collect EHR of personal lifetime health and non-health information. At present, China has established a digital resource in regional data centers, such as Wuhan digital resources (regional data centers). The regional health information systems can connect hospital HIS systems and home health care service systems so that hospitals, patients, and community health service centers are able to connect to each other with authentication.

Table 5.2 2007Q1–2009Q2 the number of Chinese online advertising of e-health (Source: iResearch Inc.)

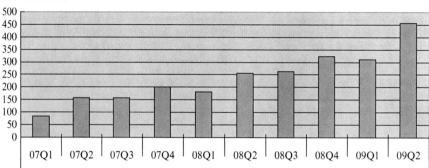

5.3.1.3   User Access and Accessibility Policies and Infrastructure

Access to e-commerce is defined by the WTO (World Trade Organization) as consisting of two critical components:

Access to Internet services
Access to e-services (Panagariya 2000).

The former deals with the user infrastructure and the latter refers to the commitments of electronically accessible services. E-health is often established with a focus on user infrastructure (Wickramasinghe et al. 2004), in particular including pharmaceutical companies. Survey shows that in China pharmaceutical companies have 30 or more computers for every 100 employees accounted for 14.55%; 20–29 every 100 units accounted for 9.1%; 10–19 every 100 accounted for 28.20%; 0–10 every 100 units accounted for 42.73%. 95.45% of the pharmaceutical companies are connected to the Internet and 80.91% have an internal LAN; 54.5% of corporate websites have a basic company profile, product descriptions, contacts, online message or customer services; 67% update their websites at least once a week. Overall, more and more enterprises increase their expenditure on infrastructure. Compared to 2003, it has increased 3% in 2004 and 5% in 2005 (data source from Operation Analysis of the pharmaceutical industry in 2004 and 2005 Development Forecast, 2005).

At the same time, web investment has also gradually increased. Table 5.2 shows that the number of Chinese online advertising of health during 2007Q1-2009Q2 based on more than 170 web-media.

The situation of hospitals HIS is as follows: In 2002, the Ministry of Health of China showed that out of 6,921 hospitals 2,179 of them built HIS, which accounted for 31%. Hospitals in the east coastal China accounted for nearly 80% of the nation. In general, China's pharmaceutical companies and hospitals are working forward to implement e-health.

In addition to pharmaceutical companies and hospitals, e-health cannot happen without the support of Internet users. China has the largest number of potential

Internet users in the world, but its Internet penetration is low. In the 2010 "Social Blue Book" reported that China's Internet penetration rate has reached 26%, which is more than the world's average. However, this penetration rate is far lower than that of the developed nations. This will be a barrier to the e-health development. The gap between rural and urban Internet penetration is still big. Fiber optic has not reached rural areas. Furthermore, education and living standards are low in rural areas, which also impacts e-health initiatives.

5.3.1.4   Governmental Regulation and Control

Government regulation aims to contribute to the healthy development of pharmaceutical e-commerce management systems, which strengthen market supervision, regulate online drug transactions, ensure information security, and safeguard the normal order of e-commerce activities. China has promulgated the "Computer Information Network and the Internet Management Interim Provisions of China" and the "Computer Information Network and the Internet Security Protection and Management Measures".

If China can further protect the privacy of the e-health information, the law will be a strong guarantee for privacy protection (Mao and Xiang 2008). For example, the "International conventions of tele-medicine and tele-health" and the United States "Health Insurance Portability and Accountability Act" (HIPPA) specifically focus on the confidentiality and privacy of electronic information management. They play a positive role in protecting the privacy of e-Health information. We assert that by combining the "International conventions of tele-medicine and tele-health" with the specific goals, China can develop appropriate national laws and regulations for e-health to guard its development.

5.3.2   Key Impact of e-Health

E-health will not only bring benefits to China, it will also have drawbacks. In this section, we discuss the effects based on the framework of Wickramasinghe et al. (2004).

5.3.2.1   Impacts of IT Education

China has a large number of consumers with a low level of IT education in rural areas, most of them are quinquagenarian. It is difficult for them to learn e-health and tele-medicine skills in a short term. The IT education and e-health are highly correlated. The development of an e-health market will lead more people to use IT technology, and the more IT education availability will support the development of e-health.

The vast majority of young people grew up in the information age. They have received an extensive IT technology education, which they use at their work. More and more young people also begin using computers, searching online and shopping online. From a long-term perspective, young people are the mainstay of the e-health market in the future. In order to develop e-health, China needs to educate the nation and increase the awareness of the concept of e-health and e-consumption.

5.3.2.2 Impact of Morbidity Rate

China is a country with a higher morbidity rate, according to the statistics of the Ministry of health of China in 2008, the hospitalization rate of residents was 0.684% and the hospital bed occupancy rate had increased to 74.6%. These statistics show that more investments are needed in medical infrastructure. The government and the public hospitals are the dominant players in the medical infrastructure, and will like to see e-health infrastructure developed HIS, EHR, and a series of supporting infra-structures. In China, e-health construction financing is primarily decided by the government's investment.

5.3.2.3 Impact of Cultural/Social Dimensions

People accept western medicine but traditional Chinese medicine has a bigger mar-ket share in China. Face-to-face therapy session with a doctor is always preferred to telemedicine. In addition, since China's two previous healthcare reforms have failed, e-health is more likely to be used as a technology-based or information-oriented direction, rather than the core of the entire medical system, and this is a challenge that e-health must address. Whether e-health can access appropriate levels of gov-ernment financing and grow quickly depends on what role it will play in the health-care reform.

5.3.2.4 Impact of World Economic Standing

China's rapid economic development provides a good opportunity for the develop-ment of e-health in China. There are a number of economic risks the Chinese e-commerce industry has to deal with. China's long-term economic risks exist (Wang 2005): economic structure is irrational; economic recovery will take time for the financial crisis. Pharmaceutical and medical market risks are accompanied with economic risks. The efficiency of the medical control system, the government medi-cal institutions, corruption, and disarrayed healthcare market are all factors that bring constraints to the development of e-health in China.

5.4 Discussion and Conclusion

According the WHO China has one of the most unfair healthcare systems in the world. One of the most surprising aspects of the system is that the majority of the expense related to healthcare is paid directly by the patient and there are few provisions for

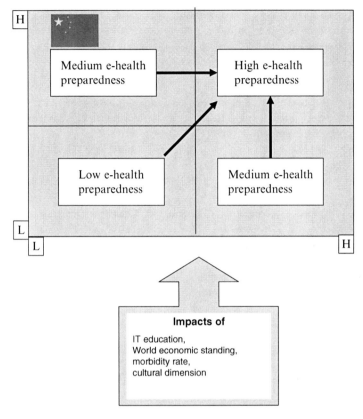

Fig. 5.2 E-health prepardness grid (Adapted from Wickramaisngeh et al. 2004)

people who cannot afford healthcare treatment. It is believed that e-health and the delivery of healthcare solutions will play a key role in addressing key problems that currently impact healthcare delivery in China including a growing ageing population, epidemics, the growing prevalence of "western illnesses" and an increasing gap between rural and urban, rich and poor. As we have described in the preceding analysis this is only possible if effective e-health initiatives are introduced and this can only occur if investment is targeted at education and training as well as the design and establishment of appropriate infrastructures across the country.

Based on the grid (Fig. 5.2) for assessing e-health preparedness (Wickramasinghe et al. 2004) we analyze China with respect to our key parameters for e-health success in an attempt to highlight the key areas. There are the four main pre-requisites above-mentioned, namely, the ICT infrastructure, the standardization policies, protocols and procedures, the user access and accessibility policies and infrastructures, governmental regulations and the role as well as the impact of IT education, the impact of the morbidity rate, the impact of the world economic standing and the impact of cultural/social dimensions. In summary, the current e-health in China has:

1. The level of the China ICT infrastructure is in its beginning phase.
2. Standardization policies, protocols and procedures are coming along.
3. It has the most netizens in the world but with a low penetration rate.
4. The government is commendable for the high level of regulations and control.

Therefore, China has a high standardization and a high government regulation, and simultaneously a low ICT infrastructure and penetration rate on PC with respect to the four pre-requisites for e-health potential. Therefore, China maps to the medium preparedness quadrant.

Figure 5.2 shows China on the e-health preparedness grid.

E-health is a realization of a people-oriented national health service and information technology management platform. Technically, e-health has not only achieved a combination of information technology and digital technology in healthcare, but also hospital information and social information. China has basically acquired the fundamental conditions for implementation of e-health, including the good governance, uniform medical diagnostic standard, hardware and software equipment and information networks, digital medical treatment equipment, manufacturing capacity, the initial EHR and electronic medical records experience. It is now vital that appropriate investment is targeted and the critical areas so that an effective e-health initiative can be realized that will indeed address the pressing problems currently plaguing healthcare delivery in China.

References

Alvarez, R. C. (2002). The promise of e-health – a Canadian perspective. *eHealth International, 1*(1), 4.

Brender, J. (2006). *Handbook of evaluation methods for health informatics.* Burlington, MA: Elsevier Academic Press Publications.

Chinese Journal of Pharmaceuticals. (2005). Operation analysis of the pharmaceutical industry in 2004 and 2005 development forecast. *Chinese Journal of Pharmaceuticals, 36*(3), I–VI.

HIS999.com. (2005). *e-health has as main objective the development of China's eleventh five-year health information technology,* Received February 6th, 2010 from http://www.his999.com/shownews.asp?id=147

Kong, W. (2009). *Chinese wireless infrastructure spending reached a peak in 2009,* Received February 6th, 2010 from http://www.isuppli.com.cn/products/china-market/0911192

Li, Y., & Duan, W. (2003). Logistics development strategy of drugs approved. *Medicine in the World,* (8), 32.

Ma, N., & Zhu, J.-H. (2005). Present condition and development of our country in hospital information system. *Information Technology,* (9), 6.

Mao, X., & Xiang, Y. (Feb. 2008). Philosophical thoughts on privacy protection in e-health age. *Journal of Wuhan University of Science & Technology (Social Science Edition), 10*(1), 32.

Mitchell, J. (2000). Increasing the cost-effectiveness of telemedicine by embracing e-health. *Journal of Telemedicine and Telecare, 6,* S16–S19.

National Bureau of Statistics of China (2009). The second national economic census the main data bulletin. Retrieved May, 2010 from http://www.stats.gov.cn/english/

Nazi, K. M. (2002). The journey to e-health: VA healthcare network upstate New York. *Journal of Medical Systems, 27*(1), 35–45.

Pan American Health Organization. (1999). *Setting up healthcare services information systems: A guide for requirement analysis, application specification, and procurement.* Washington, DC: Essential Drugs and Technology Program, Division of Health Systems and Services Development, PAHO/WHO.

Panagariya, A. (2000). E-commerce, WTO and developing countries. *The World Economy, 23*(8), 959–978.

Pharmaceutical Commerce. (2002). *Hidden opportunities for industry consolidation,* Received http://www.htsec.com/htsec/jsp/gpzx-content/content.jsp?guid={EDC4AFD3-9FD3-11D7-965B-00A0C92674A3}&type=6

The Ministry of Health of China. (2009). *The state department of the Central Committee of the Communist Party of China on deepening the views of medical and health system reform,* Received February 6th, 2010 from http://www.moh.gov.cn/publicfiles/business/htmlfiles/mohzcfgs/s7846/200904/39847.htm

The Ministry of Health of China. (2009). *Construction the platform of the Regional Health Information Guide based on health records (trial),* Received February 6th, 2010 from http://www.moh.gov.cn/publicfiles/business/htmlfiles/mohbgt/s6693/200906/41031.htm

The Ministry of Health of China. (2009). *State council on the issuance of the recent focus on medical and health system implementation plan (2009–2011) of the notice,* Received February 6th, 2010 from http://www.moh.gov.cn/publicfiles/business/htmlfiles/mohzcfgs/s7846/200904/39876.htm

The Ministry of Industry and Information Technology of China. (2009). *December 2009 operational status of China's telecommunications industry,* Received February 6th, 2010 from http://www.miit.gov.cn/n11293472/n11293832/n11294132/n12858447/12985116.html

Wang, D. (2005). *China's economic growth mode is entering a wrong path may be long-term decline,* Received February 6th, 2010 from http://business.sohu.com/20050512/n225526712.shtml

Wickramasinghe, N. S., Fadlalla, A., Geisler, E., & Schaffer, J. L. (2004). A framework for assessing e-health preparedness. *International Journal of Health, 1*(3), 316–334.

Wickramasinghe, N. S., & Goldberg, S. (2004). How M=EC^2 in healthcare. *International Journal e-health, 2*(2), 140–146.

Wickramasinghe, N. S., & Misra, S. (2004). A wireless trust model for healthcare. *International Journal e-Health, 1*(1), 60–77.

Wickramasinghe, N., Geisler, E., & Schaffer, J. (2005) "Assessing e-Health" in Spiel and Schuring Eds E-Health Systems Diffusion and Use: The Innovation, the User and the USE IT model, Idea Group, Hershey. pp. 294–323.

Xiao, S. (2005). Strategic thinking of China's promotion of e-health. *China Instrument Society of the third branch of medical devices for the first time the core of the council-cum-modern digital medical equipment and key technology research forum proceedings,* Beijing. p. 68.

Chapter 6
Improving the Process of Healthcare Delivery in an Outpatient Environment: The Case of a Urology Department

Chris Gonzalez and Nilmini Wickramasinghe*

Abstract In order to realise the healthcare value proposition of access, quality and value, it is necessary to examine existing healthcare processes to identify opportunities to re-design them and incorporate ICT (information communication technologies) to enable effective and efficient processes that do facilitate the delivery of superior healthcare. The following discusses this in the context of a urology clinic at a large hospital in the MidWest, USA.

Keywords Process re-engineering • ICT • Workflow • Urology

6.1 Introduction

In most outpatient settings waiting, delays and cancellations are sadly too common. One might be tempted to think that this is why a patient is called a patient. Both patients and providers are significantly affected by the waste of time due to waiting, delays and cancellations. Moreover, the quality and cost of health care delivery are also negatively impacted.

Quality is pillared by three different kinds of quality. The first is result quality. This is the most important, because it is responsible for patient satisfaction, which is essential for the success of healthcare institutions. The second is structural

*The author wishes to acknowledge Katharina Gaensler of the University of Cooperative Education Heidenheim, Germany for her invaluable assistance on this project.

C. Gonzalez
NorthWestern Memorial Hospital, Chicago, IL, USA

N. Wickramasinghe (✉)
School of Business IT and Logistics, RMIT University, Melbourne, VIC, Australia
e-mail: nilmini.wickramasinghe@rmit.edu.au

N. Wickramasinghe et al. (eds.), *Critical Issues for the Development*   87
of Sustainable E-health Solutions, Healthcare Delivery in the Information Age,
DOI 10.1007/978-1-4614-1536-7_6, © Springer Science+Business Media, LLC 2012

quality; which includes the conditions, required to succeed; i.e. number of employees and their skills, the infrastructure, the equipment, the organization structure and the collaboration within a team. This kind of quality is the simplest to measure. The third and easiest to impact is process quality. It includes the workflow and the information flow. If all of these three quality pillars are high, the overall quality will be also at a high level. However, if there are big differences between these then patients and providers alike will feel this imbalance and total quality will be negatively impacted.

The impression of lack of quality mostly lies in process quality problems (Kywi, 2007; Ganiban, 2004; Schnellen, 2008). But it is easy to solve these problems, because there are no big capital investments to be made. Improving the workflow lies in reducing process variation that impact flows (Institute of Healthcare Improvement 2003). While some variability is normal, other variation is not and should be eliminated. Waits, delays, bottlenecks and backlogs are not the result of lack of commitment on the part of staff. The answer to improving workflow lies in redesigning the overall, system-wide work processes that create the flow problems. Optimal care can only be delivered when the right patient is in the right place with the right provider and the right information at the right time.

To illustrate this and thereby show how it is possible to enhance quality and value in an outpatient setting the following discusses a three phase case study performed at a urology setting in a large MidWest hospital in the US. Phase 1 occurred in 2006–2007, phase 2 2007–2008 and phase 3 commenced in Oct 2008.

6.2   Background to Urology Clinic – Initial Position

In 2006, the outpatient urology department of a large MidWest hospital was convinced that quality and hence value was being compromised since its patients did not consistently move smoothly through the system. Specifically, patients on one hand and providers on the other hand were wasting too much time with waiting. This was taken as a clear sign that processes need to be improved. However moving from needing to improve processes and what to do to improve these processes was critical.

The outpatient urology department has very few emergency patients. Most of the patients that come to the urology clinic make an appointment before they come. Hence the clinic should not have to struggle with flow variation – the ebb and flow of patients arriving throughout the day – as is typical in emergency departments. So it should be possible for the urology department to control patient flow with effective scheduling. The urology clinic however does have to manage clinical variability – different patients' conditions they have to medicate and treat. In addition, they have to handle professional variability; i.e. the fact that their providers have different techniques regarding how they medicate the patients and how they organize their workflow.

Hence, some of the variability cannot be eliminated or reduced, rather it must be managed, because it is not possible to eliminate the different types of problems from which patients suffer. However, other types of variability are often caused by individual preferences and these should be reduced if not eliminated.

6.3 Preparations

There are many factors that can have an effect on the process of healthcare delivery: technical, organizational, structural, economic, human etc. The best way, to find out the reasons that cause the existing process problems was to analyze the complete urology department. In order to do this, an ethnographic research methodology was adopted and the activities of the urology clinic were critically observed and evaluated. It also was necessary to see the urology clinic from different points of views. Therefore physicians, medical assistants, medical technicians, receptionists and patients have been interviewed. For these interviews protocols and questionnaires were prepared.

6.4 Observation and Interview Results

6.4.1 Kind of Patients

In the urology department three kinds of patients appear. One is the new patient, who visits the urology clinic for the first time. It is possible that he/she has been to the Hospital before, but he/she has never visited in the urology department before. Another kind is the returning patient who visits the urology department on a previous occasion. It is possible that the reason of her/his visit is only a checkup or that she/he wants to talk to the doctor about the last medical problem or it can also be possible that she/he has a new medical problem. The third kind of patient is the patient who comes for a procedure, like a biopsy, for example. This is the only reason for his/her visit.

6.4.2 Workflow

It was not easy to clearly identify the workflow in the urology department. The first reason was that the workflow differs, depending on the kind of patients. The second reason was that there is no standard workflow, because the work is done in different ways, depending on the medical assistant and the doctor in the treatment care team. Figure 6.1 shows the approximated workflow with a new patient.

After a patient has called the urology clinic to make his/her first appointment, the urology department sends out a patient information form per mail that the patient needs to fill out (medical/social/family history, review of systems). Prior to his/her

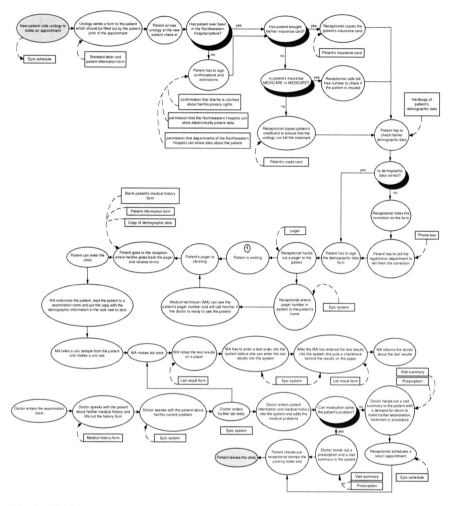

Fig. 6.1 Workflow in the urology department

appointment he/she should also call the registration department to give them his/her demographic data (address, insurance information, information about employer, in some cases information about the legal guardian).

When the patient arrives at the urology department, he/she needs to check in at the new-patient-front-desk. The receptionist hands out printed demographic data to the patient, that she/he can check if the data is correct. If the data is incorrect, the patient must use a special phone in the waiting room to call the registration department to correct the data. The receptionist will mark the errors on the printed form and the patient has to sign the form with the demographic data. If the patient has never been at the Hospital he/she needs to sign these additional forms at the check in: confirmation that she/he is clarified about her/his privacy rights, permission that the Hospital can store electronically patient data, permission that departments of the Hospital can share data about the patient. Furthermore the receptionist copies the patient's insurance card. If the patient has forgotten her/his card and the insurance is MEDICARE or MEDICAID, the receptionist can call a toll free number to check, if the patient is really insured. If the patient is insured at another insurance company, the receptionist will copy the patient's credit card to make sure that the urology can bill the patient for the treatment.

The receptionist hands out a pager to the patient and she/he will enter the pager number into the system. When the doctor is ready to see the patient, then either the doctor or the medical assistant (MA) will call the patient's pager. The patient comes back to the front desk. The receptionist hands out a copy of the demographic data, the patient information form and a blank patient medical history form to the patient that he can bring these to the doctor. Then the patient can enter the clinic.

The MA welcomes the patient and leads him to one of the three examination rooms. She takes the paper with the demographic information about the patient and puts it in the special rack besides the door. Then she takes a urine sample from the patient.

The MA makes some tests with the urine. She writes the results from the tests on a paper form. Before she can enter the results into the system, she has to enter a lab test order into the system. Then she can add the results to the order in the system, after that she makes a checkmark behind the results on the paper form and informs the doctor about the results.

Next, the doctor enters the examination room. The patient hands over the information and medical history form to the doctor. Then the doctor will have a longer conversation with the patient about his/her medical history and about his/her current problem. Depending on the patient's problem the doctor orders further lab tests. He leaves the examination room in the meantime to enter the data about the patient into the system. Depending on the tests results he will decide if he can immediately medicate patient or if he/she has to come for a second visit. Then he will hand out the patient a visit summary and in some cases a prescription or a demand for a return visit.

The patient leaves the clinic through the check-out. There the patient hands out the summary and his/her demographic data to the receptionist. The receptionist checks the summary, if another visit is required, she/he will schedule a new appointment. The demographic data are needed for the billing. Then the receptionist stamps the parking ticket and the patient can go.

6.5   Findings

The first problem is caused by unreliable patients. When patients make a first appointment, the urology clinic usually sends a form to the patients or asks them to download the form at the urology website. The patient should bring the completed form along with him/her at the time of appointment. The majority of patients don't bring the form duly completed. So they have to fill out the form in the waiting room, while the doctor is waiting.

Another problem is the inflexible scheduling. The Epic system only allows 15 min slots in scheduling. So the urology clinic usually allocates 15 min appointments for returning patients and 30 min appointments for new patients. Sometimes it is unnecessary to give a 15 min appointment to a returning patient, because the doctor knows, that he only has to talk with the patient for 5 min, for example. The rest of the time the doctor is waiting for the next patient.

The next problem is poor communication between the staff members creates waste of time. The doctor is done and ready for the next patient. The clock says that it is 10 min before the next appointment. The EPIC system shows him, that the next patient has already arrived at the urology clinic, but the doctor doesn't know, if the patient is ready for the examination or if the patient is filling out forms. So the doctor is waiting for the receptionist to forward the patient or for the medical assistant calling in the patient. Possibly the patient is also waiting for the doctor meanwhile.

Duplicate lab orders confuse the lab staff and mean needlessly waste of time for the doctor. After the examination, the doctor tells the lab staff, if he needs some blood- or uric-analysis. Then he enters the lab order into the system. The lab staff notes the verbal order on a paper and also see the electronical order on her/his screen.

There is no clear communication between the urology department and other departments throughout the hospital. This means for the patient, that he/she has to return many times which is not helpful to increase the patient's contentment. When the doctor needs an x-ray image or a CT analysis, for example, the patient has to make a new appointment with the radiology. For this appointment the patient has to come a second time to the hospital. To speak with the doctor in the urology and to continue the examination, the patient has to come a third time to the hospital.

The doctor often doesn't really know the reason for the patient's visit till he can speak personally with the patient. This often leads to unexpected extensions of the patient's visit. The doctor expects that the visit of a returning patient will take not so much time, for example, because he expects that he only has to do a regular checkup. But some returning patients have new problems, about which they want to talk to the doctor. So the doctor has to spend more time with those patients than he expected.

Yet another waste of time problem is caused by the system, because there is no account for each staff member and the urology team doesn't correctly use the shared mode functionality from the system. Here is an example: When the medical technician wants to enter results into the system, it can happen that he/she has to wait, while the doctor is using the system at the same time or if the doctor has forgotten to close the workspace.

The system's features are inadequately being used; it turned out to be another problem. While the system could take on many jobs; the crew is struggling with these jobs. Here is an example: If a patient is too late and the receptionist has waited more than 20 min she will cancel the appointment in the system. Instead the receptionist needs to check the clock the whole time; the system could automatically cancel the appointment 20 min after the scheduled time, if the patient hasn't arrived at the urology yet.

Often staff members do work, which usually is not their job, which causes confusion and a mess. For instance a doctor made a test with the patient that usually is the medical assistant's job. After the test he told the medical assistant the results of the test, while she was busy with another patient. The doctor didn't write down the results anywhere. So what happens, if the medical technician forgets the results or if she will forget to enter the results into the system?

The inexplicit division of labour also leads to a not satisfying patient support service and to additional work for the doctor. In one case a patient has arrived at the reception and he was a new patient. He needed to fill out some forms. He told the receptionist, that he has arthritis and that he can't write. The receptionist told the patient, that he shall take the blank form to the doctor, so that the doctor can fill out the form with the patient together. This is not the doctor's job and extends the time he has to spend with the patient.

Additional work for the doctor is also caused by inexplicit distribution of jobs. A new patient needs to fill out a lot of forms. The receptionist gives this filled out forms to the patient, that he/she can give them to the doctor. Later the doctor has to enter all the information from the forms into the system.

6.6 Conclusions from Phase 1

6.6.1 Suggestions for Improvement

To eliminate the bottleneck of completing and signing forms, the patients with internet access could be asked to make the appointment online. Then they could be forced to fill out the forms, as making it impossible to make a first appointment without completing the forms. The urology department also could put up a terminal in the waiting room, where the patients can fill out online forms. Both would have the positive side effect that nobody else needs to enter the data in the system later. The urology department could post the forms that have to be signed in the internet, so that the patients can download them and print them out. The patients also should be able to download the brochures ("Your Privacy Rights", for example) that they can read the information before they sign confirmations and permissions.

Another issue are the forms themselves. The urology department should redesign them, because some questions are not clear. They can ask the receptionist, he/she will know which questions are confusing for the patients, because the most of the time patients ask her/him if they don't know how to fill out the forms. The letter the urology department sends to the new patients is confusing. The letter says that the patient should be at the reception 15 min prior to her/his appointment. But on the letter is a red sticker that says the patients should be at the department 10 min prior the scheduled appointment. If someone receives a letter overcrowded with information and with a red sticker, what will this person prefer to read? What will

First visit

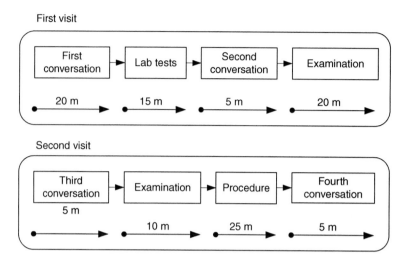

Second visit

Fig. 6.2 Exemplary and simplified standard of a medical condition's treatment

this person think is more important – letter or red sticker? And if this person decides to read both, what will he/she keep in mind?

If a patient calls to make an appointment for a return visit, the receptionist could ask the patient, why he/she wants to see the doctor – Still the same problem? Another problem? Only checkup? Or if the patient is transferred by a general practitioner, they could ask him/her about the patient's problem. If the urology department can establish the online scheduling, they could force the patients to specify the reason of their visit. The urology has to find out why the patient wants to see the doctor before he/she comes to clinic; this will be helpful to improve the time management.

Next, the urology department has to eliminate the inflexible scheduling. The Epic system should allow arbitrary time slots. If the department could find a way to find out the visit reasons of the return patients then they can introduce an intelligent scheduling. Therefore they have to establish standards depending on the patient's medical condition that they can classify the time needed for different treatments (see Fig. 6.2). Maybe they should completely reconsider their way of scheduling. There are schedules for each examination room and procedure room thinkable. Also imaginable are schedules for each staff member. This means not only schedules for each doctor but also schedules for the medical assistances, medical technicians, nurses etc.

It is very important that the urology department improves the usage of the Epic system features. At the moment they only use the system to enter and store data. But the system can assume many little jobs with which the staff is suffering at the moment. To quote an example: If a patient is too late and the receptionist has waited more than 20 min she will cancel the appointment in the system. Instead that the receptionist needs to check the clock the whole time, the system could automatically cancel the appointment 20 min after the scheduled time, if the patient hasn't arrived at the urology yet.

The system also could be used to improve the communication between the reception and the clinic. The system should show the receptionist when there is an examination room empty or when the doctor is ready to see the next patient that she/he can forward the patient to the clinic. Otherwise the system should not only show that a patient has arrived, it also should show to the clinic staff that the patient is ready to enter the clinic. The communication between the clinic staff among each other could be improved by the system, too. If they only use the system to exchange lab orders and results, they can save a lot of time while cutting down duplicate work. Anyway they have to enter the orders and the results into the system so they don't have to verbally tell each other the orders and results.

Therefore it is important that every team member has her/his own account. Then it would be possible to introduce a better user interface which is personalized and serves every team member the needed information. The lab staff only needs a list of lab orders and a user interface where she can enter the results, for example. At the moment the doctor, medical assistant, medical technician and a nurse who work in one team share only one account. This is impractical, because in this way they are not able to use the system at the same time and they cannot use the system to communicate with each other. Another aspect is that in a case of failure the urology department cannot prove who is responsible for the mistake. They should also make sure that they meet the patient's privacy rights by the way of using of the system.

To improve their healthcare delivery, the urology department should check if they can use the Epic system or another technology to improve the communication and collaboration with other departments in the hospital; so that they can finish the patient's treatment in a faster and more efficient way.

It is also important, that the urology department establishes a concrete division of labour which can only be diverged for a good reason. Therefore they need concrete work descriptions that specify which person is responsible for which task. With a business process model they could describe all steps of each jobs and who is responsible for it. If everybody knows what is his/her responsibility, the work will be done more efficiently with less confusion. First it seems that building up business processes and job descriptions is a hard work but the advantages which the department will retrieve are rewarding. It will be helpful to find out who is overloaded and who is unchallenged, so that labour can be newly distributed. The bottom line is it will be helpful to improve the contentment of the staff, to advance the healthcare delivery and to raise the satisfaction of the hospital's customers the patients which in turn extends the good reputation of the hospital. And this means more patients will opt for the Hospital when it comes to their medical condition which again means more income (see Fig. 6.3).

6.6.2 List of Recommendations

- Improve the process of completing and signing forms to eliminate this bottleneck
- Eliminate inflexible scheduling and improve an intelligent scheduling to improve the time management

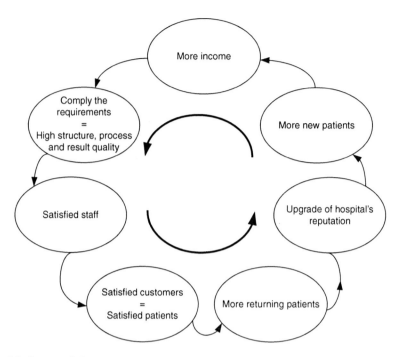

Fig. 6.3 Success circle

- Improve communication between reception and clinic to make the workflow smoother
- Eliminate doubly and needlessly work by adapting the workflow to the system in order to eliminate wasting of time
- Improve communication between the urology department and other departments to make the healthcare delivery more efficient
- Find a way to specify the reason of the patient's visit before they arrive at the urology department to improve the time management
- Try to use all features which the system has to offer to ease the daily routine
- Create system accounts for each staff member that the features the system has to offer can really be used and that the terms of HIPAA can be met
- Establish job descriptions & business processes to improve the quality of healthcare delivery
- Create medical treatment standards to lower the variability

6.6.3   Summary

The urology department can reduce the waste of time; they can improve their workflow and can raise the contentment of the providers and the patients. The bottom line is that they can advance the quality of healthcare delivery. The above listed issues can be a beginning and if the urology department tries to realize them, they will get rewarded. It is not a difficult challenge and it doesn't need a big investment! What is needed is a team – staff members who are freed of their duties for a while or an extern project team – which will reorganize the process of healthcare delivery in the urology department while they put the above listed issues into practice. However it is important to note that such changes should be effected first before any further technology solutions and e-health initiatives are introduced in order to realise the healthcare value proposition.

6.6.4 Future Research

Based on the findings from Phase I it was decided to design, develop (Phase II) and implement (Phase III) an electronic pre-visit system with multi language capability. In particular, given the high percentage of Hispanic patients a real time Spanish/English – English/Spanish system was deemed to be most appropriate. It is noted that this would be the first ever system of its kind in the US. It was envisaged that this system would be a key tool in enabling clinicians to streamline their patient work flows and thereby improve the quality of healthcare delivery. Currently the system is being implemented and tested.

References

Alberto Kywi, A. (2007). PACS Is a crowd-pleaser in healthcare. Health Management Technology, http://www.healthmgttech.com/archieves/0305/0305pacs_crowdpleaser.htm, retrieved: August 2010

Ganiban, J. (2004). "Protecting your PACS purchase" radiology today, April 2004, http://www.radiologytoday.net/archive/rt_042604p8.shtml

Inchingolo, P. (2007). Picture archicing and communications systems in today's healthcare. *Information and Technology Program Transition Studies.* http://www.tbs.units.it/EDU/GNBTS/inchin/index.html, accessed Aug 2010

Institute for Healthcare Improvement. (2003). *Optimizing patient flow – Moving patients smoothly through acute vare settings.* Innovation Series. Boston: Institute for Healthcare Improvement.

Schnellen, M. (2008). Developing a model to analyze the physic and information processes of an emergency department. In N. Wickramasinghe & E. Geisler (Eds.), *Encyclopaedia of healthcare information.* Hershey: IGI.

Smith, E. (2007). Optimizing patient care and radiologist workflow through integrated patient-realted data and image management. *Misys Healthcare Systems.* www.misyshealthcare.com, accessed Aug 2010

Wickramasinghe, N., Bali, R., & Geisler, E. (2007a). The major barriers and facilitators for the adoption and implementation of knowledge management in healthcare operations. *International Journal of Electronic Healthcare, 3*(3), 367–381.

Wickramasinghe, N., Tumu, S., & Tatnall, A. (2007b). Using actor network theory (ANT) as an analytic tool in order to effect superior PACS implementation. *International Journal of Networking and Virtual Organisations, 4*(3), 257–279.

Chapter 7
Adaptations for e-Kiosk Systems in Germany to Develop Barrier-Free Terminals for Handicapped Persons

Manuel Zwicker, Juergen Seitz, and Nilmini Wickramasinghe

Abstract At this time in Germany, the e-health sector is especially focused on the new e-health card concept, which is currently in the test stage and should be established within the next years. This e-health card will totally change the current system, because this concept allows several new functions. Some of the possible functions are compulsory for the enrollees, while other functions are optional. Examples include electronic prescriptions, electronic patient records and the emergency data of the enrollee in case of an emergency. With these new innovations, the healthcare actors are confronted not only with several advantages but also disadvantages. A sensitive aspect here is the aggregation of enrollee data, which brings some benefits, but also a threat regarding data security and access authorization. Therefore, the regulations and laws are very strict.

Because enrollees have concerns about their data, the health insurance companies have to ensure that enrollees have the possibility to check and to manage their data. Therefore, electronic kiosk systems (e-kiosks) are important, because these terminals are self-service terminals, where the enrollees can, among other things, manage their health data. Naturally, it is important that these e-kiosks are useable for all citizens, especially handicapped persons. Hence, this chapter will also identify possibilities pertaining to how these terminals can be adapted to ensure that the different groups of handicapped persons can also use these e-kiosks.

Keywords e-health card • Electronic prescriptions • Electronic health professional card • Emergency data • Electronic health record • Electronic kiosk

M. Zwicker (✉) • N. Wickramasinghe
RMIT University, Melbourne, VIC, Australia
e-mail: Manuel.Zwicker@gmx.de; nilmini.wickramasinghe@rmit.edu.au

J. Seitz
Duale Hochschule Baden-Württemberg Heidenheim, Heidenheim, Germany
e-mail: seitz@dhbw-heidenheim.de

N. Wickramasinghe et al. (eds.), *Critical Issues for the Development*
of Sustainable E-health Solutions, Healthcare Delivery in the Information Age,
DOI 10.1007/978-1-4614-1536-7_7, © Springer Science+Business Media, LLC 2012

7.1   Introduction

The implementation of the e-health card (eHC) will totally change the current healthcare system in Germany. New functions will be available and the focus will move more to the electronic-based view. These new functions include electronic prescriptions, electronic patient records and the emergency data of the individual or enrollee in case of an emergency.

In spite of these new functions though, this does not mean that there are only advantages. There are also disadvantages. Furthermore, the guarantee of data security and data protection will be a big challenge and this is naturally at great concern to enrolled patients.

E-kiosks, which are self-service terminals, have to be introduced by the health insurance companies throughout Germany so that enrolled patients can have easy access to check their medical data. However, it is important to note that these terminals must be accessible to all citizens and hence the needs and requirements of handicapped persons must also be taken into consideration. This makes the design and implementation of barrier-free e-kiosks a necessity.

This chapter will first give an overview about the German healthcare sector. Section 7.3 will explain the concept of the German eHC and will show the new possible functionality. Section 7.4 will mention the advantages and disadvantages of this eHC, whereas Sect. 7.5 will give information about data security and data protection. Section 7.6 will be focused on e-kiosks and will show possible ideas, how these terminals can be adapted for the needs of disabled persons. Section 7.7 will show an evaluation of the eHC in terms of the "e's" in e-health. Conclusions will be drawn in Sect. 7.8.

7.2   Healthcare in Germany

Healthcare is a growing industry over the last 40 years. Between 1970 and 1997 the percentage of Gross Domestic Product (GDP) spent on average on healthcare by members of the Organization for Economic Cooperation and Development (OECD) countries rose from about 5% to roughly 8% (Huber, 1999, p. 3).

Since 2000, total spending on healthcare in these countries has been rising faster than economic growth, which resulted in an average ratio of health spending to GDP of 9.0% in 2008. Challenges like the technological change, longer life expectation and population ageing will push health spending up in the future. Therefore, the growing health spending creates a cost pressure for several countries such as Germany (OECD, 2010a).

Hence, reducing these expenditures as well as offering effective and efficient quality healthcare treatment is becoming a priority globally. Technology and automation have the potential to reduce these costs (Ghani et al., 2010, pp. 113–130).

In 2008, Germany had a total expenditure on health (% GDP) of 10.5%, which was 1.5% higher than the average ratio of the OECD countries. The US spent with 16.0% the most, while France (11.2%) and Switzerland (10.7%) had also a higher value than Germany. Concurrently, Germany's total expenditure on health per capita (US$) was $3,737, whereas the OECD countries spent on average $3,060 per capita and the US with $7,538 again the most (OECD, 2010b, p. 1).

The healthcare actors in Germany are divided into enrollees, service providers (medical doctors, pharmacists, hospitals) and cost units (health insurance companies). Germany has around 82.14 million inhabitants, where around 70.23 million people have public health insurance and around 8.62 million people use a private health insurance. Furthermore, Germany has 319,697 medical doctors, 2,087 hospitals and 21,602 pharmacies, where 48,030 pharmacists work (BMG, 2009, pp. 9–133).

Hence, all these healthcare actors will be affected by the new German eHC.

7.3 The Concept of the e-Health Card

With the implementation of the e-health card (eHC), people in Germany can benefit from several new functions. Generally, the functions of the e-health card are divided into two category groups. Firstly, there is the area of administrative functions, which are compulsory for the card owners. Secondly, there is the area of medical functions, which are optional for the card holders. Both areas consist of two steps (Haarfeld, 2010).

The implementation of the e-health card in Germany begins with the implementation of the administrative functions. Therefore, in the first step of the implementation of the e-health card information about the insurance agreement and the necessity of additional payments will be stored. The data will be stored on the e-health card and can be updated for example during every consultation of a medical doctor through an online process. In addition, this first step includes data about the care provider, the personal information about the enrollee as well as the lifelong valid insurance number. Furthermore, private insurance companies can also add information about the scope of services, which a private enrollee can utilize during a stay in hospital (Haarfeld, 2010).

Moreover, the first step of the administrative area includes an insurance-coverage for the enrollee within the European Union. But the requirement here is that the appropriate countries have a social agreement among each other. The back side of the e-health card is ideal as identity card for this European Health Insurance Card (EHIC) (European Commission, 2010).

Figures 7.1 and 7.2 show the front and the back of a German eHC.

The new e-health cards are equipped with this EHIC independent from the insurance company. Therefore, the "old" E-111 forms, which were used in the past during a stay abroad in another European country, are not longer required (EU-Info Deutschland, 2010). However, these EHICs are only applicable for enrollees of a public health insurance company, because enrollees of a private health insurance

Fig. 7.1 Front of the eHC
(BMG, 2008, p. 19)

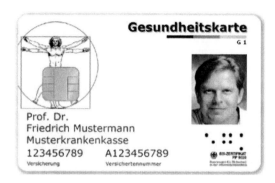

Fig. 7.2 Back of the
eHC – EHIC (BMG, 2008,
p. 30)

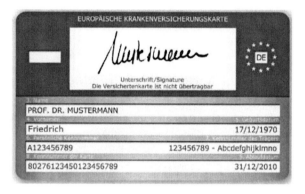

company usually have insurance-protection worldwide (Verband der privaten Krankenversicherung e.V., 2010, p. 10).

The second step of the administrative functions includes the electronic prescription (e-prescription), which is also compulsory for all involved actors of the German healthcare system. Based on this concept, it is possible to remove the nearly 600–700 million paper-based prescriptions and to process these transactions electronically. The process looks like this: At first, the doctor has to look on the insurance data of the patient. Therefore, the doctor can use the eHC of the patient and can read all the essential data with a special reading device. When the patient needs some medicine, the doctor can store the data of the decreed medicine in electronically form (e-prescription) on the e-health card or on a special server. The necessary signature of the doctor will be generated electronically with the aid of an electronic health professional card (HPC) (Die gesetzlichen Krankenkassen, 2007, pp. 1–2).

When a patient wants to redeem the electronic prescription in a pharmacy then the procedure goes in the reverse direction. Firstly, the validity of the doctor's signature will be checked. After the following presentation of the medicine through a pharmacist or another authorized staff member, the electronic prescription will become invalid and the data will be transmitted to the pharmacy's data center (Die gesetzlichen Krankenkassen, 2007, p. 2).

With the medical functions in step 3, the voluntary part begins for the enrollees and their e-health card. This means nothing more than the enrollees can decide for their own, if they want to use these additional functions or not. The main focus here is on the storage of personal health data from the enrollees. Examples are the documentation of medicine, which an enrollee has used or the storage of emergency data of the enrollee in case of emergency. Through the medicine documentation it is possible to avoid interdependencies between the individual drugs (gematik, 2010a). Furthermore, the emergency data should help the emergency doctor to medicate purposefully and effectively. For example, this could help the doctor to take allergy or chronic illness through the patient's therapy into consideration (BMG, 2010a, pp. 1–4).

The fourth and final step includes, among other things, the electronic health record (EHR). With this EHR it is possible to have access to the entire patient's data. Therefore, it is not important, if the data are stored at one place or at different places, because the patient's data can be accepted, processed and attended centrally (GVG, 2004, p. 9).

7.4 Advantages and Disadvantages of the e-Health Card

The implementation of the eHC implicates advantages and also disadvantages. At this point, it is essential to differentiate between the enrollees, service providers – here for example medical doctors and pharmacists – and cost units – here the health insurance companies.

The eHC will help the enrollees to get a higher quality of therapy. The reason is that the eHC makes data of patients available faster, which means that redundant examinations and administration of inappropriate drugs can be avoided (Medline, 2010a).

Another advantage for the enrollees is that with the storage of the health data they will receive a better overview of their health status and thus their personal responsibility will be starched. Moreover, the enrollees have great concern about their data and can therefore decide for their own, which medical data should be stored and which not. Based on the data protection and data security, the enrollees can decide which doctor for example has access (Medline, 2010a). In addition, the last 50 data accesses will be logged (gematik, 2003b, p. 17).

The service providers have the advantage that they can get a fast and extensive overview of the patient's status of health owing to the eHC. Through the documentation of the medical data redundant examinations can be avoided. Additionally, in case of an emergency the doctor can take all former examinations from other service providers into account when making his/her diagnosis (Medline, 2010b).

Furthermore, the service providers have the advantage that they can save time thanks to their optimized workflow. This time can be brought in the patient's examination and therapy (Medline, 2010b).

For the cost units, which are the health insurance companies, the eHC also brings a lot of advantages. For example, due to the reduction of redundant examinations the health insurance companies can realize cost savings. The documentation of the medicine avoid on the one hand that the patient will be examined with inadequate medicine and on the other hand this fact also results in cost savings for the health insurance companies (Medline, 2010c). As mentioned before, service providers write around 600–700 million prescriptions annually. In Germany, approximately 90% of all enrollees have a public health insurance, who will exclusively use the electronic prescription (Monetos, 2010). In addition, some of the 8.6 million private enrollees will also use this e-prescription (PKV, 2009). Based on these facts, approximately 500 million Euros can be saved every year (Scheer, 2009, p. 5).

Finally, the fact that the eHC is definitely assignable to the card holder is also an advantage for the health insurance companies. The reason is that unauthorized usage of medical services through a third party can be avoided (gematik, 2010b).

The disadvantages, which are occurring through the implementation of the e-health card in Germany, can be summarized under the point of very high implementation costs of approximately 1.7 billion Euros and 150 million Euros running costs every year (Scheer, 2009, p. 5).

7.5   Data Protection and Data Security Related to the German e-Health Card

Based on the implementation of the eHC, the medical care of the patients is believed to become better. However, it should be kept clearly in mind that the data protection and the data security have to be guaranteed, because the necessary data are personal data of the patient.

Paragraph 291a SGB V (Code of Social Law) includes precise guidelines, how the access to the individual patient data has to be arranged. These rules were developed together with the federal commissioner for data security and were regulated by law (gematik, 2010c).

The goal of the paragraph 291a SGB V is that a very high security and protection level in connection with the sensitive data of the patient and a maximum transparency for the patient can be guaranteed. For this reason, only data are allowed to be stored, which provide the medical care. Every patient, who will agree to the storage of personal medical data, will have a personal data security container, which is locked and strictly secured. Only the patients have the highness about their data. This means that the patient can decide for himself, in which amount his personal health data are allowed to be stored. This means that the patient can also decide at anytime when these data have to be deleted. Additionally, it is possible to restrict the access to these personal data and information to only selected doctors (gematik, 2008, pp. 7–8). This can be done at an electronic kiosk (e-kiosk), which will be discussed in Sect. 7.6.

The data access of a doctor or pharmacist will be realized with the two-key-principle in combination with the personal identification numbers (PINs). This means that the access to the personal data container of a patient needs two keys and

PINs. The doctor or pharmacist holds one key, which is the already mentioned electronic health professional card (HPC), and one PIN. But this key and PIN alone does not allow an access to the data container of the patient, because the second key is necessary, which is nothing more than the eHC. In addition, the patient needs to confirm the access to his data container with his PIN (gematik, 2008, p. 7). Exceptions to this procedure are the electronic prescriptions and the reading of the record of emergency data. Here the PIN of the patient is not necessary to get access to the data container.

An additional security attribute is that the last 50 accesses to the eHC will be logged on the e-health card (gematik, 2008, p. 17). Furthermore, the misuse of the eHC through a third party will be prosecuted criminally. In paragraph 307 SGB V the regulations for fines were enhanced, while paragraph 307a SGB V creates new elements of an offense in connection with the e-health card.

It is essential that all the requirements of the data security and protection will be included in the definition of the telematics infrastructure (BMG, 2010b).

7.6 Electronic Kiosks (e-Kiosks)

Section 7.5 mentioned that the enrollees respectively the patients have the highness about their personal medical data. But this can only be achieved, if the health insurance companies will install e-kiosk terminals all over the country. A definition from the Gesellschaft für Telematikanwendungen der Gesundheitskarte mbH for an electronic kiosk (e-kiosk) is that an e-kiosk is a primary system for the maintenance of applications and data through an enrollee (gematik, 2010d, p. 33).

With the usage of an e-kiosk, the enrollee can, for example, remove electronic prescriptions and administrate access rights for doctors. Furthermore, these terminals should allow the patient to activate or deactivate the voluntary applications and to read the emergency data (gematik, 2006, pp. 81–83).

The technical specifications and requirements for a barrier-free e-kiosk are not determined so far and the e-health card is at this time in the test stage (gematik, 2006, pp. 81–83). Section 7.6.1 will show the actual situation in Germany with disabled people and will mention general ideas, how e-kiosks can be barrier-free.

7.6.1 Specification for Barrier-Free e-Kiosk Terminals

Based on the information of the German Federal Statistical Office (Statistisches Bundesamt), Germany had in the year 2007 6.9 million seriously disabled persons, which were 153,000 people more than in year 2005. This means that every twelfth inhabitant, which is 8.4% of the total population, was seriously disabled. Persons are classified as seriously disabled, if they have a degree of disability of at least 50% (Statistisches Bundesamt Deutschland, 2008).

Most frequently, with 64%, these seriously adapted persons had physical disabilities. 24% of these people were handicapped because of their viscera. 14% were constrained in their movements because of restricted leg and arm functions and 13% because of their backbone and body. 5% were blind or had a visual impairment. 4% were adversely affected by hardness of hearing, disturbance of equilibrium or speech disorder. 10% were mentally and 9% were cerebral disordered. For the rest of the people the disability were not reported (Statistisches Bundesamt Deutschland, 2008).

The BGG – Behindertengleichstellungsgesetz (handicapped persons equality law) regulates the equalization of disabled persons. Paragraph 4 BGG especially defines the phrase barrier-free. Based on this, barrier-free is guaranteed when disabled persons can use the application or facility in a general common manner, without specific difficulty. Furthermore, these facilities have to be accessible and usable in principle unassisted.

Because of above mentioned information, it is essential now to have a look on e-kiosks and to develop specifications, which guarantee a barrier-free usage of the eHC and all the included functions. Because the specifications for e-kiosks are not defined through the gematik mbH so far, this chapter will be oriented on comparable solutions used for ATMs or other self service terminals. There exists a list of requirements for barrier-free self service terminals, which was defined by the senate department for integration, labor and social affairs in Berlin (Senatsverwaltung für Inneres in Berlin, 2008).

As mentioned above, 24% of the 6.9 million disabled persons in Germany were handicapped because of their viscera. This fact has no consequence for the specifications and requirements of an e-kiosk, because they have no problems with the usage of these terminals.

However, 14% of all the disabled persons in Germany were constrained in their movements because of their restricted leg and arm functions. This is a problem, because these people cannot use an e-kiosk in a usual way. For example, if these people need a wheelchair, the e-kiosk has to be adjustable in height, because when they sit in a wheelchair the standardized height of a terminal is not achievable for them. Furthermore, these height adjustments should be as easy as possible. Therefore, it is advisable to control this electronically with the aid of a switch. This switch should be placed in a position, where also people with a wheelchair can push them.

Based on the facts above, 13% of all handicapped persons had problems with their backbones and bodies. Here it is also essential, that e-kiosks are height adjustable, because these people need to stand upright. Furthermore, these terminals need a place of deposit, where these people can lay down their bags or their other baggage.

As published by the German Federal Statistical Office, 5% of the 6.9 million handicapped persons in Germany were blind or had a visual impairment. Therefore, e-kiosks should have a telephone receiver. The computer will read the enrollee's medical data and will reproduce this data to the patient by synthetic voice. Additionally, it is essential that e-kiosks will have acoustic warning signals, a Braille keyboard and Braille computer software, which will recognize this font and will transform this into standard text. Furthermore, the enrollee should have the possibility to change the size of the font according to his visual impairment. But all these measurements create a conflict related to the data security and the data protection, because people, who are blind or have a visual impairment cannot prevent the situation, that a third person will see or listen to their data. For this reason, it is necessary that e-kiosks will be isolated in special prepared areas with enough space in the surrounding area.

For the 4% of the handicapped persons, who were adversely affected by hardness of hearing, disturbance of equilibrium or speech disorder and the 10% and 9% of the disabled persons, who were mentally and cerebral disordered, are no adaptations necessary, because usually they can read the information on the display of the e-kiosk.

Another important group, who will have big problems with a classical e-kiosk, is the group of illiterates. In Germany live around four million illiterates, who have problems with reading and writing (Doebert and Hubertus, 2000, p. 8). For these people, telephone receivers are again the solution. These people will hear all the information they want by synthetic voice. An additional point for this target group is that e-kiosks need speech recognition software. This software should record all the spoken information. Furthermore, this software should also manage the e-kiosk in the point that the e-kiosk will search for the requested information and will reproduce the data by synthetic voice.

Another idea is that personal adjustments will be stored. If an enrollee inserts his/her eHC into the e-kiosk, his/her personal adjustments will be loaded and the e-kiosk will transpose his settings. This means that the e-kiosk will change the height automatically based on the preferences of the enrollee.

Finally, e-kiosks should have an integrated printer, where enrollees can print the information they want.

7.6.2 Additional Benefits Achieved Through an e-Kiosk

An e-kiosk is more than a machine, which gives information. These terminals can also be used to attract enrollees. When the enrollees will come to the health insurance company and will have a look on their medical data, this situation can be used for further affairs.

For example, e-kiosks can be featured with an integrated camera, which will make pictures (free of charge) of the enrollee and will store the pictures in a database. Because of the fact that the new eHC must have a picture of the enrollee on the front, this feature could help to save money for both enrollees and health insurance companies. Especially, socially deprived people will benefit from such a solution, while health insurance companies can reduce their administration costs (TrustTerminal AG, 2010).

Another aspect is that e-kiosks can be used to give enrollees information about for example the city, actual events and weather forecasts. Even such aspects could help to achieve a higher customer acceptance of these e-kiosks.

7.7   E's in e-Health

It is often useful to think about the "e" in e-health as having several meanings including (adapted from Eysenbach, 2001):

Efficiency – one of the promises of e-health is to increase efficiency in healthcare, thereby decreasing costs. One possible way of decreasing costs would be by avoiding duplicative or unnecessary diagnostic or therapeutic interventions, through enhanced communication possibilities between healthcare establishments, and through patient involvement. The Internet will naturally serve as a great enabler for achieving this "e" in e-health.

Enhancing quality of care – increasing efficiency; i.e., involves not only reducing costs, is not an end in and of itself but rather should be considered in conjunction with improving quality, which should be one of the ultimate goals of e-health. A more educated consumer (as a result of the informational aspects of e-health) would then communicate more effectively with their primary care provider, which will, in turn, lead to improved quality of care.

Evidence based – e-health interventions should be evidence based in the sense that their effectiveness and efficiency should not be assumed but proven by rigorous scientific evaluation and support from case histories. Web accessible case repositories facilitate the timely accessibility of such evidence and thus help in the achieving of the necessary support of a diagnosis or treatment decision. The evidence based medicine component of e-health is currently one of the most active e-health research domains, yet much work still needs to be done in this area.

Empowerment of consumers and patients – by making the knowledge bases of medicine and personal electronic records accessible to consumers over the Internet, e-health opens new avenues for patient-centered medicine, and enables patient education and thus increases the likelihood of informed and more satisfactory patient choice.

Education of physicians through online sources (continuing medical education) and consumers (health education, tailored preventive information for consumers) makes it easier for physicians as well as consumers to keep up to date with all the latest developments in the medical areas of their respective interests. This in turn is likely to have a positive impact on the quality of care vis-à-vis the use of the latest medical treatments and preventive protocols.

Extending the scope of healthcare beyond its conventional boundaries, in both a geographical sense as well as in a conceptual sense leads to enabling such techniques as telemedicine and virtual operating rooms, both of which are invaluable in providing healthcare services to places, where it may otherwise be difficult or impossible to do.

Ethics – e-health involves new forms of patient-physician interaction and poses new challenges and threats to ethical issues such as online professional practice, informed consent, privacy and security issues. However, this is not an intrinsic feature of e-health but rather a feature of the Internet technology, which is the foundation for all e-business initiatives. Therefore, e-health along with e-government, e-insurance, e-banking, e-finance and e-retailing must all contend with these ethical issues. Given the nature of healthcare, these issues could be more magnified.

Equity – to make healthcare more equitable is one of the aims of quality identified by the American Institute of Medicine (Institute of Medicine, 2001) generally and is one of the promises of e-health. However, at the same time there is a considerable threat that e-health, if improperly implemented and used, may deepen the gap between the "haves" and "have-nots"; hence, the need for a robust framework to ensure the proper implementation of any e-health initiative. In particular, some of the key issues for equity revolve around broad access and familiarity with the technology.

Table 7.1 shows an evaluation of the eHC concept in terms of the "e's" in e-health.

Table 7.1 Evaluation of the eHC in terms of the "e's" in e-health

E's in e-health	Description	Evaluation of the eHC in terms of the "e's"
Efficiency	Support efficient healthcare delivery	The eHC helps to avoid duplication or unnecessary diagnostic or therapeutic interventions.
Enhancing quality of care	Reduce incorrect diagnoses	The electronic health record, which is part of the eHC, will especially improve the communication and information exchange between the healthcare actors, which can reduce incorrect diagnoses and can thus result in a higher quality of care.
Evidence based	Support evidence based medicine	The eHC supports evidence based medicine since with the usage of the electronic health record of a patient, diagnoses and treatments from other doctors can help the doctor make his diagnosis.
Empowerment of consumers and patients	Support patients to be more active and informed in their healthcare decisions and treatments	The eHC gives patients the possibility to check their electronic health records in which their entire medical data is stored. Therefore, an e-kiosk can be used.
Education of physicians and consumers through online sources	Help physicians and patients to understand the latest techniques and healthcare issues	The eHC does not affect this issue.
Extending the scope of healthcare	Do not limit healthcare treatment to traditional boundaries	The conceptual scope of healthcare might be positively affected by the eHC, because the eHC could enable new aspects to be introduced within its purview. However, the geographical scope will be unchanged, because healthcare is already available in whole Germany.
Ethics	Including but not limited to privacy and security concerns	Related to the eHC, there are strict laws and techniques (e.g., two-key-principle), which guarantee the security and privacy of the patient.
Equity	Decrease rather than increase the gap between "haves" and "have nots"	Therefore, barrier-free e-kiosk terminals need to be defined, designed and developed.

The e-health card challenges many of these "e's" in particular "equity" so that able and disabled persons can use the system with similar ease, a point that is particularly important given that Germany had 6.9 million seriously handicapped persons in year 2007. Other considerations include empowering enrollees and ensuring the system is efficient and effective.

7.8 Conclusion

This chapter has shown that with the implementation of the e-health card, the healthcare sector and all its actors will be confronted with a lot of new functions, which are partly compulsory and partly voluntary. For example, the paper-based prescriptions can be replaced by electronic prescriptions. Furthermore, enrollees have the possibility to check their medical data centrally, because e-kiosk terminals allow enrollees to have a look at all their consolidated data aggregated from different medical doctors.

However, to date, the specifications and requirements for barrier-free e-kiosks are not developed, even though Germany had 6.9 million seriously handicapped persons in year 2007. Thus, making access and use of these e-kiosks by handicapped persons difficult or impossible. This chapter has served to show possibilities to adapt e-kiosk terminals to the needs of handicapped persons. In addition, it is important to note that the patients' medical data are very sensitive information, therefore data security and data protection play an important role.

We close by calling for more research in this area so that the e-health card will be a complete success and not create a chasm between people who can use the system and those who cannot.

References

Haarfeld, C. W. (2010). Stufenweise Einführung der Funktionen der elektronischen Gesundheitskarte. Retrieved September 14, 2010, from http://www.cw-haarfeld.de/egk/suche/showpage.php?page=stufen&sesid=EKG7-1213381815297077

Doebert, M., & Hubertus, P. (2000). *Ihr Kreuz ist die Schrift: Analphabetismus und Alphabetisierung in Deutschland*. Stuttgart: Erst Klett Verlag GmbH.

EU-Info Deutschland (2010). Die europäische Krankenversicherungskarte. Retrieved September 14, 2010, from http://www.eu-info.de/sozialversicherung-eu/5873/7355/

European Commission (2010). The European Health Insurance Card. Retrieved September 14, 2010, from http://ec.europa.eu/social/main.jsp?catId=559

Eysenbach, G. (2001). What is e-health?. *Journal of Medical Internet Research (JMIR)* 3(2). Retrieved September 16, 2010, from http://www.jmir.org/2001/2/e20/

gematik – Gesellschaft für Telematikanwendungen der Gesundheitskarte mbH (2006). Endbericht zur Kosten-Nutzen-Analyse der Einrichtung einer Telematik-Infrastruktur im deutschen Gesundheitswesen. Retrieved September 16, 2010, from http://www.gkv.info/gkv/fileadmin/user_upload/Projekte/Telematik_im_Gesundheitswesen/KNA_Endbericht.pdf gematik – Gesellschaft für Telematikanwendungen der Gesundheitskarte mbH (2008). Whitepaper Sicherheit. Retrieved September 16, 2010, from https://www.gematik.de/cms/media/dokumente/pressematerialien/dokumente_1/gematik_whitepaper_sicherheit.pdf

gematik – Gesellschaft für Telematikanwendungen der Gesundheitskarte mbH (2010a). Anwendungen der eGK. Retrieved September 14, 2010, from http://www.gematik.de/cms/de/egk_2/anwendungen/anwendungen_1.jsp

gematik – Gesellschaft für Telematikanwendungen der Gesundheitskarte mbH (2010b). Viel mehr als eine neue Krankenversichertenkarte. Retrieved September 16, 2010, from https://www.gematik.de/cms/de/egk_2/egk_3/egk_2.jsp

gematik – Gesellschaft für Telematikanwendungen der Gesundheitskarte mbH (2010c). Gesetzliche Grundlagen. Retrieved September 16, 2010, from https://www.gematik.de/cms/de/gematik/unternehmensorganisation/gesetzlichegrundlagen/gesetzlichegrundlagen_1.jsp

gematik – Gesellschaft für Telematikanwendungen der Gesundheitskarte mbH (2010d). Einführung der Gesundheitskarte: Glossar. Retrieved September 16, 2010, from https://www.gematik.de/cms/media/dokumente/gematik_ZV_Glossar_V2_8_1.pdf

BMG – Bundesministerium für Gesundheit (2008). Spezifikation der elektrischen Gesundheitskarte. Retrieved September 15, 2010, from http://www.bmg.bund.de/nn_1191726/SharedDocs/Downloads/DE/GV/GT/Gesundheitskarte/Technische_20Festlegungen_20fuer_20die_20Test verfahren/Spezifikation_20elektronische_20Gesundheitskarte/Teil-3-Aeussere-Gestaltung,templateId=raw,property=publicationFile.pdf/Teil-3-Aeussere-Gestaltung.pdf

BMG – Bundesministerium für Gesundheit (2009). Daten des Gesundheitswesens 2009. Retrieved September 16, 2010, from http://www.bmg.bund.de/SharedDocs/Publikationen/DE/Daten-des-Gesundheitswesens2009,templateId=raw,property=publicationFile.pdf/Daten-des-Gesundheitswesens2009.pdf

BMG – Bundesministerium für Gesundheit (2010a). Informationen zum Thema Notfalldaten. Retrieved September 16, 2010, from http://www.bmg.bund.de/cln_160/SharedDocs/Downloads/DE/Standardartikel/E/Glossar-Elektronische-Gesundheitskarte/Notfalldaten,templateId=raw,property=publicationFile.pdf/Notfalldaten.pdf

BMG – Bundesministerium für Gesundheit (2010b). Telematikinfrastruktur für einen sicheren Datenaustausch. Retrieved September 15, 2010, from http://www.bmg.bund.de/cln_160/nn_1168682/SharedDocs/Standardartikel/DE/AZ/E/Glossarbegriff-Elektronische-Gesundheitskarte-Telematikinfrastruktur.html?__nnn=true.

Ghani, M., Bali, R., Naguib, R., Marshall, I., & Wickramasinghe, N. (2010). Critical issues for implementing a lifetime health record in the Malaysian public health system. *International Journal of Healthcare Technology and Management (IJHTM), 11*(1/2), 113–130.

GVG – Gesellschaft für Versicherungswissenschaft und –gestaltung (2004). Managementpaper Elektronische Patientenakte. Retrieved September 16, 2010, from http://ehealth.gvg-koeln.de//cms/medium/676/MP_ePa_050124.pdf

Huber, M. (1999). Health expenditure trends in OECD countries 1970–1997. *Health Care Financing Review, 21*(2), 99–117.

Senatsverwaltung für Inneres in Berlin (2008). Katalog der Anforderungen an barrierefreie Kassenautomaten. Retrieved September 17, 2010, from http://www.berlin.de/imperia/md/content/vergabeservice/musterausschreibungen/barrierefreiekassenautomaten/rs_wtf_08_02_tabelle_anforderungen_iii.doc

Institute of Medicine – Committee on Quality of Healthcare in America. (2001). *Crossing the quality chasm: A new health system for the 21st century.* Washington, DC: National Academy Press.

Die gesetzlichen Krankenkassen (2007). Das elektronische Rezept. Retrieved September 15, 2010, from http://www.gkv.info/gkv/fileadmin/user_upload/Projekte/Telematik_im_Gesundheitswesen/2.1.7_das_elektronische_rezept

Medline (2010a). Vorteile der eGK für Patienten. Retrieved September 15, 2010, from https://www.medline-online.com/die-gesundheitskarte/vorteile-patient.html

Medline (2010b). Vorteile der eGK für Ärzte. Retrieved September 15, 2010, from https://www.medline-online.com/die-gesundheitskarte/vorteile-praxis.html

Medline (2010c). Überblick eGK. Retrieved September 15, 2010, from https://www.medline-online.
    com/die-gesundheitskarte/ueberblick.html
Monetos – Independent Information and Research on the European Private Financial Sector
    (2010). Gesetzliche Krankenversicherung. Retrieved September 15, 2010, from http://www.
    monetos.de/versicherung/gesetzliche-krankenversicherung/
OECD (2010a). Growing health spending puts pressure on government budgets. Retrieved
    September 16, 2010, from http://www.oecd.org/document/11/0,3343,en_2649_34631_455497
    71_1_1_1_37407,00.html
OECD (2010b). OECD-Gesundheitsdaten 2010: Deutschland im Vergleich. Retrieved September
    14, 2010, from http://www.oecd.org/dataoecd/15/1/39001235.pdf
PKV – Private Krankenversicherungen.de (2009). Zahl der privat Versicherten erreicht neuen
    Höchststand. Retrieved September 16, 2010, from http://www.privatekrankenversicherungen.
    de/news/00082_Zahl-der-privat-Versicherten-erreicht-neuen-Hoechststand.php
Scheer, A. W. (2009). Wie stehen die Deutschen zur elektronischen Gesundheitskarte?. Retrieved
    September 15, 2010, from http://www.bitkom.org/files/documents/BITKOM-Praesentation_
    Gesundheitskarte_22_10_2009.pdf
Statistisches Bundesamt Deutschland (2008). 6,9 Millionen schwerbehinderte Menschen in
    Deutschland. Retrieved September 17, 2010, from http://www.destatis.de/jetspeed/portal/cms/
    Sites/destatis/Internet/DE/Presse/pm/2008/07/PD08__258__227,templateId = renderPrint.
    psml
TrustTerminal AG (2010). eGK-TrustTerminal. Retrieved September 17, 2010, from http://www.
    trustterminal.com/Produkte/eKiosk/eGKTrustTerminal/tabid/64/Default.aspx
Verband der privaten Krankenversicherung e.V. (2010). Die elektronische Gesundheitskarte in der
    privaten Krankenversicherung. Retrieved September 15, 2010, from http://www.private-
    gesundheitskarte.de/broschueren_materialien/pkv_broschuere_zur_einfuehrung_der_egk.pdf.

Section II
Design and Organisation
Designing Supportive and Collaborative
Electronic Health Environments

Reima Sumoi

This section of papers has three overreaching themes: development of collaborative and sustainable electronic health platforms, the special needs of elderly, disabled or otherwise in trouble population, and peer support.

Health care is as most other industries about sharing data and processes, but especially deeply so. In all instances of care and cure, complete patient data must be available. Ironically, often this data is unavailable just for the central stakeholder, the patient or the citizen. In their article, Professor Pirkko Nykänen and Antto Seppälä work on further on the concept of citizen-centric healthcare. This concept is not born out in information systems, but its efficient implementation necessitates changes to the way how we design information systems. The citizen centric approach is also very much about power, who is the one in charge and power, and how we can empower the patients without neglecting the professional skills of health care professionals. The citizen-centric approach becomes most difficult and challenging in situations where patients are not able to take care of themselves. If we design our health care system around strong and empowered patients, what happens when they are not such ones.

In their article, Professor Jan vom Brocke, Professor Marco de Marco and Francesca Ricciardi remind us of the need for sustainable business models in all activity, including health care. As health care happens in networks, focus of development must be also on network activities. They call for innovation in network processes and introduce the concept of network embedded knowledge. Their healthy point of view is also, that while most well-off people might be at home in this networked world, the more disabled, such as elderly people, might need human support and helpers when dealing with the network-based services.

Opinions and social constructions of "truth" and behavior are born in networks. The article of Raija Halonen digs deep to the construction of meanings in the case of swine flu epidemics. The analysis shows how some topics are taken up in the discussions, and some others are forgotten, and how deeply the network discussion affects the real behavior of people. The article really shows that healthcare is not just about professional activity, but work among peers also. Consequently, the health care system should not underestimate the power and potentials of social media and networks, but should try to take all available advantage out of them.

The same topic is touched upon on the article of Tuomas Lehto. He studies the more goal-oriented and guided network support to different health care problem situations. With computer systems, persuasion can be performed effectively and in a scalable and standard way, including persuasion to more healthy living. Massive health gains can be achieved at population levels if citizen stop smoking and drinking, and move more, just to give examples. In the case of post-incident care, adherence to prescribed care instructions can make a word of difference in health results. Support gained through electronic means is usually cheap, at least when delivered to masses, positively non-intruding and standard in quality.

The problems of elderly and otherwise disabled people are also taken to focus in the article by Professors Irene Krebs, Arnim Nethe and Reetta Raitoharju. When allocating increasingly more health care activities to the net, we must also take care that those somehow disabled also have access to these services. Disabilities can include many, such as vision, hearing, moving around or motoric. With good system design and allocating proper and quality supporting devices to those needy, a lot of the problems can be solved or at least alleviated. What still more nice, services and offerings tailored for the disabled ones are most likely welcomed and appreciated by other too, such as is the case for example in building architecture. Well-off as disabled as well value sensibly structured, well-designed, clear and easy-to-access health care services on the net.

The section is one of mixed optimism and hesitation. The inevitable future of health care is in the networks, real ones supported with computer-based communication networks. This has many advantages, but the process must be supported by guidance and help to those not so much at home in the new network environments.

Chapter 8
Collaborative Approach for Sustainable Citizen-Centered Health Care

Pirkko Nykänen and Antto Seppälä

Abstract Health care systems are in transition to citizen-centered care with focus on prevention, proactive and personalized services and healthy lifestyles. Innovative technologies enable citizens' empowerment and allow them to manage their complete health and wellness. Citizen-centered tools collect life-long cross-institutional information and data from health care providers and citizens. From the health care organizations viewpoint the new paradigm implies changes in the ways how the services are produced, how they are offered for use and in the contents of the services. Research with the citizen-centered health paradigm has been active and many significant results have been achieved, for instance improvements in citizens' lifestyle, weight loss, reduction of the duration of hospitalization, better accessibility of health related information and improved communication between the care providers.

Based on our literature review we present in this chapter the approaches, achievements, barriers and challenges of citizen-centered health paradigm. We propose a new innovative approach to build the next generation, collaborative health information space that links the care providers and citizens together and helps them to access the distributed health resources any time anywhere. The visional, sustainable citizen-centered health environment offers means to gradually migrate from the current situation to a citizen-centered care environment where citizens have a participatory role in health care activities.

Keywords Citizen • Centered health care • Sustainable • Personal health record • Personal health systems • Social media • Collaborative health care environment

P. Nykänen (✉) • A. Seppälä
School of Information Sciences, Centre for Information and Systems, eHealth Research,
University of Tampere, Tampere, Finland
e-mail: Pirkko.Nykanen@uta.fi

N. Wickramasinghe et al. (eds.), *Critical Issues for the Development*
of Sustainable E-health Solutions, Healthcare Delivery in the Information Age,
DOI 10.1007/978-1-4614-1536-7_8, © Springer Science+Business Media, LLC 2012

8.1 Introduction

Health care systems around the world are facing challenges especially with availability, costs and quality of health services. Personal Health Systems 2020 Support Action (Codagnone 2009) has recognized 8 challenges that health care systems face in the future: Population ageing and other prevalence related trends (e.g. obesity), increasing income, consumerism and demand for equal and fair access, increasing capacity to cure, overshooting or mismatch in resource allocation, fragmentation and overspecialization, inflation through unnecessary costs, and fat administration. Citizens' awareness is one challenge; citizens are aware of their own health and are willing to choose services based on personal needs and preferences (Monteagudo and Moreno 2007; PricewaterhouseCoopers Health Research Institute 2005; Detmer and Steen 2006). Many of these current challenges can be solved by using ICT solutions and by developing new services that can match the organizational and structural changes in health care area (Codagnone 2009; PricewaterhouseCoopers Health Research Institute 2005; Teperi et al. 2009; Varshney 2007; Wartena et al. 2009; Hill and Powell 2009).

There are programs ongoing worldwide with the purpose to meet these challenges. We can identify some major issues that are common to most of these national health IT initiatives (McConnell 2004; Jha et al. 2008; Aaltonen et al. 2009; eHealth roadmap – Finland 2007). A general objective is to have nationally access the core patient data, i.e. patient's diagnoses, medication data, examinations, care actions and patient risk data. There is also a widely shared understanding and agreement on the contents of these core patient data. The international trend is to document the core patient data in a structured manner and for this purpose headings, classifications, nomenclatures and agreed coding systems are used. Other major issues are use of standards and secure authentication and identification of the users.

Patient data is stored locally or regionally, there are very few attempts to build a centralized national patient data archive. An exception is Finland where a national digital patient data archive is under development (eHealth roadmap – Finland 2007). A major focus generally with patient data is on easy access when and where data is needed. A clinical path, or a treatment chain can build the connection between the data entities in various systems (Adler-Milstein et al. 2009).

An important component in these national programs is a secure data transfer channel to enable patient data exchange between health care organizations and professionals, and very recently also between health professionals and patients. In most countries Internet is considered secure enough, but in some countries, e.g. in UK and Sweden special telecommunication networks have been established for health care (Iliakovidis et al. 2005; Malmqvist et al. 2005).

In most countries the national programs and initiatives put special emphasis on citizen services. The citizens should have access to their own health related data and information. There are some good examples already on these systems, e.g. in USA and UK which offer for their citizen's access to patient data which is stored in their own data bases (Aaltonen et al. 2009; Iliakovidis et al. 2005; Basch 2005). There are also commercial products already available for citizens, e.g. Health Vault and Google Health, that offer citizens tools to integrate their own health data with other wellness information for their individual needs. These examples demonstrate the ongoing shift from an organization-centered health care to citizen-centered health care where the focus is on prevention, proactive services, healthy lifestyle and personalized services for citizens.

8.2 Citizen-Centered Health Care Paradigm

Current health care systems are organization-centered and patient care processes are static and designed mostly from the physicians' viewpoint. Patient care is focusing on treatment of diseases and care is organized by specialty or intervention. Care is composed of sequences of care episodes given by various providers and this situation does not really support multi-professional and collaborative care. There is lack of communication between the participants and also many delays and queues in the processes (Teperi et al. 2009; Koop et al. 2008; Pratt et al. 2006; Ohashi et al. 2010).

In the citizen-centered care (CCC) paradigm health care systems should transform their processes in such a way that the individual citizen is placed in the middle of health care processes. Health is seen in a more holistic way where the focus is on individual's complete wellness, covering health, diseases, care, prevention, wellness and healthy lifestyle. Essential is that citizen-centered care will enable the citizen to take an active part in his/her health care processes throughout his/her lifetime anytime and anywhere (Teperi et al. 2009; Wartena et al. 2009; Pratt et al. 2006; Ohashi et al. 2010; Nykänen 2008; Tang and Lansky 2005).

The core of the citizen-centered care paradigm is to focus on preventive care, on proactive services, on early detection and diagnosis to ensure citizens personal wellness. Thus, there is a need for new citizen-oriented services covering health promotion, health maintenance and citizen education and empowerment Also health care providers should be open and able to communicate and give citizens more information on their health and wellness related issues (PricewaterhouseCoopers Health Research Institute 2005; Wartena et al. 2009; Koop et al. 2008; Ohashi et al. 2010; Continua Health Alliance 2005; Kolitsi and Cabrera 2007; Berry and Mirabito 2010).

Citizen-centered care creates a need for new kinds of interoperable and sharable networks of services which can also include other actors than health care providers. These networked services create new challenges for health care systems and care processes should become multi-professional, decentralized, distributed, easily accessible and based on personalization of care. When patient care is shared in the network of service providers there is a need to share also the patient data and care management. Currently patient data is fragmented and stored in distributed data bases and it is not easily accessible when and where needed (Varshney 2007; Pratt et al. 2006). Shared care processes need interoperable information systems to handle increasing number of information sources and participants in the patient care (Koop et al. 2008; Ohashi et al. 2010).

Since citizen-centered care model is based on the networked services and shared care management there is a need for extended communication and co-operation through processes to ensure comprehensive services. Different participants in care processes need real-time reliable information to be able to make justified decisions. The amount of health related information is increasingly growing and it is critical to have access to citizens' histories, medications, test results and clinical records but also to their lifestyle choices, behaviors and personal information (Tang and Lansky 2005; Kolitsi and and Cabrera 2007). A requirement for implementation of the citizen-centered care model is empowerment of the citizens. Citizens are not anymore passive users of services but active participants in the care processes who take responsibility of their care (Pratt et al. 2006; Kolitsi and Cabrera 2007).

Current health care services are fragmented and therefore the citizens now need to act themselves as care integrators who are responsible for the completeness of care (Monteagudo and Moreno 2007; Pratt et al. 2006).Citizen empowerment is seen as a potential tool to cut down costs in health care, because much of the responsibility is moved to the citizen (Monteagudo and Moreno 2007; PricewaterhouseCoopers Health Research Institute 2005; Wartena et al. 2009) and maintenance of wellness and prevention has better return of investment than treatment of a disease after diagnosis (Continua Health Alliance 2005; Berry and Mirabito 2010; World Health Organization (WHO) 2006).

Increased empowerment of citizens and their collaboration with service providers may improve the quality of care through improved lifestyle choices and health behaviors, better disease management, improved care coordination, and following better care recommendations. High quality information is needed to empower the citizens to make effective decisions and choices. Missing information can be damaging to citizens, their relatives and proxies and also to health care providers (Monteagudo and Moreno 2007; Varshney 2007; Center for Information Technology Leadership (CITL) 2008).

In citizen-centered care model citizens should be able to access health care from and at their homes and in everyday life, instead of visiting health care organizations. Technology makes it today possible to support the citizens' activities outside the care provider networks. These activities vary from life style and self health management to improving the life of citizens as well as managing chronic diseases (Continua Health Alliance 2005; Kolitsi and Cabrera 2007). For example chronic diseases related to the lifestyle are one of the main reasons for diseases and deaths in the developed countries (World Health Organization (WHO) 2006; Mattila et al. 2010). It would be very beneficial and cost-effective to help citizens to better manage their chronic diseases and possibly prevent these diseases by offering citizens information and support for prevention and healthy lifestyle.

8.3   Examples of Citizen-Centered Care

8.3.1   Personal Health Record

To implement the citizen-centered care model we need new tools for extended communication, collaboration and to support citizens' activities concerning their health and wellness. One of the existing tools is the personal health record (PHR).

Markle Foundation (2003) has defined attributes for PHR systems:

- Each person controls his or her own PHR,
- PHRs contain information from one's entire lifetime including information from all health care providers,
- PHRs are accessible from any place at any time,
- PHRs are private and secure,
- PHRs are transparent. Individuals can see who entered each piece of data, where it was transferred from and who has viewed it,
- PHRs permit easy exchange of information across the health care system.

These characteristics try to ensure the credibility of PHR. This definition is widely referenced to (See e.g. Monteagudo and Moreno 2007; Detmer and Steen 2006; Tang and Lansky 2005; Pagliari et al. 2007).

In the European Union research on personal health systems (PHS) is seen important. The personal health systems aim at improving and preserving the health of citizens outside the institutional care (Kolitsi and Cabrera 2007). The research focuses on wearable and portable systems, necessary tools for users, on the convergence between ICT and other technologies (e.g. biomedical sensors, micro- and nanosystems) and on connecting citizens with health care networks rather than on connecting health information systems together (Codagnone 2009).

In 2008 there were 100–200 PHR solutions already available in the USA (Center for Information Technology Leadership (CITL) 2008). The scope and nature of functions, content and information sources vary between different PHR systems but the basic idea is to give citizens access to their own health and wellness information, provide an integrated view of health and wellness including status, medical and treatment history and interactions with the providers (Markle Foundation 2003; Halamka et al. 2008; Connecting for Health 2008).

PHR systems can be divided into three different approaches. The simplest one is a standalone PHR which enables citizens to collect their information into a PHR which can be a paper-based, a portable device, a personal computer or a web based application. Standalone PHR is not connected to any other systems. The tethered approach allows citizens to view their own information from the health care providers electronic health record (EHR) and citizens do not have total control of their records. Interconnected PHR enables citizens to collect health information from multiple sources, enter their own entries, share information with different parties and totally control their own information. Interconnected PHR can produce more benefits to all stakeholders because of its interoperability with other systems (Tang and Lansky 2005; Tang et al. 2006; Detmer et al. 2008; Nykänen et al. 2009).

It is evident that PHR systems will play a major role in the change of health care systems to citizen-centered care model by empowering citizens and making health information available when and where it is needed. PHR can be seen as a technology that can improve health care delivery and the quality of care, lower the costs and help citizens' empowerment (Center for Information Technology Leadership (CITL) 2008; Markle Foundation 2003; Connecting for Health 2008; AHIMA e-HIM Personal Health Record Work Group 2005; National Committee on Vital and Health Statistics (NCVHS) 2006; Froomkin 2008). Citizens are creating (e.g. by using sensors, devices, and health diaries) and controlling their own health information, which enables the PHR model to be citizen-centered.

PHR is usually considered to include set of tools which are designed to help citizens to collect, access, coordinate, share and store their lifelong personal wellness and health information. PHR can also include decision support functions to help citizens to manage and co-ordinate their own health and wellness, and to track and manage health activities through their lifetime. Basically PHR is helping citizens to create an integrated and complete view of their health and wellness (Detmer and Steen 2006; Markle Foundation 2003; Connecting for Health 2008; Tang et al. 2006; Detmer et al. 2008; National Committee on Vital and Health Statistics (NCVHS) 2006).

The information and data in PHR is life-long and cross-institutional and it covers clinical data and information from different health care providers but there can also be citizens' own entries, observations, measurement data etc. In PHR citizens can collect their own information and manage it and possibly share it between different parties, but it is not designed to substitute the information in health care providers' information systems and in EHRs and use of PHR will not remove the legal obligations for recordkeeping from health care providers (Markle Foundation 2003; Connecting for Health 2008; Tang et al. 2006; AHIMA e-HIM Personal Health Record Work Group 2005).

The number of actors (e.g. sensors, advanced technology solutions) and stakeholders is increasing in the personal health ecosystem. Ecosystem term refers to the comprehensive system composed of PHR, integrated devices and sensors, and relevant actors and information systems in the personal health care environment. The ecosystem creates much information and data and the need for interoperability is growing (Wartena et al. 2009). Today, most sensors and information systems communicate differently and their transport mechanisms may vary. It is very challenging to create an interoperable personal health ecosystem with all of these different actors. To achieve true interoperability between different systems both structure (syntax) and meaning (semantics) of the data must be defined. Currently there are no proper standards or methods to enable real interoperability and data transfer between EHR and PHR systems (Wartena et al. 2009; Detmer et al. 2008). Without interoperability PHR systems will only be isolated information islands with limited value. PHR systems need to be integrated together with different health information systems. In the future PHR systems may even be so advanced that they have connections also to the health care delivery systems and are integrated seamlessly with other systems (Tang et al. 2006).

PHR puts new kinds of pressure also for citizens. Citizens may consider use of PHR inconvenient, difficult, or costly (Monteagudo and Moreno 2007). Citizens should be educated about PHR so they can understand the benefits of PHR and how citizen-centered health care will affect them (Tang et al. 2006). Citizens have to adopt their new roles and responsibilities related to their own health care. It is necessary to define how PHR can be part of citizens' lives and wellness management. PHR can only be successful if citizens understand potential benefits and are ready to maintain and coordinate their health information and activities with health care providers. There is also need for governmental guidelines and decisions in health care to find ways to support or reimburse the citizens' cost on using PHR systems.

8.3.2   Current Domains for Citizen-Centered Care

Chronic diseases related to lifestyle are major risks in developed countries. According to World Health Organization (WHO 2006) 70–80% of health care expenses are caused by chronic conditions. Lifestyle choices and behaviors are important for managing and preventing chronic diseases. The seven leading risk factors account for almost 60% of disease burden in Europe (World Health Organization (WHO) 2006). These factors are high blood pressure, tobacco, alcohol, high blood cholesterol, overweight, low fruit and vegetable intake and physical inactivity. All of these risk factors are closely related to lifestyle and behavior and can be managed and possibly minimized through better behavior and education. Prevention and better control of noncommunicable diseases are ways to improve the quality of life and well-being of citizens (World Health Organization (WHO) 2006).

Different tools for lifestyle, behavior and wellness management are part of the citizen-centered care model. These tools enable citizen empowerment and make it possible to manage citizens' complete health and wellness. Citizen empowerment is needed to ensure success of new models for disease management. New disease management models should help citizens to manage their complete wellness and actions to prevent diseases but also enable managing already existing diseases.

Rapid development of technology and growth of Internet use has made it possible to create pervasive health services. The goal of pervasive services is to improve citizens' lives through proactive and intelligent computing environment. Pervasive services can be used to monitor or support citizen's daily life, e.g. through sensors and devices citizens' activities (e.g. sleep, physical activity and energy expenditure) can be followed automatically and thus possibly detect emergency situations (e.g. falls, heart rate, blood glucose level) and risky situations or behaviors. Also behavior and emotion monitoring tools are being developed which can help to create more personalized care and early detection of new diseases and emergencies (Osmani et al. 2008; Mattila et al. 2008; Pulli et al. 2008). Already many mobile phones include tools to track physical activity and nutrition. Wellness systems include solutions to follow physiological measurement and development of health. Examples of developed tools are wearable devices for activity monitoring (Mattila et al. 2008), wellness diaries (Mattila et al. 2010), ECG measurement solutions for detection of cardiac syndromes (Fayn and Rubel 2010; Lee et al. 2009), tools for diabetics to measure blood glucose (Lee et al. 2009; Quinn et al. 2009), home monitoring systems (Prentza et al. 2006) and personal health records.

Home care offers many possibilities for managing chronic diseases. Continuous monitoring at home with information systems can help to improve quality of life and care. A modular home care system tailored for citizens suffering from different chronic diseases was developed in the Citizen Health System (CHS) project (Maglaveras et al. 2005). The CHS system offered citizen-focused services for measurements, communication with providers, education and interactive sessions with medical personnel to transmit measurement data or to ask advice. The CHS system supported monitoring of patients suffering from heart diseases, diabetes or obesity. The CHS project had very promising results concerning weight-loss and reducing hospitalization of heart failure patients. The CHS system was well-accepted by the citizens and physicians.

The EPI-MEDICS is a portable, intelligent and personal self-care system designed to support citizens' own management of cardiac status by providing personal ECG monitor to be used on-demand (Quinn et al. 2009). The system was designed to enable citizens to import recorded information easily to be used by health care professionals. The EPI-MEDICS was very well accepted by the providers and patients who felt more secure with such a system.

Wellness diary (WD) is an example of a mobile application which is designed to support citizens' actions on wellness management (Mattila et al. 2010). Mobile technology is suitable for wellness and self management because people usually carry the technology with them all the time, and the technology enables constant updating and immediate usage despite of the location or time. WD is a self-monitoring journal which enables recording of health and behavior related observations (e.g. activity, weight, smoking, eating, and blood pressure) which helps self-observation and behavior management. WD also gives feedback to users concerning their actions and behavior. Mattila et al. (2010) concluded that WD works quite well when it assists intervention and users get support from experts. But, users need to be properly educated about the possible benefits of using WD and self-observing. The long-term use of WD and its benefits seems to be connected to the motivation of patients and external support. Also users need interesting features which engage users, maintain their motivation, helps recovery and give more feedback. Even simple personalization of WD could help to meet the different needs of different user groups.

Aging population uses a lot of health care system resources. Independent and autonomous living is seen as a good way to reduce care costs, increase quality of life and improve efficiency of health care. Ambient assisted living (AAL) is an approach to help elderly people to manage living at home by offering them new ICT-based solutions e.g. for remote monitoring and emergency alarms and messages. AAL and independent living are trends which are affecting strongly on elderly care and transforming it towards citizen-centered care.

ICT-based applications give new ways for communication between elderly people and health care providers. The Internet gives access to health information and also enables social-networking which may give senior citizens new social relations concerning their needs and experiences about health and may offer more social activities and reduce their feeling of isolation (Frantzidis and Bamidis 2009). Needs and skills of elderly people are quite heterogeneous and new services have to be personalized according to their needs. Independent living is one example of citizen-centered care where the needs of the citizens' should be the starting point for planning of the care.

In the European Union ambient assisted living research has focused on physical and mental status of elderly people and to support independent living with the purpose to reduce costs, improve efficiency and improve quality of life by reducing institutionalization. The proportion of elderly people is growing and it is a challenge for health care systems. An example of independent living research is The Long Lasting Memories (LLM) project which combines tele-monitoring services and mental and physical training to improve detection of threats, to improve self-esteem of senior citizens and to reduce mental problems. It is based on smart home solutions and personalized training. The LLM project uses sensors to monitor the use of electronic appliances and citizens' movement to detect changes in regular movement patterns and possible emergencies (Frantzidis and Bamidis 2009; The Long Lasting Memories 2010).

The possibilities of mobile technology and broadband connections have been studied in many research projects (Frantzidis and Bamidis 2009), e.g. the AttentiaNet project which focused on independent living and reduction of social isolation, the OLDES project which focused on medical sensors and modern ICT to study lifestyle of elderly and how to improve their life quality and the ENABLE project with the focus on the needs of elderly people suffering from Alzheimer disease. ENABLE developed new services to enhance citizens' coping in daily living and components to improve memory and communication of the citizens.

Research in these domains with citizen-centered health paradigm has been active and many significant results have been achieved, e.g improvements in citizens' life style, weight loss and reduction of the duration of hospitalization. An important result from the elderly users is that they have felt more secure at home when they have had a supporting personal health system available. These results show that personal health systems may bring important benefits for the citizens and be cost-effective in the health care environment.

8.3.3 Citizen-Centered Care from the Health Care Service Provider's Viewpoint

The citizen-centered paradigm from the health service provision viewpoint means that health service providers do need to consider and analyze the citizens' needs for services and to develop services that fulfill these needs. Despite of this change in focus, the public and private health care institutions still most likely are in the future the major players and funders of health care services, though it can be expected that governments are forced to reduce the amounts of health care funding during time. This results in that fragmentation increases both across tiers of governments and within the health care service providers (GPs, primary care, secondary care) and this results in varying quality of care (Codagnone 2009; European Commission et al. 2006).

In this situation technology confident users and those who have enough economical capacities are able to buy personal health services available at consumer electronics market. More traditionalist wealthy users pay for high quality services from private organizations and those with less wealth queue for the publicly funded services adapting themselves to varying quality and waiting lists. The elderly and chronically ill may not in the future receive all services they need in the same manner as today, but the citizens will have technical devices like robots or ambient intelligence for monitoring at home to help them in long term care and rehabilitation. These citizen-services are funded by the public health organizations but their use may be controlled. The use may demand from the citizen in the future that she or he fully adopts healthy lifestyle guidelines and rules to achieve the treatments and care funded with the tax money (Codagnone 2009; Ganesh 2004).

From the health care organizations viewpoint a shift to citizen-centered care implies changes in the ways how the services are produced, how they are offered for use and finally in the contents of the services. Essential change that needs to be implemented is the extension of an organization-centered EHR with an integrated personal health record (PHR) in such a way that care provided by the health organizations, care provided by e.g. third sector actors and also the citizen's own notes, diaries and measurements from the citizen's own personal health systems are covered (Detmer et al. 2008). This kind of personal health record can improve the quality, completeness, depth and accessibility of health information and enable communication between patients and providers.

8.4   The Drivers, Barriers and Issues to Consider in Sustainable Citizen-Centered Care

8.4.1   Drivers for the CCC-Model

Current problems with accessibility, costs and quality of health care are encouraging health care systems to find more efficient ways of delivering services (Hill and Powell 2009). The cost of health care has been steadily growing proportion to GDP since the 1980s (PricewaterhouseCoopers Health Research Institute 2005) and population in Europe and USA is growing older and maintaining reasonable level of health care systems is becoming harder. As the number of retirees is growing and fewer clinicians are available there is a need for more effective use of resources (Codagnone 2009; Teperi et al. 2009; Varshney 2007; Wartena et al. 2009; Hill and Powell 2009).

Health care has been very heavily based on labor, knowledge, skills and time, today innovative. Innovative technologies make it possible to create new productive services and possibly reduce the need for massive amounts of labor and time. Diagnosing diseases, creating treatment plans, educating patients, record keeping, and communication are major time and labor consumers in health care which possibly can be enhanced by using innovative technologies and standardization (Berry and Mirabito 2010).

Health promotion and preventive services are important drivers towards citizen-centered care. They have better economical value through the ability to reduce costs by promoting healthy life style, by preventing diseases and by maintaining health than the traditional disease treatment and interventions (Continua Health Alliance 2005; Berry and Mirabito 2010; World Health Organization (WHO) 2006). Health care systems are also trying to reduce hospitalization and institutionalization by implementing intelligent home care and independent living services supported by technological solutions and by improving organizational care processes (Prentza et al. 2006; Maglaveras et al. 2005; Frantzidis and Bamidis 2009).

Technology is advancing rapidly and different sensors and devices give possibilities for citizens to track and manage their own health and wellness (Mattila et al. 2010; Osmani et al. 2008). Citizens are aware of their own health and are willing to take more responsibility of their own health (Detmer and Steen 2006). Health providers are also empowering citizens by providing them health information and giving them more responsibilities concerning their own health (Monteagudo and Moreno 2007; Wartena et al. 2009). Technological solutions and the Internet are enabling citizens to share their own health related information through different communication channels. Citizens can share their experiences and ask advices in social networks and they are very active in these today (Frantzidis and Bamidis 2009).

In the citizen-centered care (CCC) collaboration between different health care providers is necessary to enable shared, comprehensive health care. Health professionals should be able to communicate with each other and create networked services with shared care management. Different participants in the care processes need real-time reliable information to be able to make justified decisions.

Citizens' needs, preferences and skills are very heterogeneous and thus the health care delivery model needs to be very flexible and adaptable and based on individualization and personalization. Citizens need different kinds of services and support depending on their personal situation and needs. In some cases they need only a short consultation, sometimes more support or thorough advice and these can be provided by a doctor, a network of medical professionals, a nurse, a non-medical professional or by the peer support groups from the social media (Berry and Mirabito 2010). Citizen-centered care paradigm also very clearly implies the possibility to develop tailored services based on the personal needs.

From health care organizations viewpoint it is important that they install more advanced information systems which can communicate with the information systems infrastructure. Interoperability of the information systems is the key issue here. Security, privacy and confidentiality of patient data have to be ensured also in the citizen-centered care model to achieve citizens' trust on the services.

8.4.2 Barriers for the CCC-Model

The barriers for citizen-centered care (CCC) paradigm are many, mostly they are due to the current, organization- or even hospital-centered care paradigm. For the citizen-centered care the concept and processes of health care need rethinking and reengineering. In a study (Detmer et al. 2008) the following factors were identified to be the major barriers for citizen-centered care:

- Health care system culture and incentives covering physician patient autonomy hinder implementation of the CCC paradigm. Also the responsibilities of various health professionals have been tightly determined and there are concerns about liability risks, if the situation changes.
- Consumers do have concerns abo security and confidentiality of their health related data, citizens are not convinced on the confidence and trust in the changing situation.
- There is lack of technical standards for interoperability including data integration standards, common core data sets, consumer terminologies, authentication and identification processes, security and privacy standards and certification. Most existing CCC solutions are tailored and very context-dependent, and thus vulnerable for changes.
- There is lack of health IT infrastructure in many countries, mostly due to the high enterprise cost of data integration, and the mediating structures between various information systems are missing.
- Citizens have concerns about equity and usability of CCC systems and they are worried about the digital divide, existence of a racial and socio-economic disparity gap.
- There are suspicions on value realization which refers to that ICT investments in health care usually require justification based on quantifiable benefits in terms of avoided cost, improved efficiency or increased revenue. The health IT business needs to take into consideration the infrastructure and labor costs for implementation, as well as ongoing system support costs. The CCC-model with integrated PHRs is a difficult business case for cost-benefit justification, due to the lack of empirical evidence in health care and informatics literature to quantify the PHR value proposition. While many of the perceived PHR benefits accrue to citizens, it is not clear that they are willing to pay or subsidize the cost of PHRs. Although surveys show substantial numbers of citizens indicating their willingness to pay this has not yet been demonstrated in practice. Benefits such as citizen and patient satisfaction, improved communication and citizen engagement are not easily quantifiable.
- There is uncertainty on the market demand because CCC-model with integrated PHRs offer both significant potential for users and a high degree of risk for potential investors.

Lopez (2007) identified the following barriers for the CCC-model in a study: Incompleteness of the existing technical infrastructure, heterogeneity of the citizens in attitudes and knowledge, slow migration from the paper-based systems to digital systems in health care, technical difficulties in system integration due to application program interfaces, need for reengineering of work processes and procedures and concerns about data security and data privacy.

Many studies have identified critical factors for adopting electronic health records generally (Ash and Bates 2005; James 2007; Lorenzi et al. 2009) and most of these result in the following items: User attitude towards information systems, workflow impact, technical support, interoperability, expert support and communication among users.

These factors are evidently critical also for adoption of PHRs and citizen-centered care paradigm. To overcome these factors it is important to define and design the information models and data structures in such a way that they support adoption of a PHR, and redesign the underlying processes in the framework of the citizen-centered care paradigm. The PHR software architectures should be designed to implement citizen-centered processes and data and information models.

A very important concern with PHRs and citizen-centered care is the privacy and security risks. Citizen's health related data is confidential and needs to be protected from an unauthorized access and disclosure. With PHRs security and data protection issues need special attention as the citizen's health data may be in a distributed storage in a network of actors and access to that data need to be legally protected.

8.4.3 New Approaches to Consider

An innovative approach is needed to build the next generation, semantically enriched, collaborative health information space that covers both organization-centered and citizen-centered paradigms and EHR and PHR concepts respectively. The collaborative space should facilitate all stakeholders, health care providers, health professionals, patients and citizens to link, dynamically discover, effectively combine, easily and safely access the distributed health resources, data and information independent where they are provided, or needed.

An integrated PHR model is still a theoretical framework for citizen-centered health care. We need an interoperable network for new channels of communication and care management. And this points to a new tool that is clearly broader than the legal record of any provider. As traditional roles and relationships between citizens and different parts of health care delivery and financing system are fundamentally altered by a more citizen-centered framework, stakeholders may realize a variety of new benefits from interaction with PHRs.

The recent innovations in collaborative environments and social media research (Hawn 2009; Halonen 2010) can bridge the information, knowledge and collaboration gap currently existing in health care services provision and use. Collaborative environments hold considerable potential value for health care organizations because they can be used to reach stakeholders, aggregate information and leverage collaboration (De la Fuente and Ros 2009; Boulos and Wheeler 2007; Kaplan and Haenlein 2010). The collaborative environments research results support the development of a conceptual architecture that will facilitate interactive connectivity between the available health data and health information sources such as data bases, digital archives, literature or Internet for gathering and sharing adequate knowledge for making decisions in citizen-centered care. Furthermore, these advances support development of a user friendly, collaborative decision making environment.

As more and more patients already use collaborative environments and social media to track their health conditions and care, health care organizations have an opportunity to interact with the members of these online communities and to leverage data sets to inform new treatments and care pathways. Hospitals are increasingly using social media for promotional purposes and to gauge citizens' experiences with their organizations, e.g. in USA many hospitals have a social media and social networking presence to market their services and communicate to stakeholders (Hawn 2009).

In e-Business and e-Commerce more and more companies apply social media (Kaplan and Haenlein 2010) because there are many technical tools available already to support this. Social media like Facebook, LinkedIn and Twitter consist of user profiles, connections between friends and colleagues and they support communication. All these networks establish the awareness of who is there and what are they doing, they enable communication from many to many, instead of from one to one (Hawn 2009). These tools are familiar and popular to the general public, citizens, they are also easy to use and cheap to purchase, or even free to access.

The collaborative environments and social media approach offers many possibilities for citizen-centered health. Our vision from the collaborative, sustainable citizen-centered health is presented in Fig. 8.1. The vision presents a collaborative environment without borders and it is based on two collaborative virtual health spaces: (1) the citizen's personal health space, and (2) the health care organization's regulated and legally controlled health space. These two spaces build together a collaborative health environment.

The citizen's personal health space is completely controlled, maintained and managed by the citizen himself, using the tools that seem appropriate to his situation and are usable and useful for his purposes and accessible in his situation. The health organization's health space contains patient data and information which is collected and documented by health professionals in the EHRs and other relevant health information systems during the citizen's care episodes and visits. This space is for the health professionals and administrative purposes and it is legally regulated and controlled by the health organization. Citizen does not have direct access to this health space but he can link or copy his own data and information to his own personal space. This communication is one-way; the citizen cannot transmit any information from his personal space to the health organization's space. However, the citizen can give access to the health organization to the citizen's own health space if he sees this useful and beneficiary. The social collaborative environment builds thus a platform that enables communication and sharing of data and information.

Future health care, Health 2.0, is participatory. The services are enabled by information, information systems, and the community of actors that is created and collected around a person's health and wellness. This community is composed of all

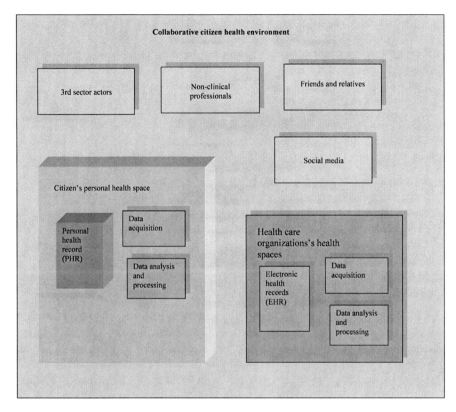

Fig. 8.1 Vision on collaborative, sustainable citizen-centered health

relevant actors needed for prevention, health care and wellness. The person himself, as a patient, as a citizen, is an active participant in this community. Thus the citizen is reshaping the health care system according to his needs and situations. These kinds of new approaches in health care change the relationship between the care givers and the care receivers.

8.5   Summary and Conclusions

Health care systems are in a transition phase, they are progressing from an organization-centered health care to a citizen-centered care, and this implies many changes on our current health care services provision, delivery and use.

Citizen-centered health care paradigm with personal health record (PHR) and personal health systems (PHS) create many challenges for health care. Froomkin (2008) found four elements of the use of PHR that create major changes in health care:

- Viewing the citizen and devices controlled by the patient build important sources of health-related data,
- Giving the citizen much greater control over health information,
- Moving personal data storage and/or queries based on personal data towards Internet-based applications,
- Permitting, even encouraging, citizens and patients to share health data via informal social networks.

Continua Health Alliance (2005) identified four considerable benefits from citizen empowerment and new models of health care:

- Improvements in citizen's lifestyles, current poor health lifestyles dramatically increase population risk for disease,
- Early diagnosis and detection reduces care costs, much costs come currently from waiting to intervene until after disease is present,
- Citizen empowerment helps the low risk populations to remain healthy by modifying personal health behaviors,
- Return on investment from wellness-focused programs has been achievable and dramatic.

CCC-based system beneficiaries are usually individual citizens but other stakeholders may also benefit from their use (Tang et al. 2006) because CCC-based systems support health care decisions and continuity of care across time and providers (National Committee on Vital and Health Statistics (NCVHS) 2006). Personal systems may also save time and money and increase the quality of care, because they may decrease duplicate testing, help to access patient records, reduce drug adverse events and improve preventive care and health management (Markle Foundation 2003; Pagliari et al. 2007).

CCC-based systems may produce benefits to individuals who wish to stay fit or are at risk and wish to maintain normal health status, to chronically ill patients, to individuals who want to live independently outside care institutions and health professionals (Codagnone 2009). The main benefit to all citizens is the access to their health information and data which they can use to support their wellness activities, e.g. management of chronic diseases, prevention, life style choices. These systems also have the potential to improve communication between the citizen and her health care provider and make it possible to create ongoing connection between the citizen and the provider so they can have a continuous care process instead of an episodic, disease focused one. Communication makes it easier for citizens and providers to ask questions, to make appointments, to request refills and referrals, and to report problems (Pagliari et al. 2007; Tang et al. 2006).

Citizen-centered care paradigm has a lot of potential for benefits but these will only be realized with widespread use (Tang et al. 2006). The health care workflows need to be changed to personalized and citizen-centered (Clarke and Meiris 2006). Partnership is essential between all stakeholders and this means new ways of making care decisions, new roles for professionals and reengineered workflows (Kolitsi and Cabrera 2007).

It is important, however, to notice that CCC-based applications are currently still a very small niche market and this is due to the barriers and gaps of socio-economic, institutional and cultural nature that the technological research will not solve by itself. The success of the approach is not only dependent on technological factors but a lot of work is needed to face the social and cultural obstacles. Policy initiatives, legislation and institutional reengineering, inter-institutional and interdisciplinary collaboration as well as support to implementation and deployment are needed to create the correct structure of incentives across the entire value chain, and to identify and sustain new business and funding models. From the health care perspective we need to increase efforts in the preventive field, to reduce healthcare fragmentation and to increase the delivery of integrated care to better inform and educate users and overcome resistances on their side and also on the side of health professionals. It is also necessary to pay attention to technical standardization and interoperability aspects of ICT (Codagnone 2009). Health care systems have to face the challenges created by new ways of working, empowered citizens and new tools.

The visional, collaborative, sustainable citizen-centered health environment offers means to gradually migrate from the current situation to a citizen-centered care environment. We are in good progress with PHS and PHR and also with health ICT infrastructures and next we need to give the citizen a participatory role in health care activities.

Acknowledgments We acknowledge the partial funding of this research by Academy of Finland through Trusted eHealth and eWelfare Space-project in the MOTIVE Research Programme 2009–2012.

References

Aaltonen, J., Ailio, A., Kilpikivi, P. et al. (2009). Kansallisen tason sähköisten potilastietojärjestelmien toteuttamisvaihtoehtojen vertailu – Kattava projekti. SITRAn selvityksiä 12, http://www.sitra.fi (in Finnish).

Adler-Milstein, J., Bates, D. W., & Jha, A. K. (2009). US regional health information organisations: Progress and challenges. *Health Affairs, 28*, 483–492.

AHIMA e-HIM Personal Health Record Work Group. (2005). Defining the personal health record. *Journal of AHIMA, 76*(6), 24–25.

Ash, J. S., & Bates, D. W. (2005). Factors and forces affecting EHR system adoption: Report of a 2004 ACMI discussion. *Journal of the American Medical Informatics Association, 12*, 8–12.

Basch, P. (2005). Electronic health records and the national health information network: Affordable, adoptable and ready fro prime time? *Annals of Internal Medicine, 143*, 227–228.

Berry, L. L., & Mirabito, A. M. (2010). Innovative healthcare delivery. *Business Horizons, 53*, 157–169.

Boulos, M. N. K., & Wheeler, S. (2007). The emerging Web 2.0 Social software: An enabling suite of sociable technologies in health and health care education. *Health Information and Libraries Journal, 24*(1), 2–23.

Center for Information Technology Leadership (CITL). (2008). The value of personal health records. *Healthcare Information and Management Systems Society (HIMSS)*, http://www.citl.org/publications/_pdf/CITL_PHR_Report.pdf. Accessed 28 Aug 2010.

Clarke, J. L., & Meiris, D. C. (2006). Electronic personal health records come of age. *American Journal of Medical Quality, 21*(3 Suppl), 5S-15S.

Codagnone, C. (2009). *Reconstructing the whole: Present and future of personal health systems,* PHS2020, European Commission, http://ec.europa.eu/information_society/activities/health/docs/projects/phs2020/phs2020-book-rev16082009.pdf. Accessed 28 Aug 2010.

Connecting for Health. (2008). *Common framework for networked personal health information: Consumers as network participants.* Markle Foundation, http://www.connectingforhealth.org/phti/docs/ConsumerNetwork.pdf. Accessed 28 Aug 2010.

Continua Health Alliance. (2005). Connected Personal Health in 2015: "Getting it Right!" – Looking back on the emergence of integrated person-centered health. Continua Health Alliance, http://www.continuaalliance.org/static/cms_workspace/CHA_WP081408v07.pdf. Accessed 28 Aug 2010.

De la Fuente, M. W., & Ros, L. (2009). A health collaborative network focus on self care processes in a personal assistant. *IFIP Advances in ICT, 307,* 759–766.

Detmer, D., & Steen, E. (2006). *Learning from abroad: Lessons and questions on personal health records for national policy.* The American Association of Retired Persons (AARP), http://assets.aarp.org/rgcenter/health/2006_10_phr_abroad.pdf. Accessed 28 Aug 2010.

Detmer, D., Bloomrosen, M., Raymond, B., & Paul, T. C. (2008). Integrated personal health records: Transformative tools for consumer-centric care. *BMC Medical Informatics and Decision Making, 8*:45, http://www.biomedcentral.com/1472-6947/8/45/. Accessed 28 Aug 2010.

eHealth roadmap – Finland. (2007). Reports of the Ministry for Social Affairs and Health, 2007:15, Helsinki.

European Commission, DG Information Society and Media, eHealth Unit (2006), Research Book of EU projects on Health. Brussels.

Fayn, J., & Rubel, P. (2010). Toward a personal health society in cardiology. *IEEE Transactions on Information Technology in Biomedicine, 14*(2), 401–9.

Frantzidis, C. A., & Bamidis, P. D. (2009). Description and future trends of ICT solutions offered towards independent living: The case of LLM project. *ACM international conference proceeding series. Proceedings of the 2nd international conference on pervasive technologies related to assistive environments.* Corfu, Greece (PETRA 09), ACM, New York, USA.

Froomkin, M. A. (2008). *The new health information architecture: Coping with the privacy implications of the personal health records revolution.* UM ELSI Group for Project HealthDesign.

Ganesh, J. (2004). E-health – drivers, applications, challenges ahead and strategies: A conceptual framework. *Indian Journal of Medical Informatics, 1,* 39–47.

Halamka, J. D., Mandl, K. D., & Tang, P. C. (2008). Early experiences with personal health records. *Journal of the American Medical Informatics Association, 15,* 1–7.

Halonen, R. (2010). Social media as a means of peer support. In R. Suomi & I. Ilveskoski (Eds.), *Navigating the fragmented innovation landscape. Proceedings of the 3rd international conference on well-being in the information society (WIS2010),* Turku, Finland (pp. 48–60). TUCS General Publication 56, August, Turku, Finland.

Hawn, C. (2009). Report from the field: Take two aspirins and tweet me in the morning: How twitter, facebook and other social media are reshaping health care. *Health Affairs, 28*(2), 361–368.

Hill, J. W., & Powell, P. (2009). The national healthcare crisis: Is eHealth a key solution? *Business Horizons, 52,* 265–277.

Iliakovidis, I., Wilson, P., and Healy, J. C. (Eds.) (2005). *eHealth. Current situation and examples of implemented and beneficial ehealth applications.* The Netherlands: IOS Press.

James, G. A. (2007). Social, ethical and legal barriers to eHealth. *International Journal of Medical Informatics, 76*(5-6), 480–3.

Jha, A. K., Doolan, D., Grandt, D., Scott, T., & Bates, D. W. (2008). The use of health information technology in seven nations. *International Journal of Medical Informatics, 77*(12), 848–854.

Kaplan, A. M., & Haenlein, M. (2010). Users of the world, unite! the challenges and opportunities of social media. *Business Horizons, 53,* 59–68.

Kolitsi, Z., & Cabrera, M. F. (2007). *Personal health systems: Deployment opportunities and ICT research challenges – Conference report.* February 12–13, 2007, Brussels. European Commission http://ec.europa.eu/information_society/newsroom/cf/document.cfm?action=display&doc_id=323. Accessed 28 Aug 2010.

Koop, C. E., Mosher, R., Kun, L., Geiling, J., Grigg, E., Long, S., Macedonia, C., Merrell, R., Satava, R., & Rosen, J. (2008). Future delivery of health care: Cybercare. *IEEE Engineering in Medicine and Biology Magazine, 27*(6), 29–38. November-December.

Lee, H. J., Lee, S. H., Ha, K. S., Jang, H. C., Chung, W. Y., Kim, J. Y., Chang, Y. S., & Yoo, D. H. (2009). Ubiquitous healthcare service using Zigbee and mobile phone for elderly patients. *International Journal of Medical Informatics, 78*(3), 193–8.

Lopez, K. (2007). Global perspective on PHRs: Consumer engagement in health information exchange in Europe & the U.S., presentation, http://www.nocalhimss.org/events/presentations/ICW-Presentation.ppt. Accessed 28 Aug 2010.

Lorenzi, N., Kouroubali, A., Detmer, D., Bloomrosen, M. (2009). How to successfully select and implement electronic health records (EHR) in small ambulatory practice settings. *BMC Medical Informatics and Decision Making 9*: 15, http://www.biomedcentral.com/1472-6947/9/15. Accessed 28 Aug 2010.

Maglaveras, N., Chouvarda, I., Koutkias, V. G., Gogou, G., Lekka, I., Goulis, D., Avramidis, A., Karvounis, C., Louridas, G., & Balas, E. A. (2005). The citizen health system (CHS): A modular medical contact center providing quality telemedicine services. *IEEE Transactions on Information Technology in Biomedicine, 9*(3), 353–62.

Malmqvist, G., Nerander, K. G., & Larsson, M. (2005). Sjunet – The national IT infrastructure for healthcare in Sweden. In: I. Iliakovidis, P. Wilson, & J. C. Healy (Eds.), *Current situation and examples of implemented and beneficial eHealth application,* (pp. 41–49). The Netherlands: IOS Press.

Markle Foundation. (2003). Connecting for health: The personal health working group final report, July 1, http://www.connectingforhealth.org/resources/final_phwg_report1.pdf. Accessed 28 Aug 2010.

Mattila, E., Korhonen, I., Merilahti, J., Nummela, A., Myllymaki, M., & Rusko, H. (2008). A concept for personal wellness management based on activity monitoring. *Second international conference on pervasive computing technologies for healthcare, PervasiveHealth 2008,* pp. 32–36, Jan. 30, 2008–Feb. 1, 2008, Tampere, Finland.

Mattila, E., Korhonen, I., Salminen, J. H., Ahtinen, A., Koskinen, E., Sarela, A., Parkka, J., & Lappalainen, R. (2010). Empowering citizens for well-being and chronic disease management with wellness diary. *IEEE Transactions on Information Technology in Biomedicine, 14*(2), 456–463.

McConnell, H. (2004). International effort in implementing national health information infrastructure and electronic health records. *World Hospitals and Health Services, 40*(1), 33–52.

Monteagudo, J. L., & Moreno, O. (2007). D2.5, Report on Priority Topic Cluster two: Patient Empowerment. eHealth ERA (http://www.ehealth-era.org/documents/eH-ERA_D2.5_Patient_Empowerment_Final_31-03-2007_revised.pdf). Accessed 28 Aug 2010.

National Committee on Vital and Health Statistics (NCVHS). (2006). Personal Health Records and Personal Health Record Systems, U.S. Department of Health and Human Services, Feb. 2006.

Nykänen, P. (2008). Requirements for user friendly personal ehealth information systems. *International council for medical and care compunetics (ICMCC) conference,* June 2008, London, UK. In: L Bos, B Blobel, A Marsh and D Carroll (Eds.), Medical care and compunetics. Studies in Technology and Informatics 137. IOS Press, Amsterdam, 367–372.

Nykänen, P., Ruotsalainen, P., Blobel, B., & Seppälä, A. (2009). Research on trusted personal health and wellness information in ubiquitous health information space. In D. Dössel & W. C. Schlegel (Eds.), *World congress on medical physics and biomedical engineering, Munchen, Germany.. IFMBE Proceedings 25/XII* (pp. 432–435). Berlin: Springer.

Ohashi, M., Hori, M., & Suzuki, S. (2010). Citizen-centric e-healthcare management based on pervasive authentication – New ICT roadmap to active ageing. *Fourth international conference on pervasive computing technologies for healthcare (PervasiveHealth),* Munich, Germany.

Osmani, V., Balasubramaniama, S., & Botvich, D. (2008). Human activity recognition in pervasive health-care: Supporting efficient remote collaboration. *Journal of Network and Computer Applications, 31*(4), 628–655. November.

Pagliari, C., Detmer, D., & Singleton, P. (2007). *Electronic personal records: Emergence and implications for the UK*. The Nuffield Trust, http://www.nuffieldtrust.org.uk/ecomm/files/Elec%20Personal%20Records%20II.pdf. Accessed 28 Aug 2010.

Pratt, W., Unruh, K., Civan, A., & Skeels, M. (2006). Personal health information management. *Communication of the ACM, 49*(1), 51–55.

Prentza, A., Maglavera, S., & Maglaveras, N. (2006). Quality healthcare management and well-being through INTERLIFE services: New processes and business models. *D2H2 1st transdisciplinary conference on distributed diagnosis and home healthcare* (pp. 109–112), 2–4 April 2006, Arlington, USA.

PricewaterhouseCoopers Health Research Institute. (2005). *Healthcast 2020: Creating a sustainable future. Pricewaterhousecoopers*, http://www.pwc.com/us/en/healthcast/past-reports.jhtml. Accessed 28 Aug 2010.

Pulli, P., Metso, A., & Zheng, X. (2008). *Ubiquitous services for senior citizens – service architecture and middleware*. Applied Sciences on Biomedical and Communication Technologies, 2008. ISABEL '08. First International Symposium on , vol., no., pp.1–5, 25–28 Oct. 2008, Aalborg, Denmark.

Quinn, C. C., Gruber-Baldini, A. L., Shardell, M., Weed, K., Clough, S. S., Peeples, M., Terrin, M., Bronich-Hall, L., Barr, E., & Lender, D. (2009). Mobile diabetes intervention study: Testing a personalized treatment/behavioral communication intervention for blood glucose control. *Contemporary Clinical Trials, 30*(4), 334–346. 1 July.

Tang, P. C., Ash, J. S., Bates, D. W., Overhage, J. M., & Sands, D. Z. (2006). Personal health records: Definitions, benefits, and strategies for overcoming barriers to adoption. *Journal of the American Medical Informatics Association, 13*, 121–126.

Tang, P. C., & Lansky, D. (2005). The missing link: Bridging the patient — Provider health information gap. *Health Affairs, 24*(5), 1290–1295. Sep/Oct.

Teperi, J., Porter, M. E., Vuorenkoski, L., & Baron, J. (2009). *The Finnish health care system: A value-based perspective*. Sitra Reports 82, http://www.sitra.fi Accessed 28 Aug 2010.

The Long Lasting Memories. (2010), http://www.longlastingmemories.eu/. Accessed 23 Aug 2010.

Varshney, U. (2007). Pervasive healthcare and wireless health monitoring. *Mobile Networks and Applications, 12*, 113–127.

Wartena, F., Muskens, J., & Schmitt, L. (2009). Continua: The impact of a personal telehealth ecosystem. *International conference on eHealth, telemedicine, and social medicine, eTELEMED '09*, Cancun, Mexico.

World Health Organization (WHO). (2006). *Gaining health – The European strategy for the prevention and control of noncommunicable diseases*. Copenhagen, Denmark: WHO, Regional Office for Europe.

Chapter 9
Strategies and Solutions in eHealth: A Literature Review

Marco De Marco, Francesca Ricciardi, and Jan vom Brocke

Abstract This study has three purposes: First, to provide a synthetic, up-to-date overview of the main emerging strategies for the health care sector in the Western developed countries; second, to understand the possible role of eHealth solutions in each of these emerging strategies; third, to understand how these emerging health care strategies and emerging eHealth solutions may be usefully applied to address one of the most important challenges for health care systems, i.e. population ageing. The overview on emerging strategies and emerging eHealth solutions provided here is based on a literature review including a wide spectrum of recent documents published on the Web about health care and eHealth. The outcome of this document search is a concept matrix linking emerging health care strategies and emerging eHealth solutions. This concept matrix is used as a framework to synthetically describe how eHealth initiatives are perceived by different stakeholders, such as investors, policy makers, insurance companies, PA bodies, researchers and academics, health care professionals, patients.

Keywords Health care strategies • eHealth • Population ageing • Health record systems • Telemedicine

9.1 Introduction

The first purpose of this study was to better understand the sentiments of health care and eHealth researchers, operators, policy makers, investors and final users, about the main trends of health care innovations in these last years. We wanted to see if it

M. De Marco (✉) • F. Ricciardi
Department of Economics and Management Sciences,
Università Cattolica del Sacro Cuore, Catholic University, Milan, Italy
e-mail: marco.demarco@unicatt.it

J. vom Brocke
Institute of Information Systems, University of Liechtenstein, Vaduz, Liechtenstein

N. Wickramasinghe et al. (eds.), *Critical Issues for the Development of Sustainable E-health Solutions*, Healthcare Delivery in the Information Age, DOI 10.1007/978-1-4614-1536-7_9, © Springer Science+Business Media, LLC 2012

is possible to extract a sort of consensus on a global basis about what are the main emerging strategies and ICT-based solutions in this sector. In the next paragraph, we will briefly describe the process of literature review through which we have tried to understand today's general sentiments about health care evolution and eHealth. Then, we will synthesize the main strategies in the eHealth sector today, on the basis of the sources we have selected. Afterwards, a list of emerging eHealth solutions will be presented, extracted from the same sources. Subsequently, we will link health care strategies to eHealth solutions: in other words, we will try to provide a synthetic but systematic description of what emerging strategies can be supported by each eHealth typical solution, and why. Finally, we will concentrate on a specific problem that is severely challenging health care systems: population ageing. We will use the strategies-solutions framework provided in the first part of this work as a guideline to propose a synthetic description of the state-of-the art of eHealth initiatives related to population ageing, and to identify some strategic areas where the developing of new business models is particularly needed.

9.2   Extracting Sentiments from the Web: Document Search Methodology

Identifying general trends for strategic choices is a necessary first step to evaluate new business models, but it is quite difficult to effectively perform such identification in a rapidly evolving field. If we look at studies published some 10–15 years ago, we can easily see that many strategies identified as winning for ICT-enabled initiatives have actually disappeared from the scenario a few years later. Of course, also the paper at hand is at risk of concentrating on ideas that will be swept away and forgotten in 5 years. To (partially) prevent our efforts from such a risk, we have chosen to conduct a preliminary investigation, aimed at screening on a wide spectrum the more recent sentiments in the eHealth community about what strategies are bound to prevail, taking into consideration not only the voices of researchers and academics, but also those of investors, policy makers, payers (such as insurance companies and Public Administration bodies), consulting firms, health care professionals, and patients.

To do so, we have chosen the following sources: the Springer online database (Springer as a publisher is particularly focused on management, new technologies and health care: http://www.springer.com/public+health?SGWID=0-40467-0-0-0); the section of the World Health Organization web site dedicated to a Global Observatory on eHealth (http://www.who.it/); one of the most popular and influent on-line patient communities (http://patientslikeme.com); a blog by a venture capitalist committed in evaluating health care start-ups (http://www.healthonomics.org); two web sites to assess how the "giants" are moving in this field, namely Google (the project "Google Health" is easily reachable via the search engine; the URL is not cited here because it is provisional for the Beta version available today) and Microsoft   (http://www.microsoft.com/hsg/   http://crm.dynamics.com/industries/healthcare-providers.aspx); and some relevant on-line resources by the European Union, and namely: the online database of the European Commission, dedicated to health (http://ec.europa.eu/information_society/activities/health/) as an aspect of the Information Society; the online database of a study group funded by the European Union, aimed at studying and assessing eHealth initiatives, with particular focus on the different strategies adopted by the different member countries (http://www. ehealth-strategies.eu/index.htm); the web site of a EU funded project, aimed at collecting and thoroughly describing eHealth practice initiatives throughout the world, and including a rich library of thousands of documents (http://www.good-ehealth.org); another EU funded web site, aimed at coordinating research in the field of eHealth (http://www.ehealth-era.org/).

The search was conducted during the summer of 2010. For each of these sources, documents published between 2005 and 2010 were taken into consideration. The documents were identified at least by title and abstract (when present); all titles that seemed relevant to answer the question "what are the 'year 2010 sentiments' about emerging strategies for health care?" were skimmed in their full-text; and those documents which resulted actually relevant to answer the research question were read carefully, taking into consideration also the writings cited in the Reference list, if published after 2005 (backward search) (vom Brocke et al. 2009).

The relevant documents (journal papers, eHealth conference proceedings, books, consulting firms' surveys, project reports, good practice reports, forum/blog posts, web advertising and promotional initiatives, web pages, web-based applications, slide shows) selected in this way were 64, starting from a pool of about 250 (the exact number depends on how single web pages or single posts in web forums are counted). For limits of space, only the most suitable, recent, clear, original and/or rich in reference list among these documents will be cited in the course of this writing, but the following synthesis results from an overall, qualitative confrontation between all the sources mentioned above.

9.3   Emerging Strategies in the Health Care Sector

The analysis of the sources described in the paragraph above allowed us to identify several trends in the current sentiments about what strategies are bound to prevail in the health care sector of Western, developed countries.

These trends may be synthetically described as follows:

1. **Improve network processes.** Health care systems are *networked systems* (Valeri et al. 2010), where very complex relationships among actors (who receives care, who decides what care is to be delivered, who pays for it, who delivers it, who evaluates it etc.) must be managed. As a consequence, innovation can't be limited to single organizations or actors (e.g. a hospital): *network processes* and *network embedded knowledge* are essential (Appelgate et al. 2001) to determine the system's performances.

2. **Develop evaluation processes**. Health care systems need ever evolving *metrics and processes to evaluate* the system's performances, as for three main aspects at least: cost control, public health and well-being performances, and customer satisfaction (Valeri et al. 2010; Blobel 2010).

3. **Develop incentives and deterrents.** In the course of health care systems evolution, strategies must be identified to *stimulate* the positive behaviors and to *deter* the detrimental ones, like corruption, negligence or waste. For example, solutions to keep unnecessary intervention rate under control are needed (Valeri et al. 2010).

4. **Enhance patient safety.** *Risk management* is going to take a pivotal role in health care systems (Stroetman 2007), as well as all the initiatives that may rise *patient safety,* improving, for example, the processes of diagnosing. Again, the role of network embedded knowledge will be crucial.

5. **Strengthen primary care.** A strong *primary care* network (responsible for all the non-specialist processes of care that may be performed before a patient is referred to a hospital, like the services of family physicians), with easy access for all, is essential for sustainable, effective and satisfying health care system (Dobrev et al. 2010).

6. **Strengthen preventive services.** *Preventive medicine* is becoming more and more important (Findley 2009). Good investments in prevention initiatives (including education, promotion, scheduled screening, coaching, public health data collection) may result in health system performances that are much better than those which could be achieved if the same funding was allocated to "ex-post" health care processes.

7. **Strengthen outpatient care.** *Outpatient care* must become more and more able to solve problems that previously requested inpatient care. Inpatient care should be devoted to highly specialized services only. All the solutions capable to reduce hospitalizations for secondary care, without damaging clinical performances, are likely to prevail. To achieve this goal, hospitals are key players: they should stop behaving as "buildings" and start behaving more and more as "territorial networks" (Mayhew and Lawrence 2006).

8. **Develop highly specialized structures.** Market competition will benefit *large and highly specialized structures.* Many small hospitals are going to be abandoned and closed. This means that strategies should be developed to effectively deliver specialized health care services *also* on a de-localized basis (Blobel 2010).

9. **Develop customer-oriented services.** Health care is bound to become more and more *customer oriented* (Smith 2001): personalization, claim management, transparency, simplicity, human interface, will be more and more important, as well as all the innovations allowing patients to save time.

10. **Develop the active role of consumers.** Our survey of web sources has confirmed that *consumers* are becoming more and more aware, demanding and willing to take control of their own health. Initiatives capable to positively develop the role of patients as active, educated members of the health care network, that choose and reward the best health care providers, are likely to enhance the quality and value of the health care system.

11. **Develop health coaching services** (Mayhew 2009). Long-term *"pull" and "push" health coaching* will become a more and more important service. It will serve the patient before (as a preventive activity) and after a disease has occurred,

through identifying potential threats, following-up, reminding, encouraging adherence to healthy behaviors, etc. (Shumaker et al. 2008).

12. **Make independent living possible.** Health care systems must concentrate on solutions that enhance *independent living* also of patients with disabilities and chronic diseases (Pomerleau et al. 2008).

13. **Protect privacy and ethics.** Health care services deal with the most important assets, i.e. life and well-being, and with the most confidential data. Every innovation in this sector, to be acceptable, must be trustworthy as for privacy protection and ethic issues.

14. **Integrate health, social and government services.** Health care is a potential catalyst for building integrated services (Dobrev et al. 2010) centered on the human person.

In addition to strategies, marking directions for future action in eHealth, also various types of eHealth solutions could be identified based on our literature review.

9.4   Emerging eHealth Solutions

In this paragraph, we identify and classify the main emerging eHealth solutions.

(a) **Distributed Electronic Health Record Systems and Associated Network Services.** These solutions (Garrido 2005) create an on-line clinical profile for each patient, where all health care related data and documents of a certain person may me stored and managed on a de-localized basis. In the context of an integrated health clinical information web-based network (Leonard 2004), health record systems may allow a dramatic simplification of many procedures (such as referrals, prescriptions, bookings, reimbursements, and the exchange of examination reports, lab results and discharge letters between the patient, the general practitioner and specialist physicians,) related to the complex networked nature of health care systems.

(b) **Administrative and Management Systems.** Support system such as financial and performance control systems, supply chain management systems, scheduling systems, billing systems, etc., which support clinical processes but normally are not used by healthcare professionals and patients during health care delivery processes (Bath 2008).

(c) **Clinical Information Systems.** Specialized tools for health professional such as, for example, computer-assisted diagnosis systems, radiology information systems, surgery training systems, pharmacy information systems (Valeri et al. 2010; Bath 2008).

(d) **Clinical Data Analysis Systems.** Specialized systems for public health researchers, such as statistical programs for analyzing infections diseases (Valeri et al. 2010).

(e) **Social Networking and Web 2.0 Systems focused on Health issues.** Web-based systems linking specific communities (e.g. parents of children suffering of a certain disease, or doctors operating within a certain health care national system). Also "traditional" health information/educational web sites are evolving towards a web 2.0, i.e. *bottom-up* and *interactive*, model.

(f) **Patient Relationship Management Systems.** Customer Relationship Management systems aimed at understanding each specific patient's needs, claims and levels of satisfaction, and at activating processes of problem solving and customer-oriented organizational innovation (Oinas-Kukkonen et al. 2008).

(g) **Telemedicine Systems**. (Dixon et al. 2008; Conley et al. 2008; Nir 2004). Personalized disease management services such as tele-radiology, tele-diagnosis, tele-consultation, remote monitoring.

9.5 Mapping Strategies and Solutions: An eHealth Strategy-Solution Matrix

Building on the analysis described above, we examined the relationship between strategies (1–14) and solutions (a–g). We were particularly interested in understanding whether each strategy is already supported by solutions, or there might be a specific need for the design of new eHealth solutions. The results are summarised in the so called Strategy-Solution-Matrix displayed in Table 9.1.

As the reader can see, all eHealth solutions may be useful to implement several strategies: there are not one-to-one links between strategies and ICT-based solutions. In other words, each eHealth solution, even if implemented for serving a single strategy in the first place (e.g. PRM may be implemented to "develop customer oriented services", strategy 9) may result in useful tools to enhance also other strategies (e.g. customer satisfaction levels measured via PRM may be used to "develop evaluation processes", strategy 2).

On the basis of these findings, we were interested in further structuring potentially promising fields of action in eHealth.

9.6 What Should eHealth Solutions Do for Emerging Health Care strategies? Different Priorities for Different Stakeholders

Looking for a kind of priority scale for the seven categories of eHealth solutions we went back to the data captured in the literature review. The sources we analyzed suggest that different stakeholder groups (investors, policy makers, payers such as insurance companies and PAs, researchers and academics, health care professionals, patients) tend to focus on different eHealth solutions as top priorities or "the next big thing".

Table 9.1 How emerging eHealth solutions (columns) may support emerging health care strategies (rows)

	(a) Health record	(b) Admn. mgmt.	(c) Clinical IS	(d) Clinical data anal.	(e) Social netw.	(f) CRM/ PRM	(g) Tele-medic.
1. Improve network processes	X	X	X	X	X	X	X
2. Develop evaluation processes	X	X	–	X	–	X	–
3. Develop incentives and deterrents	X	X	–	X	–	X	–
4. Enhance patient safety	X	–	X	X	X	–	X
5. Strengthen primary care	X	–	X	–	X	X	X
6. Strengthen preventive services	X	X	X	X	–	X	X
7. Strengthen outpatient care	X	X	X	–	X	X	X
8. Develop specialized structures	X	–	X	X	–	–	X
9. Develop customer oriented s.	X	X	–	–	–	X	X
10. Develop active role of consum.	X	–	–	–	X	X	X
11. Develop health coaching	X	–	X	X	X	X	X
12. Enhance independent living	–	–	–	–	X	X	X
13. Protect privacy and ethics	X	X	–	–	X	–	–
14. Integrate with social and gov.	X	–	–	–	X	X	–

Please refer to numbered lists in the paragraph text for a complete description of eHealth solutions (a,b,c…) and health care strategies (1,2,3…)

While our results are indeed interpretive in nature we found support for certain tendencies to be discussed in the following. Our search's outcomes could be synthesized as follows: investors tend to find the areas "a" (Distributed Electronic Health Record Systems and associated Network Services) "f" (CRM – Patient Relationship Management) and "g" (Telemedicine Systems) particularly interesting.

These findings are quite consistent with the fact that, according to a Capgemini Consulting analysis performed in 2008–2009 and described in Valeri et al. (2010), areas "a" and "g", along with those innovations in area "c" (Clinical Information Systems) specifically aimed at connecting clinical information systems to the network of Electronic Health Record Systems, are expected to be responsible for about 80% of eHealth market growth in the period 2008–2012. On the other hand, Valeri et al. (2010) provide no forecasts about expected growth of CRM/PRM. Based on our literature review we can discuss the priorities of some stakeholders in more detail:

- Policy Makers

Our investigation allowed us to provide a more thorough overview of the eHealth priorities expressed by *policy-makers*, even though this overview is substantially limited to the EU area. According to our investigations, we can say that policy-makers seem particularly focused on area "a" (Distributed Electronic Health Record Systems and associated Network Services). There is a strong consensus on the fact that a good Electronic Health Record System, based on shared standards and on strong authentication and privacy protection solutions, is a sort of essential keystone on which the whole building of a really innovated networked health care system can be built (Walker 2005; Wang 2003). Policy makers of tax-based health care systems tend to encourage the implementation of Electronic Health Record Systems provided, controlled and protected by government bodies. On the contrary, in other countries, such as the US, there is a strong tendency to rely on Distributed Health Record Systems implemented by private companies. Many major players, Microsoft and Google included, have presented their health record systems, and are competing to impose their standards.

- eHealth Payers

eHealth Payers (insurance companies, Public Administrations and organizations in charge of providing citizens with health care services) are particularly concerned with all the solutions that are expected to quickly increase efficiency. This common sentiment is confirmed by the fact that eHealth solutions more directly connected with efficiency, i.e. Administrative and Management Systems (strategy "c") and Clinical Information Systems (d) respectively accounted for 71.60% and 22.5% of the total European eHealth market in 2008. Payers, especially in countries with a tax-based health care systems, seem very scarcely interested in telemedicine systems, that accounted for a mere 0.90% of market share (Valeri et al. 2010), as well as in CRM/PRM systems, for whose market share we were unable to find quantitative data; we have just assessed that, according to our sources, these systems seem to receive more attention in the US than in Europe at the moment.

- Researchers and Academics

The sentiments of *researchers and academics* about the most important general trends in the eHealth field have been surveyed mainly through the analysis of all the issues of a specialized Springer journal (Health Care Management Science), through the analysis of the Proceedings of the First and Second eHealth Conferences (years 2008 and 2009) (Kostkova 2009; Weerasinghe 2008) and through the writings that the scholarly community submitted to the European Union to answer calls related to health care innovation and eHealth. According to these sources, scholars seem to concentrate more on eHealth solutions implying high scientific and technological specialization, such as telemedicine (h) (Weerasinghe 2008), and dense social implications, such as social networking (f). Moreover, scholars with a background in economics are interested in health care Information Systems evaluation (Bahol 2007; Goldzweig et al. 2009; Buccoliero et al. 2008; Dansky et al. 2006).

- Health Care Professionals and Patients

There is a growing interest and involving of *Health care professionals* and *patients* in social networking systems (f) explicitly dedicated to health. Many doctors, nurses, patients and their informal caregivers (e.g. parents, or children) spontaneously participate in networks that let they take major control of their own health or of their own professional issues. Apart from this, both health care professionals and patients tend to display quite passive or even skeptical behaviors as for the other eHealth initiatives, and particularly for Distributed Electronic Health Record Systems and associated Network Services (a), CRM – Patient Relationship Management (f) and Telemedicine Systems (g). In sum, exactly those eHealth solutions that investors and policy makers are more excited about are less likely to be considered important by doctors, by pharmacists and (above all) by patients; as a consequence, specific efforts must be made to have these new systems accepted and their advantages recognized in daily routines. In fact, in several successful pilot projects, Health Record Systems were distributed massively and with a "push" logic to all population, and economic incentives had to be introduced for doctors and pharmacists, to make them use the new systems and promote innovation acceptance among their patients (Dobrev et al. 2010).

Patients, in effect, may be slow in understanding all the implications of many aspects of health care innovation. Generally speaking, many factors tend to be more important than "objective" clinical excellence in order to improve customer/patient satisfaction in health care systems: patients are very positively impressed, for example, by reduced waiting times, kind nurses, nice buildings, convenient bureaucratic procedures, solicitous treatment for reducing even tolerable pain, and (often) medical remedies that relieve their symptoms without requiring lifestyle changes (Shumaker et al. 2008). This typical patient-experience-centered vision, focusing on factors that patients can easily recognize and be pleased of, may cause distortions.

For example, health care providers, if chosen directly by patients in competitive market or quasi-market systems, may choose to concentrate excessive funding in customer satisfaction "frill" initiatives, sacrificing those (also eHealth-based) improvements in clinical performances that customers are unlikely to perceive and to appreciate. In these cases, only the regulatory framework and effective information of patients (via social networks, for example) may create conditions so that health care providers keep high clinical standards, and patients make educated choices among providers.

On the other side, organizations providing tax-funded free health care may sometimes *decide* to keep customer satisfaction at a low level because if they provided patients with too convenient, satisfying and comfortable services, they would lose what they perceive as the only "barrier" that prevents an unsustainable number of patients from asking for probably unnecessary care. As a consequence, in these cases even excellent eHealth-based customer care initiatives are likely not to be accepted by health care providers, unless other, more civilized barriers against patient (and expenditure) overload are provided to replace "good old" bureaucratic bothers and uncomfortable access!

In other words, when we study health care strategies and eHealth solutions from the point of view of different stakeholders, it becomes apparent that innovation processes, to be successfully put in practice, must be founded on a sound awareness of the many, complex and contrasting interests hidden in the health care system they are faced with (Boddy et al. 2009).

So, eHealth is a *prioritizing issue* above all. It would be naïve, if not hypocritical, to say that health care systems' purpose is simply to provide the best existing clinical solutions, through the best existing customer-oriented procedures, for all. We simply have not enough money to do so; and, more importantly, we are going to have less and less money to do so in the future, because clinical solutions will become more and more refined (and expensive), whilst people will become less and less healthy. In the next paragraph, we will briefly go into this crucial issue.

9.7   Population Ageing and the Top Priorities for the eHealth Agenda

Demographic changes related to population ageing are "the top challenge" not only for health care systems, but also for pension systems in the Western world; moreover, they imply important consequences also for social and family structures and for labor markets. These facts are now widely recognized (Zweifel et al. 2009).

There is a wide consensus, too, on the fact that new technologies are expected to play a pivotal role to address such a challenge (Blobel et al. 2008).

A systematic literature review conducted in 2009 (Ricciardi 2010), through the analysis of more than 400 scholarly writings, found out that the scientific production about the role of new technologies to address the problem of ageing population is concentrated on the following ICT-based solutions mainly: computer mediated health education, stand-alone (i.e. not networked) assistive technology, social networking, and telemedicine (Myers et al. 2006). These studies are almost always conducted by scholars with the following backgrounds/approaches: medicine (as for the clinical implications of the ICT based solutions), engineering-design sciences (as for the technological aspects of assistive tools and devices), human factors (as for the study of interfaces and of their usability on the part of the elderly). Scholars with an Organizational – Information Systems background facing this problem, on the contrary, are a small minority.

As a consequence, many crucial aspects of the possible strategic role of eHealth in the challenge of ageing population have been scarcely investigated by the scholarly community so far. The writings concentrating on emerging eHealth business models (i.e. on the *ways stakeholders and actors could concretely interact to pursue their respective interests*) (Hedman and Kalling 2003) for the ageing societies are really few (Parente 2000).

In sum, the scholarly community risks to be left behind in some cutting-edge discussions on eHealth for ageing population: for example, whilst hundreds of academic writings laboriously investigate on how we could succeed in making an impaired, unwilling old person use a computer to access an eHealth service (Maddalena Sorrentino and Niehaves 2010), the world of practice is simply by-passing the problem, by enhancing the role of pharmacists, family doctors, phone call centers and younger, informal caregivers as *e-intermediaries* (Steiner 1997). In this way, networked health care services (such as e-booking or e-prescriptions) are being made available, via human interfaces, also for those who are not willing or capable to use a computer.

Using the Strategies-Solutions concept matrix described above as a reference framework, we suggest that scholars concentrate on two eHealth solutions in particular, for their potentialities to support really innovative business models in the sector of health services for the ageing society: Patient Relationship Management (solution "g") and Telemedicine (h). A third eHealth solution must be added as a priority, because, as shown in Table 9.1, it enables almost all basic and advanced network services, included PRM and Telemedicine: Distributed Electronic Health Record Systems (a).

Such tools, activated through friendly networks of e-intermediaries, seem particularly suitable to support key strategies that are expected to bring great benefits for the ageing societies: develop health coaching (strategy "11"), develop independent living (12) and integrate health, social and government services (14) (Cass Business School 2008).

9.8   Conclusions

Health care systems are among the most complex organizational networks ever created by mankind. As a consequence, the most decisive efforts to effectively innovate health care systems are not related to technological problems or to human-machine interface optimization. The core challenge for eHealth consists in *innovating network processes* and in *creating new suitable network embedded knowledge*. But processes innovation and knowledge creation must be prioritized; and the top priority now is to find solutions that keep the social and economic costs of population ageing under control, while maintaining good clinical performances and acceptable levels of customer satisfaction.

To do so, health coaching, empowered independent living and integrated socio-governmental-health distributed services are the key strategies that may significantly benefit from eHealth innovations to address health care problems related to ageing. Distributed Electronic Health Record Systems, Patient Relationship Management Systems and Telemedicine Systems seem the eHealth solutions with the most interesting prospects of value creation for the emerging business models in the next years; but the effective inclusion of the elderly in the new networked eHealth services will probably require that suitable networks of human e-intermediaries are provided.

References

Appelgate, L. M. et al. (2001). Emerging networked business models: Lessons from the field. *Harvard Business School*, (9), 801–172.

Bahol, R. (2007). Methods to evaluate health information systems in healthcare settings: A literature review. *Journal of Medical Systems, 31*, 397–432.

Bath, P. A. (2008). Health informatics: Current issues and challenges. *Journal of Information Science, 34*(4), 501–518.

Blobel, B. (March 2010). Architectural approach to eHealth for enabling paradigm changes in health. *Methods of Information in Medicine, 49*(2), 123–134.

Blobel, B., Pharow, P., & Nerlich, M. (2008). *eHealth: Combining health telematics, telemedicine, biomedical engineering, and bioinformatics to the edge: global experts summit textbook.* Amsterdam: IOS Press.

Boddy, D., et al. (2009). The influence of context and process when implementing e-health. *BMC Medical Informatics and Decision Making, 9*(9), 2009.

Buccoliero, L., et al. (2008). A methodological and operative framework for the evaluation of an eHealth project. *International Journal of Health Planning and Management, 23*, 3–20.

Cass Business School. (2008). *The economic, health and social benefits of care co-ordination for older people Cass Business School.* London: City University.

Conley, E. C., et al. (2008). Simultaneous trend analysis for evaluating outcomes in patient-centred health monitoring services. *Healthcare Management Science, 11*, 152–166.

Dansky, K., et al. (2006). A framework for evaluating eHealth research. *Evaluation and Program Planning, 29*, 397–404.

Dixon, B. E., et al. (2008). *Using telehealth to improve quality and safety: Findings from the AHRQ portfolio* (Vol. AHRQ publication no. 09-0012-EF). Rockville, MD: AHRQ Publication. December 2008.

Dobrev, A., Vatter, Y., & Jones, T. (2010). *The health information platform SISS in the region of Lombardy.* Socio-economic impact and lessons learnt for future investments in interoperable electronic health record and ePrescribing systems. EHRI Case 9, Available at www.her-impact.eu

Findley, P. (March 2009). Preventive health services and lifestyle practices in cancer survivors: A population health investigation. *Journal of Cancer Survivorship, 3*(1), 43–58.

Garrido, T. (2005). Effect of electronic health records in ambulatory care: Retrospective, serial, cross sectional study. *British Medical Journal, 330*(7491), 581–585.

Goldzweig, C. L., et al. (2009). Costs and benefits of health information technology. *Health Affairs, 28*(2), 282–293.

Hedman, J., & Kalling, T. (2003). The business model concept: Theoretical underpinnings and empirical illustrations. *European Journal of Information Systems, 12*(1), 49–59.

Kostkova, P. (Ed.) (2009). *Electronic Healthcare. Second international ICST conference*, eHealth 2009, Istanbul, Turkey, September 23–25, 2009, Revised Selected Papers. Springer.

Leonard, K. (2004). The role of patients in designing health information systems: The case of applying simulation techniques to design an electronic patient record (EPR) interface. *Health Care Management Science, 7*, 275–284.

Maddalena Sorrentino, M., & Niehaves, B. (2010). Intermediaries in E-Inclusion: A literature review. *HICSS. 43rd Hawaii international conference on system sciences*, pp. 1–10, 2010.

Mayhew, L. (2009). On the effectiveness of care co-ordination services aimed at preventing hospital admissions and emergency attendances. *Health Care Management Science, 12*, 269–248.

Mayhew, L., & Lawrence, D. (2006). The costs and service implications of substituting intermediate care for acute hospital care. *Health Services Management Research, 19*, 80–93.

Myers, S., Grant, R. W., Lugn, N. E., Holbert, B., & Kvedar, J. (2006). Impact of home-based monitoring on the care of patients with congestive heart failure. *Home Health Care Management & Practice, 18*(6), 444–451.

Nir, M. (2004). Factors affecting the adoption of telemedicine: A multiple adopter perspective. *Journal of Medical Systems, 28*(6), 671–632.

Oinas-Kukkonen, H., Räisänen, T., & Hummastenniemi, N. (2008). Patient relationship management. An overview and study of a follow-Up system. *Journal of Healthcare Information and Management, 22*(3), 24–29.

Parente, S. T. (2000). Beyond the hype: A taxonomy of e-health business models. *Health Affairs, 21*, 90–101.

Pomerleau, J., et al. (2008). The burden of chronic disease in Europe. In E. Nolte & M. McKee (Eds.), *Caring for people with chronic diseases: An health system perspective* (pp. 15–43). Maidenhead: Open University Press.

Ricciardi, F. (2010). ICTs in an ageing society: an overview of emerging research streams. In A. D'Atri et al. (Eds.), *Management of the interconnected world*. Berlin Heidelberg: Springer.

Shumaker, S. A., Ockene, J. K., Riekert, K. A., & Judith, K. (Eds.). (2008). *The handbook of health behavior change*. New York: Springer Publishing.

Smith, M. (2001). Towards a global definition of patient centred care. *British Medical Journal, 322*(7284), 444–445.

Steiner, A. (1997). *Intermediate care: A conceptual framework and review of the literature*. London: King's Fund.

Stroetman, V. (2007). eHealth for safety: impact of ICT on patient safety and risk management. Report prepared for ICT for Health Unit, *DG Information Society and Media, European Commission*, October 2007.

Valeri, L., Giesen, D., Jansen, P., & Klokgieters, K. (2010). Business models for eHealth. Available at http://ec.europa.eu/information_society/ehealth (August, 2010).

vom Brocke, J., Simons, A., Niehaves, B., Riemer, K., Plattfaut, R., & Cleven, A. (2009). Reconstructing the giant: On the importance of rigour in documenting the literature search process. *Paper presented at the 17th European conference on information systems (ECIS 2009)*, Verona.

Walker, J. (2005). The value of health care information exchange and interoperability. *Health Affairs, 25*(6), content.healthaffairs.org/cgi/content/abstract/hlthaff.w5.10.

Wang, S. (2003). A cost–benefit analysis of electronic medical records in primary care'. *American Journal of Medicine, 114*, 397–403.

Weerasinghe, D. (Ed.) (2008). *First international conference*, eHealth 2008, London, September 8–9, 2008, Revised Selected Papers. Springer.

Zweifel, P., Breyer, F., & Kifmann, M. (2009). *Health economics*. Berlin Heidelberg: Oxford University Press.

Chapter 10
Online Discussion Forum as a Means of Peer Support

R. Halonen

Abstract Today, information and communication technology has spread into our workplaces and living surroundings. In other words, the development of pervasive and ubiquitous Internet enables people to connect to services in places it was not possible a few years ago. This paper analyses and discusses social media as a means of peer support in www-based discussion forums that enable newspaper readers express their opinions and arguments in the media. At the time of swine flu approaching the country, we examined how the readers discussed the intriguing topic. During the study period, altogether 1,361 comments were given. The results reveal that people want to be heard or read and that they also seem to be eager to comfort each other.

Keywords Discussion forum • Peer support • Social media

10.1 Introduction

We'll all die. This quotation written by "Super Turbo" represents the kind of comments people write in the discussion forums today. How should readers react on that comment or how to interpret the intention behind those few words? Depending on the ongoing discussion, the interpretations may vary. However, the emergence of information and communication technology enables big audience to get their voice heard or read as Preece (1999) predicted already more than a decade ago.

In this article we investigate social media as a means of peer support in www-based discussion forums. Specifically, we tried to find out if and how a general, non-specific discussion forum is applicable as a means of peer support. In this context, peer support was seen as volunteers' actions that showed empathy and

R. Halonen
Department of Information Processing Science,
University of Oulu, Oulu, Finland
e-mail: raija.halonen@oulu.fi

N. Wickramasinghe et al. (eds.), *Critical Issues for the Development
of Sustainable E-health Solutions*, Healthcare Delivery in the Information Age,
DOI 10.1007/978-1-4614-1536-7_10, © Springer Science+Business Media, LLC 2012

comfort. In so doing, we analysed an online discussion forum where newspaper readers expressed their opinions and arguments in the media.

Internet allows synchronous and asynchronous discussion that is seen online simultaneously to a wide audience (Preece 1999; Ingram et al. 2000). While synchronous discussion permits participants to write their messages coincidentally, asynchronous discussion is built with the comments the participants send regardless of the presence of the receiver. Furthermore, the participants in electronic discussion groups can systematically select only the specific information they require or like from other members or which special knowledge they would be willing to contribute (Roberts and Fox 1998).

In mid-1990s Wellman et al. (1996) delineated that when computer networks link people as well as machines, they become social networks. They continued that members of virtual community want to link globally with kindred souls to achieve companionship, information and social support. Companionship and social support is shared with peer support (Cowie and Wallace 2000). In our paper, the free will to participate was emphasised.

From the prior literature we learn that the health sector has harnessed information and communication technology to promote healthier living already decades ago (Cowie and Wallace 2000; Solomon 2004). For example, Gustafson et al. (1999) wanted to know if patients who had been given in-home access to computers would use a specified supportive system to improve their quality of life. Even if there has been research on virtual communities on health and social outcomes for years, the virtual communities have been seen as mental health and social support interventions or focused electronic support groups (see Eysenbach et al. (2004)). Furthermore, Jadad et al. (2006) question if virtual communities are good for health or not at all.

Today, more than 200 millions hits for "health support forums" from http://groups.yahoo.com/ is a sign for the large usage of online discussion forums. However, instead of focused online discussion forums, this paper focuses on open discussion forums offered by newspapers where the discussion topics are lively and dependent on the general discussion in the society.

This paper is structured as follows. First, prior literature is presented. As a concept, "virtual community" receives a lot of attention. We also discuss peer support as a phenomenon. The empirical material is introduced with the help of descriptive quotations from the online discussions. The comments are interpreted to kind of explain why they – from all the 1,361 comments – were chosen into the paper. Finally the results are discussed and the limitations of the study are noted.

10.2   Prior Research

Despite the ever growing popularity of virtual communities, there is no consensus among researchers regarding the appropriate definition or types of virtual communities. Actually, virtual reality was suggested to become the next dominant communication medium already in mid-1990s (Biocca and Levy 1995).

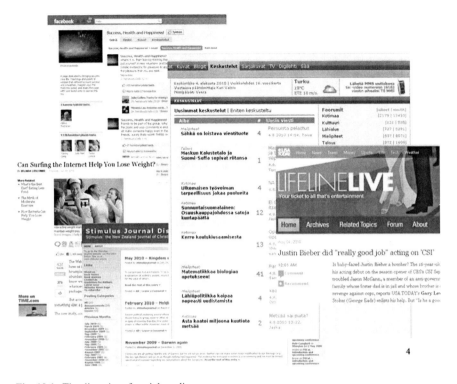

Fig. 10.1 The diversity of social media

Following Porter (2004), in this paper a virtual community is defined as an aggregation of individuals or business partners who interact around a shared interest, where the interaction is at least partially supported and/or mediated by technology and guided by some protocols or norms. This paper also acknowledges the concept introduced by Fisher et al. (2006): Virtual communities may refer to a broad range of Internet features such as chat rooms and online support groups. Figure 10.1 elucidates the diversity of social media. Furthermore, in virtual communities people find more other people with similar interests, values and beliefs than is possible in the real word. Fisher et al. (2006) highlight that the great difference compared to face-to-face interactions is the lack of sharing physical space or nonverbal and other cues that are available in traditional interaction.

To compensate lack of nonverbal cues people may include relevant emotional material in brackets. For example, people might write the following "You haven't visited us for ages (concern, worry)" and thus express their emotional feeling to the recipient (Murphy and Mitchell 1998).

Wellman et al. (1996) surmise that as people have moved indoors to private homes instead of spending time in open parks and pubs, they must more actively contact community members to remain in touch; and this contact is executed by attending computer-aided discussion groups where all members can read all messages. Adding to that, Fisher et al. (2006) note that virtual communities help meet the social needs that people are looking for when joining the community. People may be looking for positive encouragement and support. In addition, people may locate a specific virtual community that may provide them with the information or support that would comfort them in their problem or mood.

Koh et al. (2007) emphasise the need of both viewing and posting to provide a sustainable, live virtual community. However, they point out that there should be a choice for passive participation (for viewing) and a choice for active participation (posting). Participants may choose to be active or to "lurk", meaning that it is not compulsory to add own content into the discussions (Roberts and Fox 1998). Jadad et al. (2006) highlight also the questionable issue of frightened people who post their comments about diseases, making it more difficult to understand what is happening or what to do.

Prior literature has given only minor notice on the social aspects in computer-mediated communication so far (Preece 1999; Derks et al. 2007). Computer-mediated communication faces challenges compared to face-to-face communication as the means to pass on one's feelings or emotions and mood often is limited especially in cases when the communication is based on written text only (Parkinson 2008). Especially, research on peer support given in open discussion forums has received only modest attention if any.

Gustafson et al. (1999) note the benefit gained from developed information technology that offers possibilities to produce cost-effective and timely ways to deliver information, social support and skills training to specific individuals, thus multiplying professional expertise to serve many receivers. They clarify the benefits with a list of actions provided by interactive computers: First, people may have access to exactly the information they need and whenever they have questions. Second, people may ask embarrassing questions without face-to-face contact. Third, people can deal with difficult decisions at their own pace. Fourth, people may seek sources of support to help them deal with their emotional responses to health problems. Finally, people can examine how others have survived in similar problems.

In their book about peer support systems Cowie and Wallace (2000) state that peer support can emerge in a number of forms that emphasise emotional support or education and information-giving. Emotional support includes befriending, counselling-based approaches and mediation and conflict resolution. Education and information-giving support is about peer tutoring, peer education and mentoring. From these delineations, our study object was closest to information-giving and mentoring.

Solomon (2004) defines peer support as social emotional support that is offered by people who share a similar mental condition and she further categorises peer support into six classes: self-help groups, Internet support groups, peer delivered services, peer run or operated services, peer partnerships and peer employees. Self-help groups are the oldest and most pervasive models of peer support. Only the development of information technology and especially the diffusion of Internet have enabled Internet-based support groups. Indeed, while the oldest peer-to-peer groups gathered in bulletin board systems and private networks, the primary medium for virtual communities is the Internet with numerous mailing lists, newsgroups and especially discussion forums and live chat rooms (Eysenbach et al. 2004).

Online peer support groups are examples of self-help groups. In online peer support groups people with common interests gather to share experiences, ask questions, or provide emotional support and self-help (Eysenbach et al. 2004). In their systematic review of the effects of online peer to peer interactions Eysenbach et al. (2004) point out the abundance of unmoderated peer-to-peer groups in the Internet that offers great possibilities for additional research especially on non-professional-led support groups. This is also the issue our study contributes to as the newspaper discussion forum is fed by active individuals who want to get their opinions in public.

In her study of quasi-nonverbal cues in computer-mediated communication Carter (2003) notes how increasingly more people today rely on computer-mediated communication when they want to meet each other whether the purpose of the meeting is about making business or simply to form personal relationships. She continues that the traditional way people earlier perceived closeness has changed as face-to-face bonds, handshakes, bows or winks are no longer any prerequisites for creating friendships. However, people try to express their feelings also when interacting distantly, without seeing or hearing each other. Adding to that, Parkinson (2008) points out how people often need to read between the lines to imagine each other's tone of voice or nonverbal delivery, and therefore people may have suspicions of strategic manipulations.

Furthermore, the importance of social relationships in the treatment of disease and the maintenance of health and well-being has been recognised as an important aspect for decades (Cohen et al. 2000). In their study Gustafson et al. (1999) confirm that patients, who used a specified supportive system, were able to improve their quality of life with the help of the system, reduce health-risk behaviours, and use medical services more efficiently. Likewise, Brennan (1999) notes how computer networks and telecommunications provide particular support that can enhance the collaboration among clinicians, care providers and patients.

Peer support with the integration of peer relationships in the provision of health care, is an important concept of substantial significance to health scientists and practitioners today (Dennis 2003).

Jadad et al. (2006) are definite that sharing experiences and practical tips on everything from how to deal with illness to how to deal with the health system in a web-aided peer support group has benefited the correspondents. The researchers continue that the pure existence of the posted messages suggest that the benefits are real and sufficient to motivate the sending of hundreds of thousands messages about the topic.

10.3   The Study

To answer our research question we conducted a qualitative case study. A case study pays attention to the research context by considering time, social situation and location of the case (Stake 2000). In case studies, generalisation should not be the target. On the contrary, it is more essential to understand the case (Benbasat et al. 1987).

Like Preece (1999) investigated a specific discussion focused on problems with injured knee, the study at hand focused on one topic. The case was limited by time and topic, thus the focus was on contemporary events (Benbasat et al. 1987). The empirical material for the study was collected from online discussions associated with a local newspaper. The discussions were guided to follow the general principles of the newspaper and the postings to the discussion were introduced through a form provided in the www-site of the newspaper (see Fisher et al. (2006)).

It is essential to know that the comments might be published in the printed edition of the newspaper in case the correspondent had given permission for that when submitting the comments. The discussions were limited to cover a topic that was utmost topical at the time of the study, namely swine flu. However, the boundaries of the phenomenon were not clearly evident at the outset of the research and no experimental control or manipulation was used (see Benbasat et al. (1987)).

Qualitative research enables us to understand the qualitative characteristics and regularities of human beings, communities, phenomena and processes. It is central to describe how the researcher understands the research topic and how the research report is understood. Qualitative research is often reductive as the researcher makes choices of what to investigate and what to leave out (Miles and Huberman 1994). On the other hand, the researcher makes detailed observations from the real world and tries to avoid sticking into a predefined theoretical model (Yin 2003).

Content analysis is a common research method in several disciplines such as political science, social psychology and communications research. The researchers representing the disciplines agree that the analysis should be objective, systematic and quantitative. When the principles are obeyed, content analysis is a scientific, objective, systematic, quantitative and generalisable description of communications content (Kassarjian 1977). Among other things, qualitative content analysis emphasises the need for text interpretation to point out the experiences and feelings of the communicator, and – as especially in our case – to note the situation of text production (Mayring 2000). In our study, we utilised the deductive category application as we were looking for signs of peer support in the discussions. Today, interpretive research is acknowledged as a well-established part of information systems research. Web-based data from e-mails, websites and chat rooms are valuable sources for interpretive research (Walsham 2006).

In case study research, it is essential to identify the approach of the researcher, be it an outside researcher or an involved researcher (Walsham 2006). In the current study the researcher was an outside researcher as she did not participate in the discussions under study.

In the period of October 20, 2009 and November 12, 2009, a total of 1,361 comments were left in the discussion forum where swine flu was discussed in 38 separate discussions. With the help of content analysis (Mayring 2000; Silverman 2000) the study analysed how peer support was expressed in the discussions and whether there were any signs of experienced relief in the discussions.

To enable the analysis, the 38 separate discussions with their comments were downloaded on November 13, 2009 into a word document of 143 pages and 55,716 words. To ensure an analytic approach (Silverman 2000) in the analysis, the comments were first read through several times. After that, the discussions were listed and they were analysed discussion by discussion. Also, the comments were counted by discussions. Then, the comments were themed and classified and signs of peer support were searched in them. In this phase the findings were marked with different colours and markings to ease later analysis. In so doing, an interpretive approach (Walsham 2006) was applied to recognise supportive comments among the others.

10.4   Research Results

The smallest discussion included 10 comments and the largest discussion included 121 comments about the topic. The smallest discussion was about locally delivered information and the largest was about side effects of the vaccine. On November 9, 2009, people participated in 8 discussions and they posted 149 comments while on October 23, 2009, nobody commented in the discussion forum. On average, 35.8 comments were left in the discussions in the chosen period. At the time of collecting the material, it was not possible to check the time stamp of the comments. Only the date and the order of the comments were available. Neither was it possible to get any further information such as demographic details about the contributors.

The longest comment included 769 words and it was about flu, starting from the Spanish Influenza in 1918 and ending to the self help of flu. The shortest comment was *We'll all die*.

Some discussants gave their comments only once, some a few times. In the discussion forum there was one discussant (who used the nickname "Anonymous") who wrote 300 comments. However, it was not possible to find out if "Anonymous" was one person or several correspondents. The discussants also communicated with their nicknames as they called themselves for example such as "BLOND" or "Politics". As "BLOND" was always written with capitals we interpret that the nickname wanted to add special emphasis on the name (Greenwood and Isbell 2002). "BLOND" left 22 comments and "Politics" left 7 comments. Those named "Mother" or "Mom" we cannot interpret if they were all one discussant or many.

I would like to know if there are other pregnant women who don't know if one should take the vaccine or not. I'm very worried. […] What if it will be a new thalidomide etc. (October 20, 2009, "Pregnant") With this posting the active discussion about swine flu and related issues was started in the newspaper. The posting appeared reasonable, no additional emotions or opinions included.

For those who don't know: The Pandemrix vaccine includes the same amount of mercury than if you eat one Baltic herring. (November 4, 2009, "It is worth it") This comment represents a way of calming down the joint worry as the nickname completes the message by confirming the evidently funny belief of the dangerousness of the vaccine.

Ask the doctors and not the "experts" of discussion forums. (October 20, 2009, "Anonymous") Not all comments were emphatic or supportive. On the contrary, this comment briefly urges readers to seek for professional help instead of turning to the peer readers.

I wonder if they report as detailed about seasonal flu as this. Let's calm down. (October 24, 2009, "Politics") Even the chosen nickname showed that the comment was aimed to add objectivity in the discussion.

New observations from America strengthen the conception that abundant supply of vitamin D prevents and reduces swine flu. The needed daily take is 100 micrograms that is 13 times more than the official recommendation (7.5 microgram)[...]. (October 25, 2009, "Anonymous") The discussant had written the comment with bold and large font. Indeed, the discussant wanted to emphasise the message both with the chosen appearance and the written text. The discussant also used a lot of numbers to convince readers of the possessed experience and knowledge.

6% of those died in swine flu have been pregnant, i.e. pregnant women have been over-represented in the US deaths [...] I warmly recommend the vaccine to all in risk groups! (October 26, 2009, "Me") This comment represents a gentle approach that was expressed in several comments. The discussant tells facts in plain text and concludes with a nice recommendation. Also, the nick name shows no great feelings.

Could somebody email the Ministry of Health? The minister would certainly comment. (October 30, 2009, "Politics") Again, one comment was posted to seek for support from greater experience and holders of knowledge.

FAIRNESS, PLEASE! Definitely qualified health care AND IN TIME should be offered in a wealth ware society! [...] YOU CRITICS who compel to stop complaining, think a moment in your hearts ...[...] Try to find a warm thought for your peer sick people! Don't underestimate the anxiety they have because you need not perceive it. I didn't even believe that there are so many heartless people! (November 12, 2009, "xmx") This correspondent used several ways to express the strong opinion. Despite the nondescript nickname, the comment appeared to support those people that had complained in the discussions.

My deepest condolences to the family and relatives. (November 6, 2009, "Mom") After news of the first victim of the disease had been published on November 6, 2009, the discussion changed to more aggressive and emotional. This brief comment was one of the first postings and it needs no interpretation as it was simple and the nickname revealed the writer's family status.

Yes but this discussion forum is a faulty place for this. (November 6, 2009, "No-name").

Regretful cases, I'm sorry. Indeed, this discussion forum is a wrong place. Especially, as we know that there will be about 100 cases more. (November 6, 2009, "Mathias") Some people felt that a public discussion forum is not an appropriate forum to express sorrow or condolence. In addition, the discussants only rarely used a formal name instead of a nickname.

How come the discussion forum is a wrong place? I also want to express my condolences. Even if I don't know you, I want to express my empathy to you. (November 7, 2009, "John") The discussion continued despite the attempts of other contributors who also tried to stop it. There were several comments with condolences to the family. *My deepest condolences … you have been in my thoughts and prayers.* (November 7, 2009, "Mummy").

For instance, if my near relative would die, I wouldn't like that totally unknown people would express their sympathies or condolences here, whatever reason the death. (November, 7, 2009, "No-name") It seems that the same correspondent explained his or her negative comment.

I disagree. Today, many people live so alone with they burdens and experiencing their helplessness that it is only right that they can express their feelings in this kind of public forums and receive mental support, understanding, and acceptance from other living persons. This is about sharing the burden and it cannot be wrong. (November 7, 2009, "Anonymous") However, another commentator explained the justification to express sorrow and empathy also publicly.

All of us are given a certain amount of days here. When the last day comes, there's no help even from the best physicians. However, I won't take the vaccine. (November 6, 2009, "Anonymous") The comment reveals no emotional support. On the contrary, it could be interpreted to be deterministic.

I wonder if the child got Tamiflu and antibiotics? What was the medication? If none, it is an involuntary manslaughter. (November 6, 2009, "Good grief") Some comments seemed to be pure curious. This comment by "Good grief" includes also attacking elements by suggesting that a crime might have been done.

Well, what would the intravenous virus medication be? Tamiflu? Usually there is no medication for viruses. (November 6, 2009, "Anonymous") This comment did not show any sympathy for the family that had lost a child but encouraged the health care personnel.

KEEP YOUR MOUTH SHUT! Think of the relatives, no peace for grieving; is it not enough that the yellow press raves? (November 6, 2009, "Anonymous") This posting showed a powerful approach as it started with a rude dictation to be quiet. The command was also written with capitals as a sign of shouting.

All sick people should be admitted to hospital just in case. However, we have not enough places in hospitals and nursing staff to enable this … (November 8, 2009, "Retired Nurse"). Even after the reported bereavement a retired nurse wanted to calm down both those complaining for rubbish vaccination process and the overloaded vaccination personnel.

I had to queue five hours at the flu reception. Only one physician, no reasonable blood testing […] How on earth is this arrangement possible? (November 11, 2009, "Asthmatic") After the vaccinations were started, several comments complained the arrangements and organisation of the process of vaccination.

Didn't it occur in your mind that it is exceptional, pandemic … and therefore these circumstances. Kind of a war against viruses. Stop the wasted complaining. (November 11, 2009, "Anonymous") This discussant showed understanding of the difficulties and challenges that the health care personnel had to face.

Why did you go and panic there? You'd better stay at home! (November 12, 2009, "BLOND") As the health care personnel were greatly accused due to the difficulties in the vaccinations, "BLOND" felt it important to attack back.

10.5   Discussion and Conclusive Words

The research at hand analysed an online discussion forum in a newspaper to find out if there was peer support given in the discussions. The study was qualitative and it was limited by time and topic (Benbasat et al. 1987). In the period of 24 days, an active discussion was conducted online in a newspaper. On October 20, 2009 the first discussion about the influenza H1N1 was initiated in the forum and the last comments were written when the pandemic was pronounced to exist in the area. During the chosen period, 1,361 comments were posted in the discussion forum.

The first comment was posted by a pregnant woman who seemed to be concerned as in the media the flu had been told to be more serious to pregnant people and the unborn babies than to other healthy people. All the analysed 38 discussions were about the swine flu and they were partly overlapping. Therefore we interpreted that the common topic built the virtual community (Porter 2004). Adding to that, we did not separate the discussions in the analysis. Despite the partly overlapping discussion topics, the comments were separate and no duplicates were found.

Preece (1999) identified stress, uncertainty, depression, pain and frustrations in the discussions under her study. The study at hand was seeking for signs of similar emotions and several expressions were noticed as described in the earlier section. The study showed that the pandemic was widely reported in media and people were generally concerned due to the deaths around the globe. The great concern added the cohesion. However, not all discussants were worried as can see from the persuasive and comforting comments. *Let's calm down* was posted to ease the expressed worries. The discussions included numerous comments that offered instructions on how to act or behave. In this study we excluded all those comments that we could not interpret supportive or expressing any condolences. In so doing, we followed Miles and Huberman (Benbasat et al. 1987) who note the role of qualitative research and the choices made by the researchers.

Also, some comments did not show any sympathy but frustration or need for reasoning as expressed by a suggestion about asking doctors instead of writing into discussion forums. On the other hand, it was interesting to see how some discussants highlighted the healing nature of the discussion community (see also Carter (2003)).

A great change was seen in the discussions when the first death was reported in public. The correspondents expressed their sympathy and emotions. Also, when some comments appeared aggressive and rude, several comments were posted to quiet the non-supportive postings. It was interesting to note how people reacted on the condolences. Namely, there were postings that supported the grieving people but there also were postings that tended to deny the emotional expressions from the discussions. *I wouldn't like that totally unknown people would express their sympathies ...* This kind of comment can also be interpreted very sensitive despite its negative output.

It was interesting to see that the health personnel received also support, not only accusations and blames even if the positive comments were not as common. In this sense, the same discussions were able to support both those under pressure due to the difficult work load and those who had to queue for hours before they received the vaccine.

As Fisher et al. (2006) highlight the lack of cues such as facial expressions and tone of voice in computer-based interactions; we identified nonverbal cues such as emoticons (see Carter (2003)) and additional typographical appearances such as bolded text or exclamation marks in the posted comments. There were postings that included both capitals and normal font, kind of shouting some words such as *FAIRNESS, PLEASE!* to emphasise the importance in the address. Also, there were nicknames written with capitals such as "BLOND" and "PANDEMIC" that could be interpreted to include additional influence on the posting.

Following Koh et al. (2007), the discussions under study verified the need to both view and post comments in the discussion. Due to the nature of the forum being an online newspaper it is very likely that there were more lurkers (Roberts and Fox 1998) than active actors in the discussion under study. In our study it was not possible to measure the viewing but the amount of given comments talked for the active reading, too. People had to follow the discussion to be able to return quickly. Unfortunately we were not able to see the time stamps and therefore we don't know if the postings were sent in the evenings or during working hours.

Besides having own comments published in the online discussion, it was possible to see own comments published in the printed edition of the newspaper. Unfortunately we were not able to analyse if the correspondents had permitted that or not when submitting the comments. Also, we did not analyse the comments in the printed edition. Despite that, the possibility to see and let other people see personal comments might have added the amount of the posted comments (see Koh et al. (2007)).

As the empirical material in our study was downloaded from the online discussion forum after the discussion already was ended, we had no possibility to even try to find out any demographic details of the contributors. Also, when analysing the postings, we could accept the discussions as they were at the time of downloading on November 13, 2009. In case of online discussion forum there is no possibility to identify the contributors. This feature leads to the fact that there are no means to find out if one contributor used several nicknames of if one nickname was used by several contributors.

Nowadays online discussion forums are more available than ever, and the ever increasing discussions offer fruitful research material (Walsham 2006). However, in case of several parallel discussions ongoing it would be valuable to acquire also the time stamps for the postings.

In all, our study revealed that it is possible to give and get peer support publicly and anonymously. Even the experienced grief was discussed in the discussion forum. To response the expressed concern, many comments tended to be extensively informative or purely emotional (see Cowie and Wallace (2000)). However, several aggressive and less to-the-point comments were also given. Finally, we propose that more research is carried out in this area. We believe that ever more people find their ways into the online world and that the new forms of virtual communities have a lot of possibilities to make life easier.

Acknowledgements All those totally anonymous correspondents who openly posted their comments into the online discussion forum are acknowledged. The earlier version of this article was presented in the 3rd International Conference on Well-being in the Information Society and the fruitful comments of those present are warmly thanked.

References

Benbasat, I., Goldstein, D., & Mead, M. (1987). The case study strategy in studies of information systems. *MIS Quarterly, 11*(3), 368–386.

Biocca, F., & Levy, M. R. (1995). Communication applications of virtual reality. In F. Biocca & M. R. Levy (Eds.), *Communication in the age of virtual reality* (pp. 127–157). Hillsdale, NJ: Lawrence Erlbaum Associates.

Brennan, P. F. (1999). Health informatics and community health: Support for patients as collaborators in care. *Methods of Information in Medicine, 38*(4–5), 274–8.

Carter, K. A. (2003). Type me how you feel: Quasi-nonverbal cues in computer-mediated communication. *ETC: A Review of General Semantics, 60*(1), 29–39.

Cohen, S., Gottlieb, B., & Underwood, L. G. (2000). Social relationships and health. In S. Cohen, L. G. Underwood, & B. Gottlieb (Eds.), *Social support measurement and intervention: A guide for health and social scientists* (pp. 3–25). Toronto: Oxford University Press.

Cowie, H., & Wallace, P. (2000). *Peer support in action: From bystanding to standing by* (pp. 1–22). London: Sage.

Dennis, C.-L. (2003). Peer support within a health care context: A concept analysis. *International Journal of Nursing Studies, 40*(3), 321–332.

Derks, D., Bos, A. E. R., & von Grumbkow, J. (2007). Emoticons and social interaction on the internet: The importance of social context. *Computers in Human Behavior, 23*, 842–849.

Eysenbach, G., Powell, J., Englesakis, M., Rizo, C., & Stern, A. (2004). Health related virtual communities and electronic support groups: Systematic review of the effects of online peer to peer interactions. *British Medical Journal, 328*, 3–6.

Fisher, J., Mowrey, H., & Nardecchia, T. (2006). Computer mediated communication and the virtual community, Chapter 6, In Department of Communication, *Yearbook 2006* (Vol. 1, pp. 104–121).

Greenwood, D., & Isbell, L. M. (2002). Ambivalent sexism and the dumb blonde: Men's And women's reactions to sexist jokes. *Psychology of Women Quarterly, 26*, 341–350.

Gustafson, D. H., Hawkins, R., Boberg, E., Pingree, S., Serlin, R. E., Chan, F., & Graziano, C. L. (1999). Impact of a patient-centered, computer-based health information/support system. *American Journal of Preventive Medicine, 16*(1), 1–9.

Ingram, A. L., Hathorn, L. G., & Evans, A. (2000). Beyond chat on the internet. *Computers & Education, 35*, 21–35.

Jadad, A. R., Enkin, M. W., Glouberman, S., Groff, P., & Stern, A. (2006). Are virtual communities good for our health? *British Medical Journal, 332*, 925–926.

Kassarjian, H. H. (1977). Content analysis in consumer research. *The Journal of Consumer Research, 4*, 8–18.

Koh, J., Kim, Y.-G., Butler, B., & Bock, G.-W. (2007). Encouraging participation in virtual communities. *Communications of the ACM, 50*(2), 69–73.

Mayring, P. (2000). Qualitative content analysis, Forum: Qualitative Social Research, Vol. 1, No. 2. Available at: http://qualitative-research.net/fqs/fqs-e/2-00inhalt-e.htm

Miles, M. B., & Huberman, A. M. (1994). *Qualitative data analysis: An expanded sourcebook* (2nd ed.). Thousand Oaks, CA: Sage Publications.

Murphy, L. J., & Mitchell, D. L. (1998). When writing helps to heal: E-mail as therapy. *British Journal of Guidance and Counselling, 26*(1), 21–32.

Parkinson, B. (2008). Emotions in direct and remote social interaction: Getting through the spaces between us. *Computers in Human Behavior, 25*, 1510–1529.

Porter, C. E. (2004). A typology of virtual communities: A multi-disciplinary foundation for future research. *Journal of Computer-Mediated Communication, 10*(1), Article 3.

Preece, J. (1999). Empathic communities: Balancing emotional and factual communication. *Interacting with Computers, 12*, 63–77.

Roberts, C., & Fox, N. (1998). General practitioners and the internet: Modelling a 'virtual community'. *Family Practice, 15*, 211–215.

Silverman, D. (2000). Analyzing talk and text. In N. K. Denzin & Y. S. Lincoln (Eds.), *Handbook of qualitative research* (pp. 821–834). Thousand Oaks: Sage Publications, Inc.

Solomon, P. (2004). Peer support/peer provided services underlying processes, benefits, and critical ingredients. *Psychiatric Rehabilitation Journal, 27*(4), 392–401.

Stake, R. E. (2000). Case studies. In N. K. Denzin & Y. S. Lincoln (Eds.), *Handbook of qualitative research* (pp. 435–454). Thousand Oaks: Sage Publications, Inc.

Walsham, G. (2006). Doing interpretive research. *European Journal of Information Systems, 15*, 320–330.

Wellman, B., Salaff, J., Dimitrova, D., Garton, L., Gulia, M., & Haythornthwaite, C. (1996). Computer networks as social networks: Collaborative work, telework, and virtual community. *Annual Review of Sociology, 22*, 213–238.

Yin, R. (2003). *Case study research. Design and methods* (3rd ed.). London: Sage Publications.

Chapter 11
Designing Persuasive Health Behavior Change Interventions

Tuomas Lehto

Abstract In the past decade, the utilization of various technologies to change individuals' health behaviors has been a rapidly expanding field of interest. Examples of persuasive technologies can be found rather easily as there are a variety of Internet-, Web- and mobile-based systems and applications promoting healthier lifestyles. Still, the use of persuasive technology in the E-health arena is in its infancy. While the field is expanding, it is evident that more research is needed to better determine how the systems affect users' intended behaviors. This book chapter outlines several important perspectives in designing and developing persuasive health behavior change interventions. Furthermore, this chapter offers novel viewpoints, both theoretical and practical, in designing and developing health behavior change interventions. In addition, useful underlying theories and design models are identified and discussed. This type of knowledge may assist in building, deploying and evaluating behavior change support systems that are able to engage and retain large amounts of individuals, potentially enhancing population health and well-being.

Keywords Health • Behavior change • Persuasive technology • Design

11.1 Introduction

Changing people's behavior is at the heart of health promotion. In the past decade, the use of technologies to persuade, motivate and activate individuals' for health behavior change has been a quickly expanding field of research. The

T. Lehto
Oulu Advanced Research on Software and Information Systems,
Department of Information Processing Science,
University of Oulu, Oulu, Finland
e-mail: tuomas.lehto@oulu.fi

N. Wickramasinghe et al. (eds.), *Critical Issues for the Development of Sustainable E-health Solutions*, Healthcare Delivery in the Information Age, DOI 10.1007/978-1-4614-1536-7_11, © Springer Science+Business Media, LLC 2012

use of the Internet for delivering health behavior change interventions has been especially relevant. Applications and systems for preventing, assessing, and treating conditions such as alcohol problems (cf. Bewick et al. 2008), depression (van Straten et al. 2008), diabetes (Tate et al. 2003), obesity (Harvey-Berino et al. 2010), physical inactivity (Hurling et al. 2007), and smoking (cf. Shahab and McEwen 2009) have been tested in numerous controlled trials. These automated health behavior change interventions have the potential of high reach and low cost. Recent comprehensive meta-analyses provide support for their effectiveness in changing knowledge, attitudes, and behavior in the health promotion area (Portnoy et al. 2008; Webb et al. 2010).

Various terms have emerged in order to describe technology-based interventions for mental and physical health purposes: cybertherapy, digital therapy, e-therapy, Web-based therapy, eHealth, e-Interventions, digital interventions, internet interventions, computer-mediated interventions, and online therapy (or counseling), among others (Barak et al. 2009). Thus far, there is no consensus of the terminology. Barak et al. (2009, p. 5) have defined a Web-based intervention as:

> A primarily self-guided intervention program that is executed by means of a prescriptive online program operated through a website and used by consumers seeking health- and mental-health related assistance. The intervention program itself attempts to create positive change and or improve/enhance knowledge, awareness, and understanding via the provision of sound health-related material and use of interactive web-based components.

The abovementioned definition is a fine endeavor to capture the essence of *Web-based* health behavior change interventions. However, in this book chapter we will discuss Behavior Change Support Systems (Oinas-Kukkonen 2010). The definition of behavior change support systems may be more flexible than the definition presented by Barak et al. and serves the purpose of this chapter better. In addition, BCSSs are not limited to the Web, and they might run on various operating systems, platforms and devices.

On a par with health behavior change, persuasive technology has the potential for significant breakthroughs on many areas of human well-being, such as education, and environmental conservation. Examples of persuasive technology can be found rather easily as there are a variety of websites promoting healthier lifestyles. Unsurprisingly, one of the strongest domains of innovation for persuasive technology in the immediate future will be preventive health care. Still, the use of persuasive technology in the health arena is in its infancy. While the field is expanding, it is evident that more research is needed to better determine how the systems affect users' intended behaviors. Resnicow et al. (2010) point out that the first generation of patient-centered eHealth studies have concentrated mainly on answering the question of whether such programs are efficacious. They propose that the next generation of eHealth research starts to better address the questions of why, how, and for whom they work (Resnicow et al. 2010).

11.2 Behavior Change Support Systems

Oinas-Kukkonen (2010, p. 6) has defined a behavior change support system as follows:

> A behavior change support system (BCSS) is an information system designed to form, alter or reinforce attitudes, behaviors or an act of complying without using deception, coercion or inducements.

Behavior change support systems (Oinas-Kukkonen 2010) are persuasive, producing either computer-mediated[1] persuasion or computer-human persuasion BCSSs emphasize – but are not limited to – autogenous approaches in which people use information technology to change their own attitudes or behaviors through building upon their own motivation or goal. They also request a positive user experience and encourage the user engagement regularly over an extended period of time (Oinas-Kukkonen 2010).

Evidently, the design and development of BCSSs is a multifaceted issue. It links to technological services, applications, platforms, and functionality, the quality and content of information, personal goal-setting (Locke and Latham 2002) by the end-users, and social networks/environments, among other issues. In many cases, the BCSSs must be always available, they have to address global and cultural issues with a multitude of standards, habits, and beliefs. Furthermore, they have to be adaptable into a variety of domains (e.g. healthcare, education) and business models (Oinas-Kukkonen 2010).

When building BCSSs, psychological insight is needed. According to Oinas-Kukkonen (2010) several important lessons can be learned from psychological theories, including: (1) people like their views about the world to be organized and consistent (Festinger 1957); (2) persuasion is often incremental; (3) direct and indirect routes are key persuasion strategies (cf. central and peripheral route, Petty and Cacioppo 1986).

The primary research interests in BCSSs include not only human-computer interaction and computer-mediated communication, but also topics such as approaches, methodologies, processes and tools to design and develop such systems and means for examining the individual, social, and organizational impacts of them. The research underlines software qualities and characteristics, (information) systems analysis and design, and individual behavior and perceptions. Technologically, the research may address socio-technical platforms, systems, services or applications, or the software features in them, developed for persuasive purposes (Oinas-Kukkonen 2010).

Research on *persuasive technology* has been introduced relatively recently. Briñol and Petty (2009, p. 71) outline persuasion as follows: "In the typical situation

---

[1] We use the term computer for the sake of simplicity; it also includes e.g. mo-bile/smart/tracking/monitoring/wearable devices.

Table 11.1 Evolution of persuasive technologies (Adapted from Chatterjee and Price 2009)

Type (generation)	Example technology
Prescriptive systems (G1)	Phone call, brochures, CD-ROM
Descriptive systems (G2)	Web/Internet, mobile devices, sensor devices
Environmental systems (G3)	Body area networks, Context-aware real-time sensing
Automated systems (Future)	Pervasive sensing, genetic integration

Table 11.2 Outcome design matrix (Oinas-Kukkonen 2010)

	Compliance	Behavior	Attitude
Formation	Forming an act of complying	Forming a behavior	Forming an attitude
Alteration	Altering an act of complying	Altering a behavior	Altering an attitude
Reinforcement	Reinforcing an act of complying	Reinforcing a behavior	Reinforcing an attitude

in which persuasion is possible, a person or a group of people (i.e., the recipient) receives an intervention (e.g., a persuasive message) from another individual or group (i.e., the source) in a particular setting (i.e., the context)." Successful persuasion takes place when the target of change (e.g., attitudes, beliefs) is modified into the desired direction (Briñol and Petty 2009) (Table 11.1).

Webb et al. (2010) suggest that the effectiveness of Internet-based interventions is associated with (1) more extensive use of theory; (2) inclusion of more behavior change techniques; and (3) use of additional delivery modes.

Kaptein et al. (2010) argue that in order to develop beneficial programs capable of persuading individuals to change their health-related attitudes and behaviors, more insight of how different individuals respond to the persuasive strategies utilized is required. Kreps and Neuhauser (2010) call for interventions that appeal to the distinctive interests and emotions of targeted audiences to capture attention and influence behaviors (cf. 'Affective Computing', Picard 2003).

11.2.1 Types of Change

Oinas-Kukkonen (2010) categorizes behavioral changes as follows: (1) a change in an act of complying; (2) a behavior change; and (3) an attitude change. Respectively, these are called C-, B-, and A-Change, in ascending order of complexity. Different persuasive goals and strategies may be needed for applications supporting different types of changes. A design matrix can be constructed from the intended outcomes and the types of change (Oinas-Kukkonen 2010). See Table 11.2.

The designers of BCSSs should carefully consider which of these nine different goals the application will be built for as the *persuasion context* may change dramatically when moving from one slot to another (Oinas-Kukkonen 2010). Dey (2001) states that context is all about the entire situation relevant to an application and its group of users, and he defines context as any information that can be used to characterize the state of an entity. An entity may be a person, place, or object that is regarded germane to the interaction between a user and the application (including the user and applications themselves).

In our view, the ultimate goal of a behavior change support system lies within the outcome matrix. Obviously, the outcome matrix is a simplification of the matter as the intended behavior change might occur on multiple levels.

11.2.2 Examples of Health Behavior Change Interventions

In this section, we will discuss recent research endeavors of behavior change support systems in the health domain.

We have selected three very important areas for a closer view: (1) physical activity and dietary behavior change; (2) weight loss and weight management; and (3) substance abuse. Based on our experience, these are amongst the most studied areas in individual health behavior change during the past decade (cf. Lustria et al. 2009).

11.2.2.1 Physical Activity and Dietary Behavior Change

In their review, Norman et al. (2007) conclude that published studies of eHealth interventions for physical activity and dietary behavior change are in their infancy. Their results indicated mixed findings related to the effectiveness of eHealth interventions. According to these researchers, interventions that feature interactive technologies need to be refined and more rigorously evaluated to fully determine their potential as tools to facilitate health behavior change (Norman et al. 2007).

In a review conducted by Vandelanotte et al. (2007) 8 out of 15 of the trials of Web-based physical activity interventions reported positive behavioral outcomes. However, they conclude that intervention effects were momentary, and there was slight evidence of maintenance of physical activity changes (Vandelanotte et al. 2007). Neville and colleagues (2009) reviewed 12 computer-tailored interventions for dietary behavior outcomes, and reported significant positive effects on seven of the interventions. Kroeze et al. (2006) systematically reviewed the scientific literature on computer-tailored physical activity and nutrition education. They reported significant effects on 3 of 11 of the physical activity studies and 20 of 26 of the nutrition studies.

In spite of these promising results, most of the researchers advice caution in generalizing the results. For instance, Neville et al. (2009) argue that even though the evidence of short-term efficacy for computer-tailored dietary behavior change interventions is relatively strong, there is uncertainty whether the reported effects are generalizable and sustained long term. According to Vandelanotte et al. (2007) more research is required to pinpoint elements that can enhance behavioral outcomes, the maintenance of change and the engagement and retention of participants. Van den Berg et al. (2007) point out that the importance of specific components of Internet-based physical activity interventions, such as increased supervisor contact, tailored information, or theoretical fidelity remains to be determined.

Consolvo and colleagues' study of 'Houston' (2006) was one of the first attempts at developing a persuasive technology to encourage physical activity. In the study, three groups of women from pre-existing social networks shared their step counts and progress toward a daily goal with each other via their mobile phones. The prototype consisted of three elements: a pedometer, mobile phone and custom software, Houston, that was ran on the phone. Based on their analysis of the qualitative data, Consolvo et al. (2006) present "key design requirements of technologies that encourage physical activity": (1) give users proper credit for activities (cf. 'rewards', Oinas-Kukkonen and Harjumaa 2009); (2) provide personal awareness of activity level (cf. 'self-monitoring', Oinas-Kukkonen and Harjumaa 2009); (3) support social influence (cf. 'social support' category, Oinas-Kukkonen and Harjumaa 2009); and (4) consider the practical constraints of users' lifestyles (cf. 'the event', Oinas-Kukkonen and Harjumaa 2009). A more advanced mobile, persuasive technology system 'UbiFit' is presented in Consolvo et al. (2009).

'Fish'n'Steps', a social computer game (Lin et al. 2006), was designed to persuade users to take more steps each day. Each participant was assigned a weekly step count goal, which became progressively more challenging over the six weeks of the participation in the game. The user's daily step count was measured by simple pedometers. The data was linked to the different states and activity of a fish displayed in a virtual fish tank. The game utilized *competition, recognition, and cooperation* (cf. Oinas-Kukkonen and Harjumaa 2009) as an additional leverage towards the goals. The game increased participants' awareness of their physical activity status and provided motivation to increase the activity level in an engaging way (Lin et al. 2006).

Harjumaa et al. (2009) explored a prototype of a heart rate monitor (Polar FT60) that included a persuasive training program. The aim of their study was to investigate how different persuasive strategies function with different people and in relation to each other in the context of exercise behavior. The authors of the study suggest that leveraging goal setting, tracking performance, adopting social roles, along with a high overall perceived credibility influences user behavior. Short-term verbal system feedback via praise and rewards may provide additional persuasive effect. They also emphasize that even if the product is designed for a homogenous target group, small individual differences between users may weigh in persuasion. It may be wise to select a set of persuasion principles and use them together rather than rely on one principle only. In turn, persuasion principles are interlinked. Thus, the effect of persuasion principles may be "more than the sum of its parts" (Harjumaa et al. 2009).

11.2.2.2   Weight Loss and Weight Management

One of the most vibrant areas within health behavior change research has been Web-based software systems promoting weight loss and weight management. These Web-based services are illustrative examples of BCSSs in the eHealth space.

Recent research suggests that the Web may be a highly viable channel for delivering weight loss and obesity interventions across diverse populations. Web-based weight control applications have the potential to achieve outcomes similar to other lifestyle treatment options. Several randomized trials have demonstrated Web-based weight-loss interventions to be efficacious for short-term weight loss. However, online programs have not accomplished weight losses of the magnitude typically produced by traditional individual and or group treatment approaches. These findings should be interpreted with caution, however. According to Bennett and Glasgow (2009) most randomized controlled trials in this particular domain have been relatively small and underpowered, suffering from high levels of attrition and occasionally reporting change in only secondary outcomes, e.g., knowledge and self-efficacy, rather than primary outcomes, e.g., behavior change. Tsai and Wadden (2005) argue that minimal evidence still exists for recommending the use of commercial Internet-based interventions. Also, Womble and colleagues (2004) found in their study that a commercial Internet-based weight loss program produced only minimal weight loss and was not as effective as a traditional manual-based approach. Harvey-Berino et al. (2004) reported that participants assigned to an online weight maintenance program sustained similar levels of weight loss over 18 months compared to individuals who continued to meet face-to-face.

Bennett and Glasgow (2009) summarize that greater results in weight loss are typically observed with such Web-based weight-loss interventions that are highly structured, provide support from a human counselor, utilize tailored materials, and promote a high frequency of website logins. Krukowski and colleagues (2008) share this view by concluding that structured interventions comprising behavior therapy components, interactive and dynamic website features, and synchronous communication produce the most significant weight losses.

The current generation of online weight loss interventions takes advantage of a set of varying software components, such as self-monitoring functionality, food diaries, body mass index calculators, support forums, and coach messaging (Lehto and Oinas-Kukkonen 2010). See Table 11.3. Yet, it is unclear which of these features, either in isolation or collectively, are associated with the greatest magnitude of weight loss.

Lehto and Oinas-Kukkonen (2010) investigated the utilization of various persuasive features on six weight loss websites. The Persuasive Systems Design Model (Oinas-Kukkonen and Harjumaa 2009) was applied to extract and analyze persuasive

Table 11.3 Typical content in weight loss websites

Content	Example
Health-related advice	Nutrition, diet, physical activity, exercise, weight loss, and weight management advice
Self-monitoring tools	Food/activity/weight logs and trackers, body mass index and calorie counters, diaries, reminders, feedback
Social/peer influence components	Blogs, forums, groups, instant messaging, chat rooms, e-mail/inbox, competitions/challenges, social media connectivity, public recognition
Expert components	"Ask an expert", expert blogs, expert moderation on forums/chat rooms
Rehearsal and simulation	Workout builders, video workouts, exercise planners

system features found in the sites. The evaluated sites provided relatively good primary task support and strong social support. However, there were weaknesses in both dialogue and credibility support.

The results of their study indicate that there is room for improvement in both designing and implementing Web-based interventions for weight loss.

11.2.2.3 Substance Abuse

A digital therapy intervention for smoking cessation, 'Happy Ending', has been shown to be efficacious in previous randomized controlled trials (Brendryen et al. 2008; Brendryen and Kraft 2008). Happy Ending is a fully automated system and delivered by using the Internet and mobile phone. The intervention builds on multiple theories: self-regulation theory, social cognitive theory, cognitive–behavior therapy, motivational interviewing and relapse prevention. The arrangement of the content matches to psychological processes that people undergo at specific points of time in a process of therapy-supported self-regulation. The design of the intervention is novel in that it combines four delivery modes (SMS, Interactive Voice Response, e-mail, and Web). Happy Ending blends "just-in-time therapy" and a tunneling strategy. The two forms of just-in-time therapy are a craving helpline, and the relapse prevention system based on a daily assessment of the target behavior (Brendryen et al. 2010).

Lehto and Oinas-Kukkonen (2009) studied persuasive features (Oinas-Kukkonen and Harjumaa 2009) in Web-based alcohol interventions. They suggest that the evaluated websites were not very persuasive. Nevertheless, all evaluated sites successfully demonstrated trustworthiness, expertise, and surface credibility. Primary task support principles were utilized relatively poorly in many of the sites. Interestingly, and perhaps rather worryingly, tailoring was applied in only one of the sites. There were also notable differences between the evaluated sites. For instance, some sites placed more emphasis on online social support than others. Many of the sites did not offer any online social support. The authors believe that providing (expert-moderated) support groups as a part of a technology-based intervention is a very important aspect of such interventions. There are several techniques (e.g. instant messaging, chat rooms, discussion forums, social networks) readily available to facilitate communication between peers. In anonymous online support groups, the participants may overcome the feeling of being stigmatized, and time and location are no longer obstacles for participation.

11.2.2.4 Summarizing the Examples

Thus far there is limited evidence on the effectiveness of behavior change support systems. Researchers have been cautious about the generalizability of the results. Finding e.g. optimal theories, strategies, and delivery modes require further research. Both rigorous evaluations of existing health-related behavior change systems, and experimental/pilot studies with creative approaches are called for.

Atienza and colleagues (2010 p. 86) make an excellent remark that "health information technology does not occur in a vacuum, but rather technologies exist within social systems." In order to widespread adoption, dissemination, and extended use of technology-based health interventions to take place, it is incumbent on researchers to investigate not only how the interventions affect individuals, but also how individuals interact with technology and each other (Atienza et al. 2010).

11.3 Design and Theory Issues

A large number of health information system projects fail. Most of these failures are not due to flawed technology, but rather due to the lack of systematic considerations of human and other non-technology issues in the design and implementation processes (Zhang 2005, p. 1)

Attempts to create persuasive systems often fail, because many projects are too ambitious being set up for failure. For example, a design team might select a difficult behavior as the target, e.g. smoking cessation, but without having ever before created such a persuasive system the success rate might be low (Fogg 2009b). Thus, designing systems that aim at behavior change requires thorough understanding of the problem domain, the underpinning theories and strategies of persuasive systems design. Usually an interdisciplinary team of professionals is called for. According to Kuziemsky et al. (2007) the primary challenge for information system design in healthcare is to interconnect the medical, technical and social contexts.

Consolvo et al. (2009, p. 414) emphasize that "lifestyle behavior change is a long-term endeavor that pervades everyday life, including the social world. If done poorly, the technology is likely to be abandoned; therefore a principled approach for its design is needed".

Kreps and Neuhauser (2010) have identified four main directions for designing eHealth interventions to attain their full promise for promoting health. According to them, eHealth interventions must be (1) interactive, encouraging and involving; (2) effective, transparent, and interoperable; (3) dynamic, personally engaging; and have (4) high reach, and adaptability. Glanz and Bishop (2010) warrant for creativity. In their view, interventions should be "as entertaining and engaging as the other activities with which they compete".

Pagliari (2007) argues that designing effective eHealth systems involves applying expertise from diverse fields. Such advantageous interdisciplinary collaboration, with the ultimate goal of achieving transdisciplinary working, may be alleviated by increasing familiarity with each others' terminologies, theories and methods. Moreover, "mutual trust and respect for each others' aims, epistemologies, and contextual drivers, as well as a willingness to step outside traditional working boundaries" is required (Pagliari 2007).

Some might argue that behavior change technologies should be designed for action, not persuasion. In our view, however, persuasive behavior change support systems ultimately aim at both, motivating and facilitating (and maintaining) change.

According to Oinas-Kukkonen (2010), many BCSS design issues are general software design issues rather than specific to BCSSs only. These include, but are not limited to, usefulness, ease of use, ease of access, high information quality, simplicity, convenience, attractiveness, lack of errors, responsiveness, high overall positive user experience, and user loyalty.

11.3.1 Examples of Persuasive Design and Analysis Tools

In *Fogg Behavior Model* (FBM), behavior is a product of three factors: motivation, ability, and triggers, each of which has subcomponents (Fogg 2009a). The FBM asserts that for an individual to perform a target behavior, she must (1) be sufficiently motivated; (2) have the ability to perform the behavior; and (3) be triggered to perform the behavior (Fogg 2009a). Fogg underscores that these three factors must take place at the same moment, otherwise the behavior will not happen. According to Fogg (2009a), the FBM is useful in analysis and design of persuasive technologies. The FBM may also helps teams work together efficiently since the model gives enables people to share thoughts about behavior change (Fogg 2009a). See also Fogg's eight steps in early-stage persuasive design (Fogg 2009b).

Persuasive Systems Design Model (PSD Model) is a recent conceptualization (Oinas-Kukkonen and Harjumaa 2009) mainly for designing and developing persuasive systems. Thorough analysis of the persuasion context (the intent, event, and strategy of persuasion) is needed to discern (in)opportune moments for delivering the messages (Oinas-Kukkonen and Harjumaa 2009). The PSD model consists of a set of design principles under four categories: (1) primary task; (2) human-computer dialogue; (3) perceived system credibility; and (4) social influence. The design principles in the primary task category focus on supporting the user's primary activities. Design principles related to human-computer dialogue aid in achieving the goal set for using the system. The perceived system credibility design principles relate to how to design a system so that it is more credible and thereby more persuasive. The design principles in the social influence category describe how to design the system so that it motivates users by leveraging social influence (Oinas-Kukkonen and Harjumaa 2009). The greatest benefit of the PSD model may be achieved when it is applied together with a sound behavior change theory or a model, such as the *Elaboration Likelihood Model* (Petty and Cacioppo 1986).

Design with Intent (DwI) means design that is intended to influence or result in certain user behavior – it is an attempt to describe many types of systems (products, services, interfaces, environments) that have been strategically designed with the intent to influence how people use them (Lockton et al. 2008; Lockton et al. 2009). The Design with Intent Toolkit[2] consists of a wiki and 101 design patterns (cards),

---

[2] http://www.danlockton.com/dwi/. Accessed Aug 25, 2010.

which are grouped according to eight 'lenses' bringing divergent disciplinary perspectives on behavior change.

There are also a number of other examples of design strategies. Consolvo et al. (2009) have proposed a set of design strategies for technologies motivating lifestyle behavior change. They propose eight design strategies: (1) abstract and reflective; (2) unobtrusive; (3) public; (4) aesthetic; (5) positive; (6) controllable; (7) trending/ historical; and (8) comprehensive. The authors state using theory and findings from recent persuasive technology research to extend existing design goals.

Based on their systematic review, Lustria et al. (2009) has presented strategies used in computer-tailored online behavioral interventions. The organizing heuristic includes two main categories: implementation strategies and message tailoring strategies. The first category hosts three subcategories: (1) general implementation strategies; (2) modalities; and (3) tools for building self-regulatory skills. The latter category includes (4) tailoring criteria and (5) tailoring mechanisms.

Ritterband et al. (2009) has conceptualized *A Behavior Change Model for Internet Interventions*. The model has two main objectives: informing future development; of Internet interventions and helping to predict and explain behavior changes produced by those (Ritterband et al. 2009).

RE-AIM (Reach, Effectiveness, Adoption, Implementation, Maintenance) is used to report results or compare interventions, it is also a design/planning tool and as a method to review intervention studies (Glasgow et al. 1999).

11.3.2 Design Science Approach

According to Hevner et al. (2004) two paradigms command much of the research in the Information Systems discipline: *behavioral science* and *design science*. The first attempts to develop and verify theories that explain or predict human or organizational behavior. The latter is aiming for enhancing the boundaries of human and organizational capabilities by devising novel artifacts. Both paradigms are "foundational to the IS discipline, positioned as it is at the confluence of people, organizations, and technology" (Hevner et al. 2004, p. 75).

Design science is a discipline oriented to the creation of successful artifacts, which may be, for instance, constructs, models, methods, or instantiations. Peffers and colleagues (2007) have proposed the design science research methodology (DSRM). The DSRM process model is presented in Table 11.4.

The process is structured in a nominally sequential order. It is not assumed that one would always proceed from step 1 through activity 6. The process may actually be initiated at virtually any step. *A problem-centered approach* might be feasible if the idea resulted from observation of the problem or from suggested future research (e.g. in a paper from a prior project). *An objective-centered solution* could be prompted by an industry or research need that can be addressed by developing an artifact. *A design- and development-centered* approach would arise from the existence of an artifact that has not yet been formally supported as a solution for

Table 11.4 DSRM process model (Adapted from Peffers et al. 2007)

Activity	Explanation	Resources required (e.g.)	Possible research entry points
1. Problem identification and motivation	Define problem Show importance	Knowledge of the state of the problem and the importance of its solution	Problem-centered initiation
2. Define the objectives for a solution	What would a better artifact accomplish?	Knowledge of the state of problems and current solutions, if any, and their efficacy	Objective-centered solution
3. Design and development	Determining the artifact's desired functionality and its architecture and then creating the actual artifact. Artifacts may be constructs, models, methods, or instantiations	Knowledge of theory that can be brought to bear in a solution	Design and development centered initiation
4. Demonstration	Find suitable context. Use artifact to solve the problem (this could involve its use in experimentation, simulation, case study, proof, or other appropriate activity)	Knowledge of how to use the artifact to solve the problem	Client/context initiated
5. Evaluation	Observe how effective, efficient Iterate back to design	Knowledge of relevant metrics and analysis techniques	
6. Communication	Scholarly and professional publications	Knowledge of the disciplinary culture	

the explicit problem domain in which it will be applied. Such an artifact might have come from another research domain, it might have already been used to solve a different problem, or it might have appeared as an analogical idea. Lastly, a *client-/context-initiated* solution may be derived from observing a practical solution that worked, resulting in a design science solution if researchers (designers) work backward to exercise rigor to the process retrospectively (Peffers et al. 2007).

We believe that researchers and designers of eHealth interventions, or BCSSs, may benefit from this type of novel, yet formal, approach. The DSRM is intended as a methodology for research, even so, there would appear to be no reason it could not be used in practice (Peffers et al. 2007).

11.3.3 Underpinning Theories

There is no unified theory or model to inform eHealth development to promote behavior change (Neuhauser and Kreps 2003; Pingree et al. 2010). Nevertheless, a number of prominent health behavior theories and models have informed the design of health behavior change interventions (Tufano and Karras 2005). These theories and models have their origins in the disciplines of psychology, sociology, communication, and medicine, and they call on research in persuasion, social marketing, and relational communication (Neuhauser and Kreps 2003).

According to Glanz and Bishop (2010) the most often used theories of health behavior are *Social Cognitive Theory* (Bandura 1991, 1998), the *Transtheoretical Model* (Prochaska et al. 1997), the *Health Belief Model* (cf. Janz and Becker 1984; Rosenstock et al. 1988), and the *Theory of Planned Behavior* (Ajzen 1991). This notion is supported by many researchers (e.g. Neuhauser and Kreps 2003; Norman et al. 2007; Webb et al. 2010). For instance, in a recent extensive systematic review (85 studies) conducted by Webb and colleagues (2010) only three theories were used by three or more studies to develop the intervention; social cognitive theory, the transtheoretical model, and the theory of reasoned action/planned behavior. In a review by Norman et al. (2007) the majority of studies explicated the theoretical underpinnings of the intervention designs, and transtheoretical model and social cognitive theory were the most common theories used.

Glanz and Bishop (2010) argue that reviews of studies on an array of health behaviors have indicated that theory-based interventions are more effective than those not using theory. In Webb and colleagues' (2010) review and meta-analysis, interventions differed considerably in their use of theory, but more comprehensive use of theory was associated with larger effect sizes. They suggest that "this finding is consistent with assertions that interventions can benefit from using behavior change theory and extends the evidence base to interventions delivered on the Internet".

According to Fishbein and Cappella (2006), theories of (predicting) behavior change are valuable since they aid in identifying the determinants of any given behavior, which is a crucial first phase in the development of successful interventions to change behavior. Atienza et al. (2010) stress the need for identifying, clearly delineating and explicitly testing of which theories and constructs are most pertinent for a specific research topic or area (e.g., smoking cessation, obesity prevention), under what circumstances (e.g., environments, locations, time periods), and for which individuals or groups.

Pingree and colleagues (2010, p. 103) hypothesize that "given the wide variety of purposes and techniques of e-health, there will probably never be a single general theory of e-health". Nevertheless, they point out that this should not lead to the opposite extreme of applying a set of lower-level theories to explain different facets of a single intervention. They suggest that researchers should strive to apply or develop comprehensive theories to cover the complexity of their interventions. They maintain that "Ideally, this work should be a starting point for e-health development: identify the outcome(s) to target, then some mechanisms known to causally affect them, and work backwards to design the e-health intervention to activate at least some of those mechanisms (Pingree et al. 2010, p. 103)". We suggest that this type of approach is closely related to design science (see Sect. 3.2).

Glanz and Bishop (2010, p. 412) offer a contrasting view: "The strongest interventions may be built from multiple theories. When combining theories, it is important to think through clearly the unique contribution of different theories to the combined model."

Cappella (2006) maintains that behavior change and information processing theories are not two distinct traditions of theorizing about attitude processes, but are complementary. Thus, these theories not plainly answer different questions, rather answer complementary questions (Cappella 2006).

O'Keefe (2001) posits that there are three general kinds of theories have informed work on persuasion: (1) theories of attitude; (2) theories of voluntary action; (3) and theories of persuasion proper. The first two are not directly connected to persuasion, but have proved influential in shaping understandings of persuasion processes (O'Keefe 2001).

O'Keefe (2001) proposes reasons why there has not been more rigorous integration of the variable-analytic and applied-research findings within the different theoretical frameworks. He argues that one possible explanation is the width of academic fields in which persuasion-relevant research is conducted. He also points out that researchers are not encouraged to look abroad for relevant work, and that the research literature is scattered. He criticizes extant theoretical frameworks for failing to address a wide range of relevant issues. For instance, although emotional and visual aspects of persuasion are clearly important, theoretical models so far have not been designed to focus on such aspects. O'Keefe (2001) calls for more expansive frameworks, taking up a broader range of matters and engaging relevant work across disciplinary boundaries.

Fishbein has proposed an integrative model of behavior (see Fishbein and Yzer 2003; Fishbein and Cappella 2006) that attempts to bring together a number of theoretical perspectives.

Brewer and Rimer (2008) note that disappointing outcomes for some health behavior change interventions should urge us to consider the use of persuasion strategies. We share their view, that several established persuasion theories, including the *Elaboration Likelihood Model* (Petty and Cacioppo 1986), *Heuristic Systematic Model* (Chen and Chaiken 1999), and the *Unimodel* (Kruglanski and Thompson 1999) merit more attention.

11.4 Conclusion

This chapter has discussed several important perspectives in designing and developing persuasive health behavior change interventions. Clearly, designing such interventions is a demanding task. Based on the current state of related research, we suggest that several challenges (even obstacles) in designing persuasive health behavior change interventions are remaining. These include, but are not limited to: (1) lack of unified theory; (2) lack of interdisciplinary awareness, communication and efforts; (3) lack of accepted design models; (4) lack of common terminology; and (5) lack of evidence of individual contributing factors/components. We concur with Resnicow and colleagues (2010, p. 101) who state that "a better understanding of what is inside the black box of e-health interventions will lead to more empirically informed and ultimately more effective programs."

The chapter makes contribution at several levels. First, it introduces persuasive technology and behavior change support systems to the eHealth research community. Second, it offers several novel viewpoints, both theoretical and practical, in designing and developing health behavior change interventions. Third, it presents many theories and design models by other researchers, thus being a useful starting point for researchers and designers. Finally, the chapter addresses, though briefly, an important aspect of information systems research that has not yet gained attention in the eHealth community, that is design science research. As mentioned previously, we believe that researchers and designers in the eHealth domain may benefit from this type of approach. Some might consider our stance technologically deterministic. However, we do not simply claim that the use of technology, no matter how persuasive, is enough in health behavior change endeavors. Even so, understanding and using persuasive technology may prove to be valuable in such efforts.

Obviously, there are some limitations to the study. The amount of different facets and groups of interest in the eHealth space is overwhelming. For instance, cultural, economic, emotional, ethical, and privacy considerations were beyond the scope of this single chapter. Additionally, issues concerning evaluation, integration (e.g. into existing healthcare systems) and dissemination of eHealth interventions were excluded.

To conclude, this chapter was motivated by the need to explore the current state of persuasive health behavior change interventions, in research and practice. The chapter has merely scratched the surface of a large umbrella called eHealth. As demonstrated, there is a lot of future work to be done. Future research needs to address a multitude of open questions beginning with 'what', 'how' and 'why'. As persuasion should be incremental, we believe that this diverse and highly fascinating research area benefits the most when building on small successes.

Acknowledgments The author would like to thank Professor Harri Oinas-Kukkonen for guidance of the research and for comments on this book chapter. The author wishes to express his gratitude to the Graduate School on Software and Information Systems (SoSE) and the SalWe Research Program for Mind and Body (The Finnish Funding Agency for Technology and Innovation grant 1104/10) for funding parts of this research.

References

Ajzen, I. (1991). The theory of planned behavior. *Organizational Behavior and Human Decision Processes, 50*(2), 179–211.

Atienza, A. A., Hesse, B. W., Gustafson, D. H., & Croyle, R. T. (2010). E-health research and patient-centered care examining theory, methods, and application. *American Journal of Preventive Medicine, 38*(1), 85–88.

Bandura, A. (1991). Social cognitive theory of self-regulation. *Organizational Behavior and Human Decision Processes, 50*(2), 248–287.

Bandura, A. (1998). Health promotion from the perspective of social cognitive theory. *Psychology & Health, 13*(4), 623–649.

Barak, A., Klein, B., & Proudfoot, J. G. (2009). Defining internet-supported therapeutic interventions. *Annals of Behavioral Medicine, 38*(1), 4–17.

Bennett, G. G., & Glasgow, R. E. (2009). The delivery of public health interventions via the internet: Actualizing their potential. *Annual Review of Public Health, 30*, 273–292.

Bewick, B. M., Trusler, K., Barkham, M., Hill, A. J., Cahill, J., & Mulhern, B. (2008). The effectiveness of web-based interventions designed to decrease alcohol consumption–a systematic review. *Preventive Medicine, 47*(1), 17–26.

Brendryen, H., Drozd, F., & Kraft, P. (2008). A digital smoking cessation program delivered through internet and cell phone without nicotine replacement (happy ending): Randomized controlled trial. *Journal of Medical Internet Research, 10*(5), e51.

Brendryen, H., & Kraft, P. (2008). Happy ending: A randomized controlled trial of a digital multi-media smoking cessation intervention. *Addiction, 103*(3), 478–484. discussion 485–476.

Brendryen, H., Kraft, P., & Schaalma, H. (2010). Looking inside the black box: Using intervention mapping to describe the development of the automated smoking cessation intervention 'happy ending'. *Journal of Smoking Cessation, 5*(1), 29–56.

Brewer, N. T., & Rimer, B. K. (2008). Perspectives on health behavior theories that focus on individuals. In K. Glanz, B. K. Rimer, & K. Viswanath (Eds.), *Health behavior and health education: Theory, research, and practice* (pp. 149–162). San Francisco: Jossey-Bass.

Briñol, P., & Petty, R. E. (2009). Persuasion: Insights from the self-validation hypothesis. In M. P. Zanna (Ed.), *Advances in experimental social psychology* (pp. 69–118). New York: Elsevier.

Cappella, J. N. (2006). Integrating message effects and behavior change theories: Organizing comments and unanswered questions. *Journal of Communication, 56*(s1), S265–S279.

Chatterjee, S., & Price, A. (2009). Healthy living with persuasive technologies: Framework, issues, and challenges. *Journal of the American Medical Informatics Association, 16*(2), 171.

Chen, S., & Chaiken, S. (1999). The heuristic-systematic model in its broader context. *Dual-process theories in social psychology*, 73–96.

Consolvo, S., Everitt, K., Smith, I., & Landay, J. A. (2006). Design requirements for technologies that encourage physical activity. *Paper presented at the proceedings of the SIGCHI conference on human factors in computing systems*, Montreal, Quebec, Canada.

Consolvo, S., McDonald, D. W., & Landay, J. A. (2009). Theory-driven design strategies for technologies that support behavior change in everyday life. *Paper presented at the proceedings of the 27th international conference on human factors in computing systems*, Boston, MA, USA.

Dey, A. K. (2001). Understanding and using context. *Personal and ubiquitous computing, 5*(1), 4–7.

Festinger, L. (1957). *A theory of cognitive dissonance*. Stanford: Stanford University Press.

Fishbein, M., & Cappella, J. (2006). The role of theory in developing effective health communications. *Journal of Communication, 56*(s1), S1–S17.

Fishbein, M., & Yzer, M. (2003). Using theory to design effective health behavior interventions. *Communication Theory, 13*(2), 164–183.

Fogg, B. (2009a). A behavior model for persuasive design. *Paper presented at the proceedings of the 4th international conference on persuasive technology*, Claremont, California.

Fogg, B. (2009b). Creating persuasive technologies: An eight-step design process. *Paper presented at the proceedings of the 4th international conference on persuasive technology*, Claremont, California.

Glanz, K., & Bishop, D. B. (2010). The role of behavioral science theory in development and implementation of public health interventions. *Annual Review of Public Health, 31*, 399–418.

Glasgow, R. E., Vogt, T. M., & Boles, S. M. (1999). Evaluating the public health impact of health promotion interventions: The re-aim framework. *American Journal of Public Health, 89*(9), 1322–1327.

Harjumaa, M., Segerståhl, K., & Oinas-Kukkonen, H. (2009). Understanding persuasive software functionality in practice: A field trial of polar ft60. *Paper presented at the proceedings of the 4th international conference on persuasive technology*, Claremont, California.

Harvey-Berino, J., Pintauro, S., Buzzell, P., & Gold, E. C. (2004). Effect of internet support on the long-term maintenance of weight loss. *Obesity Research, 12*(2), 320–329.

Harvey-Berino, J., West, D., Krukowski, R., Prewitt, E., VanBiervliet, A., Ashikaga, T., & Skelly, J. (2010). Internet delivered behavioral obesity treatment. *Preventive Medicine, 51*(2), 123–128.

Hevner, A., March, S., Park, J., & Ram, S. (2004). Design science in information systems research. *MIS Quarterly, 28*(1), 75–105.

Hurling, R., Catt, M., De Boni, M., Fairley, B. W., Hurst, T., Murray, P., Richardson, A., & Sodhi, J. S. (2007). Using internet and mobile phone technology to deliver an automated physical activity program: Randomized controlled trial. *Journal of Medical Internet Research, 9*(2):e7. http://www.jmir.org/2007/2/e7/

Janz, N. K., & Becker, M. H. (1984). The health belief model: A decade later. *Health Education Quarterly, 11*(1), 1–47.

Kaptein, M., Lacroix, J., & Saini, P. (2010). Individual differences in persuadability in the health promotion domain. In T. Ploug, P. Hasle, & H. Oinas-Kukkonen (Eds.), *Persuasive technology* (pp. 94–105). Lecture notes in computer science. Berlin/Heidelberg: Springer.

Kreps, G. L., & Neuhauser, L. (2010). New directions in ehealth communication: Opportunities and challenges. *Patient Education and Counseling, 78*(3), 329–336.

Kroeze, W., Werkman, A., & Brug, J. (2006). A systematic review of randomized trials on the effectiveness of computer-tailored education on physical activity and dietary behaviors. *Annals of Behavioral Medicine, 31*(3), 205–223.

Kruglanski, A., & Thompson, E. (1999). Persuasion by a single route: A view from the unimodel. *Psychological Inquiry, 10*(2), 83–109.

Krukowski, R. A., Harvey-Berino, J., Ashikaga, T., Thomas, C. S., & Micco, N. (2008). Internet-based weight control: The relationship between web features and weight loss. *Telemedicine and e-Health, 14*(8), 775–782.

Kuziemsky, C. E., Downing, G. M., Black, F. M., & Lau, F. (2007). A grounded theory guided approach to palliative care systems design. *International Journal of Medical Informatics, 76*(Suppl 1), S141–S148.

Lehto, T., & Oinas-Kukkonen, H. (2009). The persuasiveness of web-based alcohol interventions. In Godart Claude, Gronau Norbert, Sharma Sushil, & Canals Gérôme (Eds.), *Software services for e-business and e-society* (IFIP advances in information and communication technology, pp. 316–327). Boston: Springer.

Lehto, T., & Oinas-Kukkonen, H. (2010). Persuasive features in six weight loss websites: A qualitative evaluation. In T. Ploug, P. Hasle, Harri Oinas-Kukkonen (Eds.), *Persuasive technology*, (pp. 162–173). Lecture notes in computer science. Berlin/Heidelberg: Springer.

Lin, J., Mamykina, L., Lindtner, S., Delajoux, G., & Strub, H. (2006). Fish'n'steps: Encouraging physical activity with an interactive computer game. In P. Dourish, & A. Friday (Eds.), *Ubicomp 2006: Ubiquitous computing*, (pp. 261–278). Lecture notes in computer science. Berlin/Heidelberg: Springer.

Locke, E. A., & Latham, G. P. (2002). Building a practically useful theory of goal setting and task motivation. A 35-year odyssey. *American Psychologist, 57*(9), 705–717.

Lockton, D., Harrison, D., Holley, T., & Stanton, N. A. (2009). Influencing interaction: Development of the design with intent method. *Paper presented at the proceedings of the 4th international conference on persuasive technology*, Claremont, California.

Lockton, D., Harrison, D., & Stanton, N. (2008). Design with intent: Persuasive technology in a wider context. In H. Oinas-Kukkonen, P. Hasle, M. Harjumaa, K. Segerståhl, & P. Øhrstrøm (Eds.), *Persuasive technology* (pp. 274–278). Lecture notes in computer science. Berlin/Heidelberg: Springer.

Lustria, M. L., Cortese, J., Noar, S. M., & Glueckauf, R. L. (2009). Computer-tailored health interventions delivered over the web: Review and analysis of key components. *Patient Education and Counseling, 74*(2), 156–173.

Neuhauser, L., & Kreps, G. (2003). Rethinking communication in the e-health era. *Journal of Health Psychology, 8*(1), 7.

Neville, L. M., O'Hara, B., & Milat, A. J. (2009). Computer-tailored dietary behaviour change interventions: A systematic review. *Health Education Research, 24*(4), 699–720.

Norman, G. J., Zabinski, M. F., Adams, M. A., Rosenberg, D. E., Yaroch, A. L., & Atienza, A. A. (2007). A review of ehealth interventions for physical activity and dietary behavior change. *American Journal of Preventive Medicine, 33*(4), 336–345.

O'Keefe, D. J. (2001). Persuasion. In T. O. Sloane, S. Bartsch, T. B. Farrell, & H. F. Plett (Eds.), *Encyclopedia of rhetoric* (pp. 575–583). Oxford: Oxford University Press.

Oinas-Kukkonen, H. (2010). Behavior change support systems: A research model and agenda. *Persuasive Technology*, Vol. 6137, 4–14.

Oinas-Kukkonen, H., & Harjumaa, M. (2009). Persuasive systems design: Key issues, process model, and system features. *Communications of the Association for Information Systems, 24*(1), 28.

Pagliari, C. (2007). Design and evaluation in ehealth: Challenges and implications for an interdisciplinary field. *Journal of Medical Internet Research, 9*(2), e15.

Peffers, K., Tuunanen, T., Rothenberger, M., & Chatterjee, S. (2007). A design science research methodology for information systems research. *Journal of Management Information Systems, 24*(3), 45–77.

Petty, R., & Cacioppo, J. (1986). The elaboration likelihood model of persuasion. *Advances in Experimental Social Psychology, 19*(1), 123–205.

Picard, R. (2003). Affective computing: Challenges. *International Journal of Human Computer Studies, 59*(1–2), 55–64.

Pingree, S., Hawkins, R., Baker, T., duBenske, L., Roberts, L. J., & Gustafson, D. H. (2010). The value of theory for enhancing and understanding e-health interventions. *American Journal of Preventive Medicine, 38*(1), 103–109.

Portnoy, D. B., Scott-Sheldon, L. A., Johnson, B. T., & Carey, M. P. (2008). Computer-delivered interventions for health promotion and behavioral risk reduction: A meta-analysis of 75 randomized controlled trials, 1988–2007. *Preventive Medicine, 47*(1), 3–16.

Prochaska, J., Johnson, S., & Lee, P. (1997). The transtheoretical model of behavior change. *American Journal of Health Promotion, 12*(1), 38–48.

Resnicow, K., Strecher, V., Couper, M., Chua, H., Little, R., Nair, V., Polk, T. A., & Atienza, A. A. (2010). Methodologic and design issues in patient-centered e-health research. *American Journal of Preventive Medicine, 38*(1), 98–102.

Ritterband, L. M., Thorndike, F. P., Cox, D. J., Kovatchev, B. P., & Gonder-Frederick, L. A. (2009). A behavior change model for internet interventions. *Annals of Behavioral Medicine, 38*(1), 18–27.

Rosenstock, I., Strecher, V., & Becker, M. (1988). Social learning theory and the health belief model. *Health Education & Behavior, 15*(2), 175.

Shahab, L., & McEwen, A. (2009). Online support for smoking cessation: A systematic review of the literature. *Addiction, 104*(11), 1792–1804.

Tate, D., Jackvony, E., & Wing, R. (2003). Effects of internet behavioral counseling on weight loss in adults at risk for type 2 diabetes: A randomized trial. *Journal of the American Medical Association, 289*(14), 1833–1836.

Tsai, A. G., & Wadden, T. A. (2005). Systematic review: An evaluation of major commercial weight loss programs in the united states. *Annals of Internal Medicine, 142*(1), 56–66.

Tufano, J. T., & Karras, B. T. (2005). Mobile ehealth interventions for obesity: A timely opportunity to leverage convergence trends. *Journal of Medical Internet Research, 7*(5), e58.

van den Berg, M. H., Vliet Vlieland, T. P. M., & Schoones, J. W. (2007). Internet-based physical activity interventions: A systematic review of the literature. *Journal of Medical Internet Research, 9*(3):e26. http://www.jmir.org/2007/3/e26/

van Straten, A., Cuijpers, P., & Smits, N. (2008). Effectiveness of a web-based self-help intervention for symptoms of depression, anxiety, and stress: Randomized controlled trial. *Journal of Medical Internet Research, 10*(1), e7.

Vandelanotte, C., Spathonis, K. M., Eakin, E. G., & Owen, N. (2007). Website-delivered physical activity interventions a review of the literature. *American Journal of Preventive Medicine, 33*(1), 54–64.

Webb, T. L., Joseph, J., Yardley, L., & Michie, S. (2010). Using the internet to promote health behavior change: A systematic review and meta-analysis of the impact of theoretical basis, use of behavior change techniques, and mode of delivery on efficacy. *Journal of Medical Internet Research, 12*(1), e4.

Womble, L. G., Wadden, T. A., McGuckin, B. G., Sargent, S. L., Rothman, R. A., & Krauthamer-Ewing, E. S. (2004). A randomized controlled trial of a commercial internet weight loss program. *Obesity Research, 12*(6), 1011–1018.

Zhang, J. (2005). Human-centered computing in health information systems. Part 1: Analysis and design. *Journal of Biomedical Informatics, 38*(1), 1–3.

Chapter 12
Accessibility in the Web for Disabled People

Irene Krebs, Arnim Nethe, and Reetta Raitoharju

Abstract Accessibility in the context of the internet has been researched repeatedly in the last years and there are many treatises on this issue. The rapid development of computers and particularly internet software technologies in the Web 2.0 is the reason that a lot of this literature is outdated and the described methods are not applicable anymore. But especially these new technologies are very attractive to disabled people because they offer an interactive access to a lot of services to which can be very helpful. These possibilities should not be inaccessible for a minority just because of an insufficient technical realisation.

This thesis aims at providing a basis for further discussion on cutting-edge methods for accessible web technologies and offers a set of instructions to successfully realise accessible concepts in internet projects according to the Web Content Accessibility Guidelines 2.0 (WCAG).

Keywords Disabled people • Accessibility • Web • Barrier-free Systems • Web technologies

I. Krebs (✉)
Prof. Dr.-Ing., academic staff
Industrial Information Systems, Brandenburg University of Technology Cottbus,
Konrad-Wachsmann-Allee 1, D-03046 Cottbus
e-mail: krebs@iit.tu-cottbus.de

A. Nethe
Prof. Dr.-Ing. Habil.,extraordinary professorship
Biomedical Equipment Technology, Brandenburg University of Technology Cottbus,
Konrad-Wachsmann-Allee 1, D-03046 Cottbus

R. Raitoharju
Dr.Sci, Principal lecturer
Information technology (Health informatics), Turku University of Applied Sciences,
Joukahaisenkatu 3 C, 20520 Turku

N. Wickramasinghe et al. (eds.), *Critical Issues for the Development*
of Sustainable E-health Solutions, Healthcare Delivery in the Information Age,
DOI 10.1007/978-1-4614-1536-7_12, © Springer Science+Business Media, LLC 2012

12.1   Introduction

Accessibility in the internet is topic of discussions ever since the beginning of the World Wide Web. A common awareness on accessibility failed to arise out of these efforts and discussions and does not exist until today, neither between developers nor users.

> Do you have an idea what is meant with the term "accessible website"? The response to this question was stated with a clear no of 78% of the interviewees (TNS EMNID 2009).

This shows clearly that in terms of accessibility a lot of work still has to be done. The low recognition of the term accessibility does not result out of the fact that a minority is affected by it. In the survey it was demonstrated that even 92% of all interviewees have left at least once an e-commerce website due to the fact that the usage was complicated and not at all customer friendly. All sections of the population had been presented in the survey. That means that almost all internet users had been affected once by barriers in the internet. In Germany meanwhile all sections and age groups of the population do use the internet; they differentiate regarding their way of using the internet as well as the time they spend and the frequency in which they use it. Therefore barriers or obstacles might occur and be problem to everyone. It might happen that an obstacle complicates the usage of a service in the internet or even makes it impossible to use. In rough economic times it is essential for a company not to lose customers because of defective developments in their online shops or online services. Beside the turnover for the single business that the company loses it is possible that it also loses the customer that receives better service from a competing company and forever turns his back to our company.

In the internet it is impossible for a company to interfere while the client is online with a personal consultation. That could lead to the fact that the potential but also frustrated client leaves the website. This scenario might happen as well in the case of governmental projects. In this sense especially the internet presentation of public institutions of the federal and state governments as well as local authorities needs to be analysed more intensively. The German Federation and the states are obliged to guarantee the accessibility to their products and services according to the equality law (Federal government 2002). But still, there are improvements to be made, especially in the review of new offers. Through the enhancement of the web 2.0, where internet users are engaged to participate actively, new internet applications of the Federal government are evolving. Here people can vote, discuss and do a lot of things more to take actively part in the creation of the German democracy and the European Union. The aim is to review the criteria of accessibility in new developments already in the planning and realization phase and once introduced and offered to internet users to stick to these criteria.

Beside the increase of private internet users the number of internet users at work rises considerably. According to the Federal Office of Statistics already 51% of companies communicate through the internet and have a paperless and fully electronic realization of their processes. These figures do represent a challenge for accessibility on the one side but also opportunities on the other. An offer of service that is easily accessible to all people would increase the amount of users while reducing the number of users going the conventional way. For example a visually impaired employee could fill out fully accessible pdf-documents on the computer which is almost impossible for them with documents in paper form.

12.2 Basics

The motivation results from the fact that the term accessibility is still weakly distributed and that the awareness on it needs to be increased remarkably. No speaking about the real possibility that everybody could be affected by these problems and barriers personally in the future. Especially developers of so called Rich Internet Applications (RIA) should in detail deal with the topics of user-friendliness and accessibility. RIA offer the users an added value in using the internet while operating intuitively. For that reason we will later on consider the differences and common ground of these two terms. Today already 29% of all men in the age group 55 and older use the internet on a daily basis or almost every day. In 2009 33 million people had been aged 55 or older. This number will raise until 2020 to 39 million people while at the same time the overall number of the population will decrease (Statistisches Bundesamt 2009c). Another 5 years later the age group of 20–54 will be already smaller than the one of 55 and older. Statistisches Bundesamt 2009b These numbers demonstrate clearly that due to a demographic change adaptation and changes in internet offers need to be realized. At this point it is important to mention that the public use of the internet, especially of the World Wide Web, has only started at the beginning of the 1990s. These generation that grew up with the WWW will be having an important impact on the statistics of the ageing population that means the number of "older" internet user will increase rapidly in a comparably short period of time. These changes need to be considered in common web standards that are creating the basis today for the World Wide Web of the coming years. It is obvious that the technology cycle of HTML standards are very long and therefore the development towards accessibility is nothing that can be realized on a short term basis.

Beside the consideration of the age groups the number of severely disabled people in 2007 amounted up to 6.9 million from which 348,000 had been blind or visually impaired people (Federal Office of Statistics 2009c, p. 8) For all these people the article 3 clause 3 of the basic law is in force: "No person shall be disfavored because of disability." Statistisches Bundesamt" 2009d Until today unfortunately only regional and federal authorities are obliged due to regulations to transpose this also in the internet. Of course disabled people will be meeting barriers almost every day in their lives but to eliminate them where they arise just because of bad planning or insufficient knowledge seems a realistic objective.

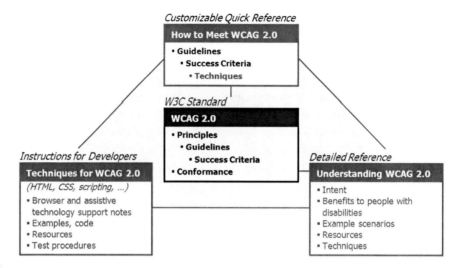

Fig. 12.1 Detailed structure of WCAG 2 document (World Wide Web Consortium 2008)

12.3 Accessibility and Usability in the Web

Accessibility has to guarantee an access for all people. It describes the situation of any place or any medium. Accessibility therefore is given when everybody has access to this place or this medium, independently in which way this person has a limitation. The German Industry Standard (DIN) has found a definition in the expert report #124 on "Creation of accessible products" that fits for everybody:

> "… Characteristics of a product that can be used if possible by all people in every age group with different abilities in an almost equal way and without any assistance." (With "fully accessible" it is not just meant being free of obstacles in a physical sense (please see DIN 33942) but rather accessible, reachable and usable) 11 German Industry Standard 2002.

The Web Content Accessibility Guidelines (WCAG) are guidelines for a fully accessible internet that had been established by the World Wide Web Consortium (W3C) (Hille and Kunde 2002). The W3C is a worldwide association of scientist and experts that works particularly hard for standards in the web and develops them. Although the WCAG 2 had only been adopted in December 2008 its development had been done much earlier. Due to several errors in the WCAG 1 a new draft of the follow-up version had been published already in January 2001.

The WCAG 2 had been created with the demand not only to address HTML developers but also decision makers, purchasers, teachers, pupils and students. For that reason the structure of the WCAG 2 is created in a way that the requirements for accessibility had been divided into global principles, general guidelines, success criteria and techniques. This way information on the general idea of accessibility until technical details and typical mistakes (World Wide Web Consortium (2008) are being communicated in a target oriented way. In the W3C standard of the WCAG 2.0 (Fig. 12.1) specific technologies are not yet mentioned. The W3C standard explains generally the requirements of accessible web sites. In "Techniques for WCAG 2.0" developers can find details of the realization, specific instructions for solutions and detailed explanation of mistakes.

A clear standardization of accessibility is only possible if specific techniques and technologies are being defined. Quick changes and developments of the information technologies make that impossible, as already demonstrated with the problems of the WCAG 1. It would be useful here if the Web Accessibility Initiative checks regularly the new standards according their compatibility of accessibility and gives regularly advice for future versions of these standards. Even if permanent up- to-date technical standards would be developed by an expert committee of the W3C, the updates would need to be disseminated permanently. The transformation into laws, regulations and test periods for that is still very time-consuming. With an adequate expenditure this could be changed. Unfortunately in the field of accessibility it is not expected to happen. A better automation of these procedures would have a similar effect while having considerably less costs. Defined regulations published by the W3C in a language like XML that can be adapted automatically in existing manual or automatic tests. The document of the WCAG 2 of the W3C with the requirements and techniques could be a first step for such an approach.

After the perceived success of the eEurope 2002 action plans the topic accessibility as main goal in the following eEurope 2005 had been given up. The focus has been set at fields like e-government, e-health, e-learning and e-business with no special regard to accessibility. In the action plan the speech is about e-inclusion. Despite the integration of the Web Accessibility Initiative (WAI) guidelines into the EU-legislation accessibility is not explicitly called. Rather digital divide is addressed. That means a general division of the society into parts of population with better access to the internet and to information and having advantages in the information society respectively. "Better" access can mean a higher access speed, but also fewer barriers for the usage of the web. In the update of the action plan of 2004 it had been recognized that there are intervention needs in the fields of digital integration and of digital accessibility in particular. For that reason "priorities have to be reassessed at the background of their thorough analysis." (European Commission, 2004, p.28) The final benchmarking report does not refer to that and does not present any related results. But it addresses the digital divide between the social strata as well as between the different European regions. Only the follow-up programme of the Europe 2005 action plans, the i2010 strategy postulates accessibility as a main objective. The recent study of the European Commission about the accessibility of websites has used the WCAG 1 and WCAG 2-criteria for a test of 102 websites from ten EU countries. This study which has been published in December 2009 has drawn comparative figures from the years 2008 and 2007. All tests have been carried out at the same basis. The comparability has been guaranteed by analysing for each country six ministries and six websites of public interest. Finally only 102 from 120 websites could be assessed. Some of the selected sites where expired, others have not been accessible or could not be analysed with the chosen testing methodology. Finally, none of the websites has successfully passed the complete automatic and manual tests (Table 12.1).

Table 12.1 Web accessibility WCAG 1.0 compliance levels, including "marginal" fails (Commission of the European Communities 2009)

Year	% of sites that passed automatic and manual testing	% of sites that passed automatic testing only	% of sites that marginally failed automatic testing	% of sites that failed (more than marginally)
2009	0.0	22.5	14.7	62.8
2008	2.9	20.0	18.1	59.0
2007	3.6	11.8	15.5	69.1

12.4   Conclusions

In general the compliance with technical and social standards in various fields is observed and respected, in particular in Germany. Equality can be found as a key word everywhere. But many people associate the meaning of the word accessibility with a wheelchair ramp. Companies have started to analyse how to enlarge the target groups and how to develop new businesses in the global competition. All people, potential clients, who meet any obstacles using the internet – no matter from which reasons – for information, for online shopping or for the use of e-government services are excluded by the companies or by the state. No company can risk losing customers, especially not in economically hard times. The exclusion of a considerably big group of people from these services can be simply avoided by the use of accessibility-technologies already starting from the conception and the development phase.

Related tests can reflect only the initial or the current state of the websites. Later changes, i.e. affected by Java-Script, hardly can be evaluated with the present approach. At this point we see a potential for further research: to analyse the accessibility of a website not only in its actual state, but also to anticipate it for each of the possible different states.

Accessible websites and web applications lead to new standards in the internet and they offer many proven advantages for companies. These facts clearly should be communicated by public initiatives. In times of economic crisis and mass unemployment projects for the improvement of the accessibility of the internet have no first priority. Nevertheless it is a big challenge of the information society to facilitate and to support the participation at the social life to everybody.

References

Bundesregierung. (2002). *Gesetz zur Gleichstellung behinderter Menschen (Behinderten-gleichstellungsgesetz – BGG).* http://www.gesetze-im-internet.de/bgg/BJNR146800002.html. Accessed 16 Dec 2009.

Commission of the European Communities. (December 2009). *Study on Web accessibility in European countries.* http://ec.europa.eu/information_society/activities/einclusion/library/studies/web_access_compliance/index_en.htm. Accessed 10 Mar 2010.

Deutsche Industrienorm. (2002). *DIN-Fachbericht 124 Gestaltung barrierefreier Produkte.* Berlin: Beuth.

Hille, C., & Kunde, B. (2002). *barrierefrei kommunizieren: Behinderungskompensierende Techniken und Technologien für Computer und Internet.* Meißen: Technischer Jugendfreizeit- und Bildungsverein (tfjbv) e.V., 2006.

Statistisches Bundesamt. (2009b). *Informations-Gesellschaft in Deutschland: Ausgabe 2009.* Statistisches Bundesamt. Wiesbaden: Statistisches Bundesamt, 2009. – ISBN 978-3-8246-0868-3.

Statistisches Bundesamt. (2009c). *Statistik der schwerbehinderten Menschen: Kurzbericht. Wiesbaden: Statistisches Bundesamt.* http://www.destatis.de/jetspeed/portal/cms/Sites/destatis/Internet/DE/Content/Publikationen/Fachveroeffentlichungen/Sozialleistungen/SozialSchwerbehinderte2007pdf.psml. Accessed 16 Dec 2009.

Statistisches Bundesamt. (2009d). *Unternehmen und Arbeitsstätten: Nutzung von Informations- und Kommunikationstechnologie.* Wiesbaden: Statistisches Bundesamt.

TNS EMNID. (April 2009). *Bekanntheit des Begriffs "Barrierefreie Websites".* http://www.stiftung-barrierefrei-kommunizieren.de/upload/bilder/aktuelles/barr1509.pdf. Accessed 23 Jan 2010.

World Wide Web Consortium. (December 2008). *The WCAG 2.0 documents.* http://www.w3.org/WAI/intro/wcag20.php. Accessed 13 Feb 2010.

Section III
The Importance of People in E-Health: Lest We Forget

Rajeev K. Bali

Introduction

This brief chapter serves as an introduction to the section of the book dealing with people-focussed issues surrounding E-Health. Much has been written about its efficacy but the vast majority of the literature seems to focus on the technical, that is: the role of information and communication technologies (ICTs).

E-Health allows healthcare stakeholders, via the judicious use of ICTs, to access healthcare and clinical information both locally and at a distance (Mitchell 1999). Being a knowledge-based activity, the core of E-Health focusses on Knowledge Management (KM), itself a skilful blend of people, process and technology (Bali et al. 2009).

People Focus

E-Health implementation in contemporary entities may require a change to the existing organizational culture in place. This change will both enable and facilitate full adoption of the E-Health precepts allowing for complete integration across functional domains with due regard to business processes, human factors, motivation and contemporary and future technologies (including new social media).

The three components (people, process and technology) has been compared to a three-legged stool; if one is missing, then the stool will collapse (De Brún 2005). It has been contended that one leg (people) is more important than the others. An organisation's primary focus should be on developing a knowledge-friendly culture and knowledge-friendly behaviours among its people, which should be supported by the appropriate processes, and which may be enabled through technology (De Brún 2005).

Various individuals are involved in providing E-Health delivery including healthcare professionals, specialists, nurses, pharmacists, medical assistants, administrators and other related healthcare staff. Theses are the users who will use the ICT in their daily routine in dealing with patients and it may well be that many of them possess limited ICT skills. Many may well be set in their existing ways and existing work processes may well have been ingrained into their daily lives for decades. Any purported change in their routine daily workflow is bound to be viewed with some degree of hostility and resistance. In addition, relatively poor awareness about ICT projects has further compounded the problems and challenges for implementing information systems at healthcare facilities. Proactive initiatives, such as providing training and short courses on ICT and medical informatics knowledge, are critical. Healthcare professionals need to embrace ICT as a mainstream tool for the future healthcare system, especially via the adoption of telehealth and telemedicine in improving healthcare delivery to citizens (Wootton and Craig 1999; Maheu 2001).

If the ultimate goal of E-health is to improve patient outcomes, all of the inherent components must be measured against the benchmark of patient need in order to achieve system-wide objectives of safety and effectiveness (Epstein 2000, 2005; Arora 2003).

The Chapters

The chapters in this section focus on the essential human (people and patient) aspects of E-Health.

Bleuer et al. write about a new KM-based software project which incorporates effective representation models in order to reduce knowledge gaps. The use of the MeSH Index (Medical Subject Headings) combines with user-led knowledge gap identification results in an intelligent and functional solution.

Bos offers a comprehensive review of human-based issues for E-Health. A paradigm shift is required to achieve a trustworthy relationship between patients and healthcare providers. New technologies and the continued growth of social media will help herald the arrival of more informed and empowered patients.

Hannan continues the theme of empowerment and offers "before and after" hypothetical vignettes to illustrate how patients can effectively access their own healthcare records. In combination with changes in healthcare and IT, patient record access helps to build a "Partnership of Trust" between patients and healthcare professionals.

Bali et al. present three clinical cases (breast screening, maternity services and Crohn's disease) in order to demonstrate both the effect of E-Health but, more specifically, the importance of the human dimension within them.

Finally, *Popovich* introduces a case study which models the exchange of immunization records between provider-based electronic health records and state immunization registries, and demonstrates the potential for increased provider revenue.

References

Arora, N. K. (2003). Interacting with cancer patients: The significance of physicians' communication behavior. *Social Science & Medicine, 57*(5), 791–806.

Bali, R. K., Wickramasinghe, N., & Lehaney, B. (2009). *Knowledge management primer*. USA: Routledge.

De Brún, C. (2005). Principles and processes of knowledge management. Knowledge Management Specialist Library. www.library.nhs.uk/KNOWLEDGEMANAGEMENT/ViewResource.aspx?resID=94013. Accessed 13 Sept 2010.

Epstein, R. M. (2000). The science of patient-centered care. *Journal of Family Practice, 49*(9), 805–807.

Epstein, R. M., Franks, P., Fiscella, K., Shields, C. G., Meldrum, S. C., Kravitz, R. L., et al. (2005). Measuring patient-centered communication in patient-physician consultations: Theoretical and practical issues. *Social Science & Medicine, 61*(7), 1516–1528.

Maheu, M. M. (2001). *E-Health, telehealth, and telemedicine: A guide to start-up and success*. San Francisco: Jossey-Bass.

Mitchell, J. (1999). *From telehealth to e-health: The unstoppable rise of e-health*. Canberra: Department of Communications, Information Technology and the Arts.

Wootton, R., & Craig, J. (1999). *Introduction to telemedicine*. London: The Royal Society of Medicine.

Chapter 13
Knowledge Management: Often Neglected but Crucial to eHealth

**Juerg P. Bleuer, Daniele Talerico, Kurt Bösch,
Vincent Lampérière, and Christian A. Ludwig**

Abstract Suva (Swiss National Accident Insurance Fund) is the most important carrier of obligatory accident insurance in Switzerland. Its medical division initiated a knowledge management project called InWiM. "InWiM" is the acronym for "Integrierte Wissensbasen der Medizin" which can be translated as "Integrated Knowledge Bases in Medicine". The project is part of an ISO 9001 certification program and comprises the definition and documentation of all processes in the field of knowledge management as well as the development of the underlying ITC infrastructure. The knowledge representation model used for the ICT implementation regards knowledge as a multidimensional network of interlinked units of information. The model allows annotations for a narrative description of the nature of the units of information (e.g. documents) and the cross-links as well. Information retrieval is achieved by means of a full implementation of the MeSH Index, the thesaurus of the United States National Library of Medicine (NLM). InWiM manages not only publications but also keeps track of "knowledge gaps", i. e. areas where sound knowledge is missing. Knowledge gaps are indexed with MeSH terms in a similar way to publications. This improves knowledge management: In particular it is possible to search and find knowledge gaps and solutions covering the same or a similar topic, thus allowing adequate collating and it prevents duplication of work. Furthermore, literature search strategies for the NML are predefined and do not need every time to be reinvented from scratch.

J.P. Bleuer (✉)
Healthevidence GmbH, Berne, Switzerland
e-mail: bleuer@healthevidence.ch

D. Talerico • K. Bösch • V. Lampérière • C.A. Ludwig
Suva, Lucerne, Switzerland
e-mail: daniele.talerico@suva.ch; kurt.boesch@suva.ch; vincent.lamperiere@suva.ch;
christian.ludwig@suva.ch

N. Wickramasinghe et al. (eds.), *Critical Issues for the Development
of Sustainable E-health Solutions*, Healthcare Delivery in the Information Age,
DOI 10.1007/978-1-4614-1536-7_13, © Springer Science+Business Media, LLC 2012

Keywords Knowledge Management • Information Storage and Retrieval • Databases, Bibliographic • PubMed • Medical Subject Headings • Evidence-Based Medicine • Insurance, Accident

13.1 Introduction

Although the majority of eHealth initiatives focus on health records management and interoperability of healthcare IT systems, knowledge management remains one of the corner stones for high quality and cost-effective health care delivery. Medicine often faces the problem of a diversity of opinions about the facts of a case. The coexistence of doctrines results in insecurity about the appropriateness of any actions and concerns doctors and patients as well; additional costs may be another negative effect. In the late 1970s, a working group at McMaster University, Hamilton, Ontario, started to develop new concepts for clinical decisions. Later, this work emerged in a worldwide movement, called Evidence-based Medicine (EBM) (Evidence-Based Medicine Working Group 1992). David Sackett defined evidence-based medicine as "the conscientious, explicit, and judicious use of current best evidence in making decisions about the care of individual patients" (Sackett et al. 1996). But before you can make "explicit and judicious use of current best evidence", you are in need of the current best knowledge. Given the fact of today's information overflow, an enterprise wanting it's healthcare professionals to practice Evidence-based Medicine needs an appropriate knowledge management infrastructure.

Since ever, insurance medicine aims at high quality health care delivery but focuses at the same time on the cost-effectiveness of interventions. This may be one of the reasons why knowledge management IT-infrastructure gained ground in particular in the domain of insurance medicine. Another reason may be the fact, that in insurance medicine, divergent opinions not only affect curative procedures but they also bear the risk of different decisions about financial aspects, e.g. whether a health problem is covered by the accident insurance or not. Patients perceive divergent decisions in this field as injustice and lawsuits may be the consequence. Furthermore, from an ethical point of view, such divergence in verdicts is unacceptable.

13.2 The InWiM Project

Suva (Swiss National Accident Insurance Fund) is the most important carrier of obligatory accident insurance in Switzerland. It is an independent, non-profit-making company under public law and mainly insures companies in the secondary business sector, i.e. industrial, trading and commercial enterprises. Suva's services comprise not only insurance but also prevention, case management and rehabilitation. Prevention focuses on occupational and leisure-time safety as well. In order to ensure the most effective treatment for all patients, Suva's medical division supports doctors working in inpatient and outpatient care with comprehensive case management and with conciliar advice. Two Suva clinics provide inpatient rehabilitation.

In 2002, Suva started the InWiM project. InWiM is an acronym and stands for "Integrierte Wissensbasen der Medizin", which can be translated as "Integrated Knowledge Bases in Medicine". The project is part of an ISO 9001 certification program and comprises the definition and documentation of all processes in the field of knowledge management as well as the development and the implementation of the InWiM knowledge management application. The latter makes all the functions available that are needed to collect, generate, administer and distribute information and knowledge.

13.3 Data, Information and Knowledge

In everyday language, people often do not differentiate between the terms "data", "information" and "knowledge" and many different definitions for these terms can be found in the literature. InWiM adopts the definitions of Rehäuser et al. (1996). According to them, the term "data" refers to symbols that represent a fact or statement of event without any relation to other data. The term "information" is used for data in context. "Knowledge" is achieved through the process of linking pieces of information together based on logical thinking. Schreyögg and Geiger call this an "approach to knowledge inspired by information theory" (Schreyögg and Geiger 2007).

In general, knowledge management systems do not deal with pure data. At the time when data is subject to knowledge management processes, it has already been put in some sort of context. Therefore, it is more appropriate to use the term "information". In practice, there is no strict border between information and knowledge. It is useful to consider the way from information to knowledge as a continuum. The following example may illustrate this: one single scientific publication will give the reader information about a specific issue. If he considers several studies and puts the results and conclusions in relation, he will gather more and more knowledge about the subject of these studies. Eventually some authors will write reviews about studies and someday, somebody will summarize all the publications including the primary, secondary and tertiary literature. Along the way, information is transformed into knowledge. Provided that the reviews are properly done, the knowledge gets sounder and sounder with each review.

It may be helpful in this context to distinguish the term "knowledge" as we understand it here from the meaning in everyday language, where knowledge has the connotation of "truth" which distinguishes it from "belief". Knowledge in the context of information theory however, does not imply correctness. Knowledge and information may be wrong or right. In order to point out that some knowledge is reliable, one may speak of well-established knowledge. Evidence-Based Medicine goes further and denotes the reliability with levels of evidence and grades of recommendation respectively (Canadian Task Force on the Periodic Health Examination 1979). E.g. evidence is considered to be sound if it is supported by multiple studies of high methodological quality (Oxford Centre for Evidence-based Medicine 2009).

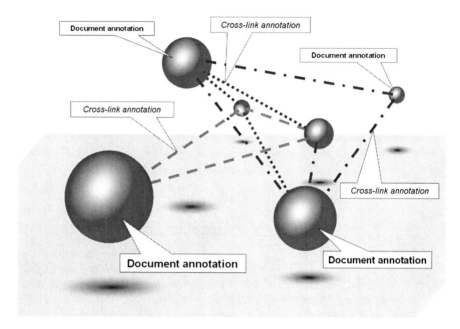

Fig. 13.1 Multidimensional cross-links between documents (information units). Information units are shown as *balls*. The *lines* represent cross-links, depicting the various dimensions of link-ups. Annotations permit comments both on the cross-links as well as on the individual documents

13.4   The Underlying Knowledge Management Model

According to Schreyögg and Geiger, "knowledge" is understood as a result of linking pieces of information together by means of brain work. This implies that knowledge is subjective: Personal knowledge can be seen as an individual network of interlinked pieces of information. It is important to see that such a personal knowledge network is multidimensional. The latter results from the fact that information can be interlinked from different points of view. The following example may illustrate this: Let us assume that we have some studies investigating the effect of different surgical techniques in joint surgery. It will make sense to link all the papers that report on the same technique on different joints as well as those which investigate different techniques at the same joint. Additional links may denote judgments about study quality, demographical issues, etc. Figure 13.1 illustrates how units of information (e.g. publications of studies) are linked together in multiple dimensions. In contrast to the hyperlink technology in the World Wide Web, all links are bidirectional: the target knows the source of the links. The links are therefore called cross-links.

The "inspired by information theory" understanding of knowledge (Rehäuser et al. 1996), implies that knowledge always has to be seen in context (Rehäuser et al. 1996;

Steinmüller 1993; Von Krogh and Koehne 1998). A model, which claims to be able to depict knowledge as a network of cross-linked units of information must therefore include meta-information not only for the units of information (e.g. documents) but also for each cross-link. Meta-information not only includes the name of the author, date, version, etc. but also free text annotations, which allow for a narrative description of the point of view under which a specific cross-link was established.

If we adopt the model that personal knowledge can be seen as a multidimensional network of information, corporate knowledge can be regarded as the synthesis of all personal knowledge networks in an institution: This means that each user can store his units of information (e.g. documents) and that these documents are visible for all other users. Each user can then construct as many cross-links as needed which include not only his own but also units of information from other users. Annotations can be added to cross-links and units of information as well: the number of annotations is not restricted, neither per document nor per cross-link. All annotations are visible not only to the author but to all users.

13.5 Information Retrieval

Information retrieval is achieved by means of the MeSH Index (Medical Subject Headings), the thesaurus of the United States National Library of Medicine (NLM). MeSH is a controlled vocabulary with over 26,000 descriptors (2011) and it is based on concepts (National Library of Medicine 2011): Each MeSH term denotes a specific concept which refers to a well defined object in the real world. This approach makes MeSH much more valuable than the simple use of cues which always goes along with ambiguity in meaning. MeSH terms are hierarchically structured with superordinate concepts and subordinate concepts thus allowing appropriate representation of real world objects within the scope of healthcare and research.

The InWiM implementation of MeSH supports all features including subheadings and limits. It allows users to search the in-house document repository as well as to access the online literature service of the NLM (www.pubmed.org) through the same graphical user interface.

13.6 User Participation: Reporting of Knowledge Gaps

The term "knowledge gap" has different meanings: Tichenor, Donohue and Olien used it already in the 1970s to denominate differences in knowledge between groups with different socio-economic status (Tichenor et al. 1970). In this publication, it means "area of lack of knowledge" and not the difference in knowledge between groups of individuals.

It was again David Sackett who pointed out the importance of identifying knowledge gaps when practicing and teaching EBM: He stated that "... to guide the learner in transforming knowledge gaps into well-built clinical questions" is one of four key steps in teaching how to ask questions for EBM (Straus et al. 2000). As the philosophy of EBM is the foundation of Suva's knowledge management efforts and namely the InWiM project, the skill in "transforming knowledge gaps into well-built (clinical) questions" is trained in the framework of continuous medical education and Suva doctors are encouraged to localise and report knowledge gaps.

However, asking clinical questions makes only sense if somebody will answer them. This answer is what we call a "knowledge solution". Knowledge solutions may vary in extent and comprehensiveness: Depending on the subject, they may answer simply a particular question or contain profound scientific treatises (e.g. evidence-based guidelines). Furthermore, a knowledge solution may cover only a certain aspect of a reported knowledge gap or answer more than one reported clinical question resulting in a somehow fuzzy n:m relation between knowledge gaps and knowledge solutions.

Over time, knowledge gap reports can become numerous in an enterprise with more than 200 users which makes it difficult to keep track of open, fully or partially answered questions, knowledge solutions under way etc. and their mutual dependencies. Facing the need of an appropriate management tool, the reporting and management process for knowledge gaps was modelled and a software module called "knowledge gap manager" was developed: Knowledge gaps are defined as entities identified and reported by employees with the help of a web based reporting tool. In order to facilitate further processing each reported knowledge gap allows for indexing with keywords according to its content. The same applies for knowledge solutions, where indexing with keywords is implemented as well. Given the full implementation of MeSH in the InWiM application, it was self-evident to use MeSH terms for indexing. However, with regard to knowledge gaps not all MeSH terms and features make sense. That is why MeSH terms where restricted to the "Disease Category" tree. This part of the MeSH index covers all diseases and allows mapping of issues to specific health problems.

13.7   Comparison and Outlook

InWiM has several innovative features: The cross-link feature is innovative not only because of the bidirectional link-up but also for the possibility to ad annotations. Main stream document repositories in general limit annotations to documents only.

As far as the authors are aware, InWiM is currently the only implementation worldwide – except for the NLM and its national representatives – which supports all MeSH features for in-house retrieval.

The same applies to the management of knowledge gaps: The InWiM knowledge management application is the first one with such functionality and a paragon is therefore missing. Compared to asking questions by email or phone, the solution has several advantages, especially with regard to the MeSH feature. This allows a "semantic capture" of an issue at the beginning of its life cycle, just when the corresponding question arises and facilitates handling at every further stage of processing: In particular it is possible to search and find knowledge gaps and solutions covering the same or a similar topic, thus allowing adequate collating and it prevents duplication of work. Furthermore, literature searches in the NLM (www.pubmed.org) are predefined and do not need every time to be reinvented from scratch.

The InWiM application is running now in Version 2.0. Current users include doctors and other healthcare professionals at Suva. It is planned to use InWiM not only as an intranet application but to open it for access over the internet in order to support professionals in inpatient and outpatient healthcare. Later, patients will also have access, thus making insurance medicine transparent and decisions understandable for lay persons.

Acknowledgments The authors would like to thank all the members of the project group for their work and valuable input: Klaus Bathke, Erich Bär, Viktor Bydzovsky, Fiorenzo Caranzano, Massimo Ermanni, Bruno Ettlin, Pius Feierabend, Roland Frey, Franziska Gebel, Carlo Gianella, Raphael Good, Ulrike Hoffmann-Richter, Roland Jäger, Sönke Johannes, Bertrand Kiener, Hans Kunz, Jürg Ludwig, Wolfgang Meier, Bettina Rosenthal, Jan Saner, Rita Schaumann-von Stosch, Felix Schlauri, Holger Schmidt, Fred Speck, Klaus Stutz, Benno Tobler, Felix Tschui, Walter Vogt.

References

Canadian Task Force on the Periodic Health Examination. (1979). The periodic health examination. *Canadian Medical Association Journal, 121*, 1193–1254.

Evidence-Based Medicine Working Group. (1992). Evidence-based medicine. A new approach to teaching the practice of medicine. *Journal of the American Medical Association, 268*, 2420–2425.

National Library of Medicine (2011). Fact Sheet. Medical Subject Headings (MeSH). National Library of Medicine. http://www.nlm.nih.gov/pubs/factsheets/mesh.html. Acessed 27 September 2011.

Oxford Centre for Evidence-based Medicine. (2009). Levels of evidence. http://www.cebm.net/index.aspx?o=1025. Accessed 27 September 2011.

Rehäuser, J., Krcmar, H., & Schreyögg, G. (1996). *Wissensmanagement in Unternehmen*. Berlin: Walter de Gruyter.

Sackett, D. L., Rosenberg, W. M. C., Gray, J. A. M., Haynes, R. B., & Richardson, W. S. (1996). Evidence-based medicine: What it is and what it isn't. *British Medical Association, 312*, 71–72.

Schreyögg, G., & Geiger, D. (2007). Wenn alles Wissen ist, ist Wissen am Ende nichts?! Vorschläge zur Neuorientierung des Wissensmanagements. In A. Zeuch (Ed.), *Management von Nichtwissen im Unternehmen*. Heidelberg: Carl Auer.

Steinmüller, W. (1993). *Informationstechnologie und Gesellschaft: Einführung in die Angewandte Informatik*. Darmstadt: Wissenschaftliche Buchgesellschaft.

Straus, S. E., Richardson, W. S., Rosenberg, W., Haynes, R. B., & Sackett, D. L. (2000). *Evidence-based medicine: How to practice and teach EBM* (2nd ed.). Edinburgh: Churchill Livingstone.

Tichenor, P. J., Donohue, G. A., & Olien, C. N. (1970). Mass media flow and differential growth in knowledge. *Public Opinion Quarterly, 34*, 159–170.

Von Krogh, G., & Koehne, M. (1998). Der Wissenstransfer in Unternehmen: Phasen des Wissenstransfers und wichtige Einflussfaktoren. *Die Unternehmung, 5*, 235–252.

Chapter 14
Patient Empowerment: A Two Way Road

Lodewijk Bos

Abstract This paper will deal with the patient related aspects of e-Health. The use of computing and networking has become an essential element in recent and future developments in health and care. Devices that lead to self-management, access to electronic records, decision support, social networks and social media are some of the major aspects.

The production and availability of data and information will lead to a paradigm shift in the physician-patient relationship based on the addition of their respective experiences. To make this into a relationship of trust requires insight into the needs of both patients and caregivers.

How do caregivers deal with possible knowledgeable patients; how can they assist to increase the patient's knowledge; how will they (have to) react to patient record access. On the other hand, what will be the responsibility of the knowledgeable patient; what are his rights to be informed.

Keywords Patient empowerment • Telemedicine • mHealt • EHR • Social media • eHealth

14.1 Introduction

In the context of this chapter it is important to look at definitions of the terms e-health and patient empowerment. Next we will take a closer look at the tools that are provided by e-health, namely the internet, electronic health records (EHRs) and digital homecare. Finally we will deal with the most important aspect of patient

L. Bos (✉)
President ICMCC,
Utrecht, The Netherlands
e-mail: lobos@icmcc.org

N. Wickramasinghe et al. (eds.), *Critical Issues for the Development*   203
of Sustainable E-health Solutions, Healthcare Delivery in the Information Age,
DOI 10.1007/978-1-4614-1536-7_14, © Springer Science+Business Media, LLC 2012

empowerment, information as access to relevant and adequate information is the first step to patient empowerment.

14.1.1 e-Health

One of the first definitions of e-health was given by Gunther Eysenbach in 2001:

> e-health is an emerging field in the intersection of medical informatics, public health and business, referring to health services and information delivered or enhanced through the Internet and related technologies. In a broader sense, the term characterizes not only a technical development, but also a state-of-mind, a way of thinking, an attitude, and a commitment for networked, global thinking, to improve health care locally, regionally, and worldwide by using information and communication technology. (Eysenbach 2001)

That there was a need for such a definition is shown by the fact that according to Google scholar, this article has been cited 286 times (Google Scholar 2010). In his article, Eysenbach mentions ten "e's which together perhaps best characterize what e-health is all about". One of those e's is:

> **Empowerment** of consumers and patients – by making the knowledge bases of medicine and personal electronic records accessible to consumers over the Internet, e-health opens new avenues for patient-centered medicine, and enables evidence-based patient choice.

By mentioning those 10 e's Eysenbach avoids doing what in 2005 Oh et al. do, taking the "e" as abbreviation of "electronic": electronic health. "we used the search query string *eHealth OR e-Health OR electronic health*" (Oh et al. 2005).

In 2005 Oh et al. and Pagliari et al. (2005) made overviews of the meaning of the word e-Health.

> Our analysis suggests that there is significant variability in the scope and focus of existing definitions of eHealth both within the research literature and relevant sources on the World Wide Web. In terms of its functional scope, most definitions conceptualize eHealth as a broad range of medical informatics applications for facilitating the management and delivery of health care. Purported applications include dissemination of health-related information, storage and exchange of clinical data, interprofessional communication, computer-based support, patient-provider interaction and service delivery, education, health service management, health communities, and telemedicine, among others.
>
> Overall, the definitions suggest a general excitement and optimism about the potential of this rapidly evolving field to improve health care processes and patient outcomes, and many clearly identify projected benefits such as improved clinical decision making, efficiency and safety. (Pagliari et al. 2005)

Oh et al. conclude with: "Questions remain about how the differing concepts and understandings of the term eHealth affect different stakeholders. What do people expect from eHealth? Do patients want eHealth? Do health care providers want eHealth? How does eHealth change the relationships, understandings, and interactions within the health care system? Time, patience, and further research will provide at least provisional answers to these questions, and to the myriad of questions still unasked" (Oh et al. 2005).

The focus within the use of the word e-Health remains mainly on non-patient stakeholders, very often application-driven (Wickramasinghe et al. 2005), albeit patient–related, either in chronic diseases, behavioural changes or health disparities (Lintonen et al. 2008; Ahern et al. 2006; Gibbons 2005).

For this chapter e-Health will be defined with an adaption from the 2001 definition by Eng (2001):

> The use of information and communications technology, especially the internet, to improve or enable health and healthcare.

14.1.2 Patient Empowerment

For years patient empowerment has been subject of thinking and research. First discussions started in the mid-1990s (Saltman 1994). In 2004, Salmon and Hall published a very interesting study on the subject with a somewhat skeptical view:

> We therefore suggest that, in imposing patient empowerment on clinical care, medicine unwittingly opposes patients' interests. The accounts of patients' perspective that are currently available suggest that patients do not generally embrace empowerment. In emphasizing research into how to empower patients at the expense of research into what patients feel like when they have been 'empowered', medicine paradoxically continues the tradition of assuming that 'doctor knows best'. Unless the balance of research is reversed, academic and political statements that 'patient empowerment … has put patients in charge of their medical destiny', or that 'by offering choice, patients will be given the chance to control their own destiny' will continue to construct a framework for clinical care that obfuscates rather illuminates patients' needs. (Salmon and Hall 2004)

Real definitions of patient empowerment are hard to find. "The term "patient empowerment" describes a situation that citizens are encouraged to take an active part in their own health management. Patient empowerment is considered as a philosophy of health care that proceeds from the perspective that optimal outcomes of health care interventions are achieved when patients become active participants in the health care process. It makes emphasis in the importance of individual involvement in health decision making." (Monteagudo and Moreno 2007)

Bos et al. have created a definition of patient empowerment taking into account the recent developments in the use of ICT, on which we will elaborate more in this chapter

> Patient 2.0 Empowerment is the active participation of the citizen in his or her health and care pathway with the interactive use of Information and Communication Technologies. (Bos et al. 2008)

14.2 Internet

Information and Communication Technology (ICT) has as one of its most important components the internet which in its turn has become one of the main drivers of e-health (Lupiáñez-Villanueva et al. 2009).

Building the first computers we never imagined that they would become the tool enabling one of the biggest shifts in society. It is comparable to the invention of the printing press which allowed common people to have access to the bible (and other texts) in the vernacular and to be independently informed, under the condition that you knew how to read.

The internet has opened the gates of information. But more important, being based on computer technology it is a two-way process. A typewriter does not allow you to read what you wrote a year ago from the machine itself; your (classical) TV set does not allow you to react to the news it brings you. The computer allows you to do just that through the internet; the individual has almost overnight become a both passive and active user. Although not yet seen by many, the internet could mean the end of the classical consumer, as the word consumer assumes intake-only.

So the internet allows us not only to consume information, but to add to it our own and, even more important, our own experience, the way persons act with and react to information. This will help people to realize that the basis of information is data. And the chip, the technology that allowed the creation of the computer, has enabled possibilities to gather data in unprecedented ways and quantities.

> All the actors in health care systems are facing the rise of the Network Society; a society whose social structure is made up of networks powered by microelectronic-based information and communication technologies, and a new technological paradigm: Informationalism, based on the augmentation of the human capacity for information processing and communication made possible by the revolution in microelectronics, software, and genetic engineering. (Lupiáñez-Villanueva et al. 2009)

The result of the above-mentioned developments is a society that has the ability to empower people, to iron out differences based on century old informational disparities. The new access to information also enables a new way of communication, helping people to realize that only in the rarest occasions their condition/problem is truly and a hundred percent unique, that there always is another person who has been or is in a similar situation able to help with their experience. And vice versa. Modern technology allows us to seek and hopefully find this person.

These new technologies will be of essential assistance in achieving a new perception in health and medicine, the patient as a partner in their health and wellbeing related processes by offering the citizen the tools to assume that position.

> Through secure and practical ICT based tools and services citizens can take greater control of their health: whether it be making an appointment online with their doctor, or getting a second opinion on test results, or learning how to take preventive measures to stay healthy. This is a feasible step and can make a real difference for the efficiency of health systems, and for patients' lives. (Kroes 2010)

Most will have read the above paragraphs assuming "internet" being used as a synonym to "World Wide Web". But they are not the same. "This is not a trivial distinction. Over the past few years, one of the most important shifts in the digital world has been the move from the wide-open Web to semiclosed platforms that use the Internet for transport but not the browser for display. It's driven primarily by the rise of the iPhone model of mobile computing, and it's a world Google can't crawl, one where HTML doesn't rule. And it's the world that consumers are increasingly choosing, not because they're rejecting the idea of the Web but because these dedicated platforms often just work better or fit better into their lives (the screen comes to them, they don't have to go to the screen). The fact that it's easier for companies to make money on these platforms only cements the trend. Producers and consumers agree: The Web is not the culmination of the digital revolution" (Anderson and Wolff 2010).

14.2.1 Web 2.0: Health 2.0

The interactive use of information creates the web as a platform combined with: the power to harness collective intelligence; users adding value; innovation in assembly (O'Reilly 2005). This phenomenon has become known as Web 2.0.

> What seems clear is that Web 2.0 brings people together in a more dynamic, interactive space. [...] Web 2.0 is primarily about the benefits of easy to use and free internet software. For example, blogs and wikis facilitate participation and conversations across a vast geographical expanse. Information pushing devices, like RSS feeds, permit continuous instant alerting to the latest ideas in medicine.
> The web is a reflection of who we are as human beings – but it also reflects who we aspire to be. In that sense, Web 2.0 may be one of the most influential technologies in the history of publishing, as old proprietary notions of control and ownership fall away. An expert (that is, doctor) moderated repository of the knowledge base, in the form of a medical wiki, may be the answer to the world's inequities of information access in medicine if we have the will to create one. (Giustini 2006)

The core elements of Web 2.0 are wikis, blogs and podcasts (Kamel et al. 2006) as well as social networks. They form ways to inform both patients and professionals.

Web 2.0 has been the start of a whole range of 2.0 concepts, amongst others Health 2.0.

> Health 2.0 defines the combination of health data and health information with (patient) experience through the use of ICT, enabling the citizen to become an active and responsible partner in his/her own health and care pathway. (Bos et al. 2008)

Although the "creation" and discussion on Health 2.0 started around 2008, it already has freed itself from its Web 2.0 roots and has the tendency, following the remarks by Anderson and Wolff (2010), to become an application driven world (Bos 2010).

14.3 Digital Homecare

Digital Homecare is a collection of services to deliver, maintain and improve care in the home environment using the latest ICT technology and devices. Assistive technology, telemedicine, mhealth, rehabilitation, are all contained within digital homecare. (Yogesan et al. 2009)

> Digital homecare is now finding its way into patients' and clients' homes. It is a new form of care provision. It bridges the distance between the client/patient and his care providers,

both in terms of spatial distance and in terms of distance in time. This new form of care enables the client/patient to remain at home, and yet receive good quality care. Another benefit of digital homecare is that it allows the demand for care to be satisfied at an afford-able price. (Meijer 2009)

Ensuring the patient to be able to stay home during his cure and care process as much as possible has multiple benefits. Research has shown that patients recover quicker when receiving home care in a familiar environment (Rahme et al. 2010); for elderly it is not advisable to transfer them into an unfamiliar environment (Gaßner and Conrad 2010); financial benefits are also considerable (CBI 2009).

14.3.1 Telemedicine

Literally thousands of studies have been published on the use of telemedicine for all kinds of chronic diseases, assistive technologies and monitoring of cure processes. Many of those show the benefits of the use of telemedicine. In primary care the appli-cation of teleconsultation is a good example, especially in rural areas, as it allows the GP to "move" the point-of-care to the patient's home at the same time providing the GP with access to specialist knowledge. "In the most common situation (613 out of the 927 requests), GPs usually would have prescribed a visit to the patient. However, after teleconsultation, only seven appointments were actually required in order to better evaluate the patients' conditions through a face-to-face visit. The majority of these specialist consultations implied a lower need of hospital resources. In 397 cases, no actions were indicated, with a consequent relevant cost saving. On the contrary, six patients effectively needed hospitalisation and 22 patients were in such critical conditions requiring urgent admission to EDs." (Zanaboni et al. 2009)

Other areas in which telemedicine is quickly gaining importance are dermatol-ogy (van der Heijden et al. 2010), psychiatry (García-Lizana and Muñoz-Mayorga 2010) and stroke (Johansson and Wild 2010).

Still, there seems to be a limited use of these new resources and technologies (Whitten et al. 2010). "Our research indicates that the needs of patients are not or not fully met by ICT instruments offered by caregivers. From a patient's perspective it means fewer possibilities in self-management of his illness.

The institutionalised care organizations are not equipped to tackle the escalating chronic disease burden or health issues which might prevent such diseases through encouraging different lifestyles. A new approach is needed in the co-operation of caregiver and patient: the co-creation of health.

Co-creation of health leads to a different way in health service delivery. The design of systems, the content needed, the approach in using these resources all have to be changed.

Only by doing all of the aforementioned items one can truly speak of Patient Empowerment as it is meant to be" (Meijer and Ragetlie 2007). "An important sug-gested reason is the lack of a mature legal framework for the accountability in a distributed and high-technology-based healthcare system, which new organizational and social elements. The distance between e-health promises and reality of the majority of e-health systems is other relevant argued cause. Near all commercial and even research systems present serious functional deficiencies, such as a poor interoperability and non-accomplishment of information standards and normalization of codes" (Prado-Velasco et al. 2009).

14.3.2   Sensors

Sensors have been essential in the improvement of monitoring technology.

Pills that contain a sensor can be combined with sms technology to send relevant conditional information to physicians (Bruce 2007).

"Smart clothing", i.e. the convergence of leading-edge textiles design and manu-facture with a combination of communications, computing and sensor technologies (Manning and Kun 2009) offers a completely different way of independent living and self-management. These wearables can be used to monitor bodily functions (Gravitz 2010), in fall-risk detection (Giansanti et al. 2009) or as walking assistance for Parkinson patients (Bächlin et al. 2010).

But it can and will also bring some relief to hospitals: "Wearable technology may provide an integral part of the solution for providing health care to a growing world population that will be strained by a ballooning aging population. By providing a means to conduct telemedicine – the monitoring, recording, and transmission of physiological signals from outside of the hospital – wearable technology solutions could ease the burden on health-care personnel and use hospital space for more emergent or responsive care" (Rutherford 2010).

14.3.3   mHealth

The development of mobile technologies, more specific health applications for cell and smart phones (mHealth) have changed the outlook for telemedicine and digital homecare (mHealth Initiative).

The increasing use of cellphones makes them a growingly important tool for health. Text messaging has become a major communication feature, as 72% of adults and 87% of teen users in the US text (Lenhart 2010). It is used in many appli-cations already, be it for asthma control (Prabhakaran et al. 2010), medication adherence (Merrill 2010) or for checking the quality of drugs in developing coun-tries (Cheng 2010).

A 6 month study at the George Washington University (USA), starting May 2010, Dr. Neal Sikka looked at the accuracy of wound diagnostics with the aid of cellphone images. In this study, "researchers recruit people who have arrived at the hospital with cuts, skin infections, rashes and other flesh wounds." Patients use their own camera phones to document their injuries. After filling out a questionnaire about their medical history and symptoms, they send the images to a secure e-mail account. All images are downloaded and stored on a secure hard drive.

"We'll look at their picture along with the questionnaire and make a diagnosis," Sikka said. Researchers use a PC to zoom in and focus on specific parts of the photo. Then the doctor will see the patient to see if the cellphone diagnosis was accurate.

"The initial data is encouraging," Sikka said. "The study will continue through October, but so far, he says, about 90 percent of diagnoses are accurate. Sikka said camera phones with at least three megapixels, autoflash and autofocus work well" (Tamura 2010).

However in more serious cases like skin cancer diagnoses, "for the important subgroup of malignant pigmented lesions, both diagnostic and management accuracy of teledermatology was generally inferior to clinic dermatology and up to 7 of 36 index melanomas would have been mismanaged via teledermatology" (Warshaw et al. 2009). Nevertheless, "evidence is continuing to gather which proves its position in a supportive role both to primary care and in enabling timely and appropriate treatment to our patients as part of a fully integrated service" (Halpern 2010).

14.4   Social Networks

Social networks are an elementary part of Web 2.0 and especially Health 2.0. Web 2.0 is often used interchangeably with "social media" or "user-generated content" (Spallek et al. 2010). They exist for professionals, like SERMO in the USA (with a membership of 115,000 physicians) (Sermo 2010), for patients, e.g. PatientsLikeMe but more general networks like Facebook or Twitter also allow active exchanges between the two groups and sharing of experience and satisfaction which "could be a quality improvement or accountability experiment, the results of which may be broadcast to others via knowledge-sharing sessions with patients and provider organizations." (Born et al. 2009)

> Professionals are connected to the Internet and make an intensive use of it, mainly for questions related to the search and consultation of information. The use of the Internet as a communication tool with other health care professionals is widespread, but it is still unusual to communicate with patients or to produce health information for them. The increase of the information flow available on the Internet has not been accompanied by an increase of the interaction which is still constricted to face-to-face meetings. In spite of this, most professionals positively value the relevance of the contents available on the Internet and they do not consider that the patient's search for information is negative either for the professional–patient relationship, for health outcomes or for patients' health management. However, just a very small percentage of professionals recommend their patients to consult health information on the Internet or even talk about the Internet during face-to-face meetings. Furthermore, results suggest that also a small percentage of patients are pushing the use of the Internet in their relationship with the health care professional. (Lupiáñez-Villanueva et al. 2009)

Especially patient networks are seen as important sources of information and research and as valuable representation of the growing concept of e-patients.

However, numbers do not support the immense buzz about these patient internet groups.

PatientsLikeMe is a well-known organization within the US health 2.0 scene. It is even considered one of the leading online communities. Nevertheless, only 79,000 people have joined the community, worldwide, 41,000 of them in the US (PatientsLikeMe 2010). The fact that they say to focus on less common diseases (although chronic fatigue syndrome and HIV don't seem to fit those criteria) cannot be the explanation of those relatively low numbers, nor their policy on how they deal with data (PatientsLikeMe Facebook 2010).

Nevertheless, these networks can become a very important element in the support of people with so called orphan diseases. In the words of one of the leading Australian economists, Nicholas Gruen: "It enables people to identify their symptoms and their disease and go into a data rich environment in which they keep a record of their medications and can also be put in touch with all sorts of people with similar conditions. This creates obvious human social benefits, which has been done on the net before but it also creates a completely alternative set of possibilities" (Sweet 2010). Chronic diseases are covered relatively well, both in available information and networks. Rare diseases however are not despite the large numbers of people involved, either as patient or as relative. "Rare diseases affect a limited number of individuals (defined as no more than one in 2000 individuals in the European Union and no more than about one in 1,250 in the USA), but the number of disorders that fit this definition is very large (>5,000 according to WHO). Therefore, the number of patients affected by a rare disease could be about 30 million in Europe and 25 million in North America. The true burden of rare diseases in Europe and elsewhere is difficult to estimate, since epidemiological data for most of these diseases are not available." (Schieppati et al. 2008)

> With social media we can aggregate across space and across the world and create a safe environment for support. Although there may be only 10 people in greater New York with a certain disease, there may be 250 people across the world.[1] (Chen 2009)

Nonetheless, first signs of the importance of online communities become apparent. In 2007 the anti-diabetic drug Avandia (GlaxoSmithKline) was associated with a significant increase in the risk of myocardial infarction and with an increase in the risk of death from cardiovascular causes that had borderline significance (Nissen and Wolski 2007). A new report (2010) says patients began discussing the risks of GlaxoSmithKline diabetes drug Avandia in online forums and blogs well before a meta-analysis linked it to higher heart-attack risk (Iskowitz 2010).

Recent research indicates that so-called clustered online social networks can influence behavioral changes and therefore promote good health practices people are quicker to change when they hear the message from more than one source (Centola 2010; Reuters 2010).

---

[1] Observation by Dr. Sand, Beth Israel Deaconess Medical Center in Boston, MA.

14.5 Social Media

Another aspect of Web 2.0 is the rise of the so-called social media. Social media are defined as: "a group of Internet-based applications that build on the ideological and technological foundations of Web 2.0, and that allow the creation and exchange of user-generated content" (Kaplan and Haenlein 2010). The best known examples are Facebook and Twitter, but also phenomena like blogs and wikis are part of it.

These new forms of communications have the potential to enhance exchange of information and ideas between the various stakeholders in health. Much so, that in 2009 a strong discussion has emerged whether medical professionals and their patients should "be-friend" on *Facebook* (Jain 2009; Pho 2010). These new media show a novel approach towards privacy and openness from all and any user. "The rapid growth and accessibility of social networking websites has fundamentally changed the way people manage information about their personal and professional lives. In particular, it has been suggested that interaction in virtual communities erodes elements of responsibility, accountability and social trust that build tradition-ally meaningful communities. The purpose of this study was to investigate how undergraduate medical students use the social network website Facebook, and to identify any unprofessional behaviour displayed online. [...] The majority of respon-dents did have a Facebook account and admitted there were photos they found embarrassing on the site. Over half of the respondents reported they had seen unpro-fessional behaviour by their colleagues on Facebook. Although students say that they are aware of the UK's General Medical Council (GMC) guidance, unprofes-sional behaviour is still demonstrated on the site" (Garner and O'Sullivan 2010).

Twitter, famous for its short communications and the ability to tag the messages, is increasingly considered a data mining source, to "be used to gather important real-time health data by creating a 'mashup,' which combines health status updates with location-based information. To track outbreaks, for example, it would be rela-tively easy for a health organization to enable people to submit Twitter status updates with symptoms and location data using a predefined format so that the updates are machine readable and easily mapped" (Scanfeld et al. 2010).

Blogs can be important tools in supplying health information. David Colquhoun, professor of pharmacology at University College London is quoted to have said: "On a blog I can just give my view. It's obviously that – and people can take it or leave it. Also, bloggers often seem to be better at investigative journalism than jour-nalists are. All sorts of facts about dodgy practices appear on blogs long before they reach the regular magazines or papers; that is both fun and useful, I think. [...] Blogs are an enormous step towards real democracy, though the price for that is that every madman and quack can do the same. Indeed, that is what makes it so impor-tant for people with knowledge, expertise, and honesty to fight back and draw a line in the sand at the tide of nonsense that engulfs us. The papers don't fulfil that role at all well – and in fact often exacerbate it." (Coombes 2007)

But not only professionals do blog. Patients do as well. Unfortunately there is hardly any research done on the subject of blogging patients. A search for "blog

AND patient" in PubMed delivers six results (11 September 2010). However it is safe to assume, that most blogs by patients deal with their experiences related to either their condition(s) or their caregiver/care facility. These blogs should play an essential role as narrative addition to EHRs or as ODL (see below).

Finally we have a short look at *wikis*. "A wiki is a website that allows the easy creation and editing of any number of interlinked web pages via a web browser using a simplified markup language or a WYSIWYG text editor. Wikis are typically powered by wiki software and are often used to create collaborative wiki websites, to power community websites, for personal note taking, in corporate intranets, and in knowledge management systems" (Wiki 2010). Wikis have always been subject of discussion. "Wikipedia's medical entries – as has been reported with other entries on other issues – are not reliable for the simple fact that they are prone to manipulation, as is all Wikipedia content" (Pho 2009). "Basically, because of the openness and rapidity that wiki pages can be edited, the pages undergo an evolutionary selection process not unlike that which nature subjects to living organisms. "Unfit" sentences and sections are ruthlessly culled, edited and replaced if they are not considered "fit", which hopefully results in the evolution of a higher quality and more relevant page. Whilst such openness may invite "vandalism" and the posting of untrue information, this same openness also makes it possible to rapidly correct or restore a "quality" wiki page" (Kamel et al. 2006).

In 2010 research indicates that Wikipedia is achieving a relatively high level of reliability (Friedlin and McDonald 2010; Rajagopalan et al. 2010; Leithner et al. 2010).

14.6   Electronic Health Records

An EHR is a container of links to all medical information about the citizen stored at hospitals, GP practices, pharmacies, independent lab and exam facilities, etc. (the Electronic *Medical* Records), together with the input from devices and paramedics. In addition, the citizen must be able to add his input (comments, over-the-counter-drug use, lifestyle, etc.), to make corrections as well as to decide who is going to see which part of his data and if/how his de-identified data will be used. These two elements (medical and patient provided) combined create an Electronic *Health* Record (Bos et al. 2008).

What differentiates an EHR from an EMR is the fact that patients can add their own information. Only when medical data are combined with the physician's observations and decision as well as the patient's experience, an EHR becomes meaningful and a part of the Web 2.0 concept.

EHRs can play an important role ensuring the patient with supply of information that is at the same time relevant, trustworthy and comprehensible. In the words of Wiljer et al.: "This study suggests that providing patients with access to their personal health information through a PHR may have a positive impact on their experience. Other studies have demonstrated that providing patients with access to personal health information online is feasible. Studies have also suggested that providing patients with access to this information online has the potential to reduce the time that patients wait for results, to empower patients to better manage their care, to improve decision making and to improve communication between health care providers and patients. At the same time, concerns have been raised about the potential harm that this access could have on patients and their families. The concerns range from patients accessing information without understanding the clinical significance of the results, to misunderstanding the information, and receiving bad news without the appropriate clinical or educational support, causing anxiety and undue distress for patients and providers alike. The results from this study suggest that providing access to personal health information may not impact negatively on patient anxiety" (Wiljer et al. 2010).

It remains questionable how effective access to EHRs/PHRs or patient portals is. At the Australian Health e-Nation Conference in 2010, Morton Elbaek Petersen, chief executive of Denmark's ehealth portal, said that, with 80% having secure access to their own EHR, only 10% of the population actually log into the system to access their personal electronic healthcare records (Gliddon 2010). In the UK access to the Summary Care Record and the use of the online personal health organizer HealthSpace had been disappointingly low (Greenhalgh et al. 2010). In 2008 it was reported that 40,000 patients at Beth Israel Deaconess have PHRs, but only 42 patients have added any information to those files (Vesely 2008).

14.7   Health Information

Web 2.0 is the logical consequence of the societal move from the information to the knowledge society that started early in the first decennium of the twenty-first century. Knowledge, defined by information + experience, can be created through the new tools that now enable citizens, i.e. patients to communicate their experiences.

> While knowledge is one of the keys to forming a Partnership of Trust, another is the possession of the skills necessary to apply that knowledge for the benefit of the partnership. Many of the required skills may already be possessed and practiced by the partners – honesty, candour, tact, discretion, courtesy and mutual respect. Others may need to be developed. Patients, for example, may need to gain the confidence to ask questions of the doctor if he or she does not understand what is being explained about the condition, its cause, effects or treatment. When patients feel trusted by the doctor, patients are more ready to express their worries without being concerned about being disbelieved or dismissed as being silly. In addition to this, an informed patient, after some discussion of the condition with the doctor, may feel it necessary to question the conclusions reached by the doctor. In this circumstance, courtesy and tact will be particularly important on the part of the patient when raising the issue and the doctor who responds to it. Both need to recognise that it is possible and legitimate to disagree without the intrusion of any tension or offence between them. (Hannan and Webber 2007)

Since Hannan introduced his partnership of trust concept, a new term has become popular, Participatory Health, "a cooperative model of health care that encourages and expects active involvement by all connected parties (patients, caregivers, healthcare professionals, etc.) as integral to the full continuum of care. The 'participatory' concept

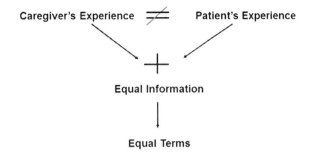

Fig. 14.1 Partnership on equal terms

may also be applied to fitness, nutrition, mental health, end-of-life care, and all issues broadly related to an individual's health." (Society for Participatory Medicine).

The basics of these concepts are sharing and trust. Sharing of information, data, experience and a mutual trust based on that sharing. Of course, the caregiver's experience differs from the patient's, however they have to share those experiences to come to a real partnership, a partnership on equal terms (Fig. 14.1).

This can only be achieved by sharing the same data and therefore the same information. The patient's search for information is driven by curiosity about his own condition. They therefore need access to their own data, the same data that are available to their care provider i.e. their own EHR.

> Medical knowledge is becoming increasingly specialised and there is an inevitable 'competence gap' between medical doctors and their patients. Through online information sources, citizens can to some extent bridge this 'competence gap' by informing themselves about disease prevention and healthy lifestyles, various health problems and treatment options. This can have an empowering effect and allow patients to exercise a certain degree of choice. (ESDIS 2006)

> As health care moves towards a patient-centered model and information becomes an integral part of health care, information integration becomes a critical point. People should have easy access to their own medical records and to any information they need in order to make decisions about their own health care. This constitutes a great challenge at the moment, which requires a means to interconnect and interrelate information from various sources which are relevant to one person and create a personal virtual health space containing links to all the health information a person owns or is interested in. (Karkalis and Koutsouris 2006)

An important element is the fact that the user is actively searching for information, especially in the field of health information. Obtaining information from the Web is often the basis for making health decisions and is thus an influential force.

> While the percentage of adults who go online (79%) has not changed significantly for several years, the proportion of those who are online and have ever used the Internet to look for health information has increased to 88% this year, the highest number ever.

- Fully 81% of all Cyberchondriacs[2] have looked for health information online in the last month. And 17% have gone online to look for health information ten or more times in the last month. On average, Cyberchondriacs do this about 6 times a month.

---

[2] Cyberchondriacs: people using the Internet to look for information about health topics [Harris].

- Very few Cyberchondriacs are dissatisfied with their ability to find what they want online. Only 9% report that they were somewhat (6%) or very (3%) unsuccessful. And only 8% believe that the information they found was unreliable.
- Just over half (53%) of all Cyberchondriacs report that they have discussed information they found online with their doctors.
- Half (51%) of all Cyberchondriacs say they have searched for information on the Internet based on discussions with their doctors. (The Harris Poll #95 2010).

These numbers are for the United States. They may differ considerably when looking at other countries. In Spain, 53.8% of those who are online look for health-related information[3] (Sevillano 2010).

As the above numbers show this kind of self-education is becoming increasingly important and offers a significant opportunity for patients to become actively engaged in their own care (Bos 2007). During the pre-Internet era, medical information was published in medical textbooks and journals only, whereas patients can now gain access to citations of more than 20 million (bio)medical articles online (Pubmed). Indeed, many patients are now helping to inform their doctors on the latest research and treatments. In 2001 Gerber and Eiser postulated that the Internet age offers opportunities to improve the patient–doctor relationship by sharing the burden of responsibility for knowledge. They also underlined the necessity for research to identify the effects on the patient–doctor relationship, as well as the effects on patient and doctor satisfaction and on health outcomes especially since healthguides[4] provides a common set of clinically based guidelines (Gerber and Eiser 2001).

In 2005, Blanch et al. concluded that "First, although the Internet has not replaced physicians as the primary source of medical or health information for patients, patients trust the Internet as an additional information source and would like their physicians to recommend specific websites. This observation strongly supports the Information Rx project from the American College of Physicians and MedlinePlus, which is providing physicians with pre-printed prescriptions with checkboxes to help physicians recommend reputable websites to their patients. Second, patients report that health searches on the Internet help to decrease anxiety, improve understanding and doctor–patient communication, and have had a positive effect overall on the doctor–patient relationship. Though doctors show some concern that searching the Internet is a sign of low trust in the provider, patient responses do not bear that out. Doctors and patients differ greatly on their problem-specific fund of knowledge. Many physicians do not communicate clearly, due to time constraints and differences in education level, which can strain the doctor–patient relationship. The Internet allows patients to have

[3] El 53.8% de los internautas hace búsquedas relacionadas con temas de salud y bienestar, según datos de 2009 del Instituto Nacional de Estadística (INE).

[4] The Map of Medicine represents the state of the art in health 1.0. The map, intended for clinical use, is a web-based visual representation of evidence-based patient care journeys covering 28 medical specialties and 387 pathways. A patient version of the map, called Healthguides, is now being created by more than 500 doctors and nurses to give patients the same in-depth clinical information as used in the NHS, in easy to follow charts. http://www.mapofmedicine.com/.

some of their questions answered that were not addressed during visits, which seems to be generally good for the doctor–patient relationship. Third, better studies need to be performed, with more robust methods." (Blanch et al. 2005)

The access to health information on the WWW causes a change in the patient-health professional relationship. "Until recently, many health professionals felt that patients were unable to cope with bad news and should be therefore kept ignorant of many details of their illness. However, with the easy access and availability of information through the Internet many patients are no longer satisfied with this attitude. They want to be fully informed and be part of the treatment decision making." (McMullen 2006)

> Physicians perceived it as good that Internet-informed patients generally have better knowledge of health-related issues. This increased knowledge made it easier for them to begin an interaction about health-related problems. Moreover physicians reported that they discuss health-related issues on a more elaborate level with Internet informed patients compared to other patients.[ ] Physicians considered consultations with Internet-informed patients problematic if patients insisted on an inadequate interpretation of Internet information. In some cases physicians were confronted with patients who tried to validate their irrational view while ignoring the physician's expertise. In these situations physicians tried to explain the correct interpretation of the health-related Internet information, which was described as a time-consuming procedure.[ ] Physicians have experienced a change in their professional role in recent years since the introduction of health-related Internet information during consultations. This role can be described as a partner of the patient, who is nowadays more involved in the consultation and in medical decisions. (Sommerhalder et al. 2009)

A Capstrat-Public Policy Poll from as recent as April 2010 confirms that physicians are still the main source of information (Capstrat 2010) (Fig. 14.2).

Wiljer et al. 2010 also state that 86% of participants 'agreed' or 'strongly agreed' that having reliable information approved from the hospital would make them feel more able to make decisions about their treatment and disease (Wiljer et al. 2010).

However, the internet delivers information in abundance and its quality can be disputed.

> In 2005, the criteria perceived as the most important indicators of quality and usefulness for health Web sites among non-professional and professional groups of users: (1) availability of information, (2) ease of finding information/navigation, (3) trustworthiness/credibility and (4) accuracy of information. Both non-professional and professional users, in Europe and the USA, favor academic/university sites (89.4%, n = 1,403) and sites sponsored by medical journals (88.9%, n = 1,394), closely followed by government agencies (86.1%, n = 1,395). We have also observed that a significant number of Web users, about 25% of a sample of 1,386 persons from all over the world, lack confidence in sites sponsored by pharmaceutical manufacturers and commercial, mainstream media organizations. (http://www.hon.ch/Survey/Survey2005/res.html)

> In this regard, it remains important to continue research on how individual patients and their families use the web, and increasingly, interactive and social web applications, for health-related purposes. What information, in its different forms, is retrieved and created in this changing online environment and how is this information further combined with information from other sources in order to aid individual decision-making? Research should also address differences in use of applications between different types of patients, and between patients and professionals. Finally, it is important to pay more attention to how institutions and physicians can better utilize these web applications to provide information environments that further support improved health for their patient populations. (Adams 2010)

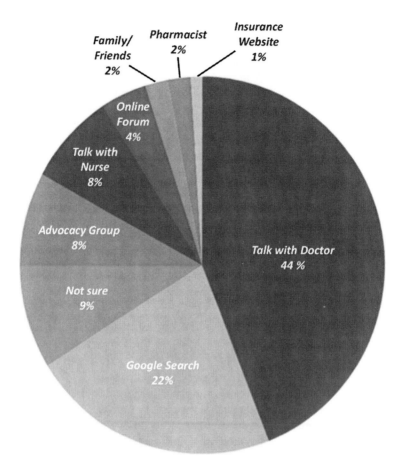

Fig. 14.2 Percentage of respondents ranking the following sources as the most influential source the last time they sought health information (Capstrat-Public Policy Poll, April 2010)

But also for health professionals the abundance of information has become a burden. A poll in 2010 shows that professionals rely ever more on non-scientific information but do focus on online information specifically targeted towards them, like MedScape (PrNewswire 2010).

14.7.1 Information Therapy

To achieve an optimal exchange of information, a physician should supply his patient with information, a principle called Information Therapy (Ix): "the prescription of the right information to the right person at the right time as part of the process of care. The concept changes the role of consumer health information from one where information is "about" the patient's care to one in which the information is a key part of care. It is part of the therapy, and hence the name information therapy. An Ix is relevant, specific information for each patient's moment in care. For short, we call each information prescription an 'Ix' just as a medication prescription is generally known as an 'Rx'" (Kemper et al. 2010).

Coberly et al.: "The findings suggest that patients respond favorably to a physician-directed, condition-specific email prescription, initiated in the context of a routine clinic visit, that relies on health information from a comprehensive Internet-based resource (such as MedlinePlus). Patients who reported they visited the Internet site and used MedlinePlus were satisfied with the health information they received and were enthusiastic about its future use. Further strategies are needed to encourage patients to 'fill' an information prescription, to clarify specific targeted Internet sites, and to integrate information prescriptions into a provider's workflow to ensure compliance" (Coberly et al. 2010).

14.7.2 Observations of Daily Living

Another aspect is the direct data input from the patient (ODL). "Observations of daily living (ODLs) are recordings that people make of selected activities and events that occur in the course of their day. Collecting and using ODL data – information on sleep, diet, exercise, mood, adherence to medication regimens – is an area of PHR development that is genuinely user-directed, both in the kind of information that is contained in the record and the health-related activities that stem from it" (Project HealthDesign 2009). "Thanks to smartphones and wireless monitoring devices, experts say, it is getting much easier to capture such data and summarize it in easy-to-read graphics and charts for patients and physicians" (Landro 2010). As mentioned before, patient blogs should be considered as well.

However, all these acquired data need to be stored. The ideal place would be an EHR, as these observational data (either machine or human produced) can then be combined with clinical data and medical observations. To manage these data and, in case of data provided by devices directly to select them, knowledge management and biostatistics will become important areas of research and application.

Especially in areas like orphan diseases but also in public health, the management and (secondary, anonymized) use of these data is extremely important. "In other fields – genetics, banking and retailing – data management is a valuable skill. People are trained and develop careers in the field. In public health research, data management is the poor cousin of analysis. Undervalued and underfunded, inadequate data management undermines the rest of the scientific enterprise. One review in the United Kingdom of Great Britain and Northern Ireland found that many of the variables collected in epidemiological studies were never cleaned and coded, so they could not be used even by the primary researchers, let alone shared. In complex population-based surveys in developing countries, data management and analysis skills are in even shorter supply, so a higher proportion of data probably goes to waste" (Pisani and AbouZahr 2010).

Although Pisani and AbouZahr focus their article on data from researchers and governments, this will be increasingly applicable to physicians and especially patients as either or both will become "owners" of the data contained in EHRs. The same is true for the "output" from online communities like PatientsLikeMe.

14.8   Conclusion

"Remember being empowered is a state of mind, the internet is a tool on that journey" (http://twitter.com/ReginaHolliday/status/24337346433 2010). This was a tweet (Twitter message) from Regina Holliday,[5] one of the leading voices in the US patient empowerment movement. And of course she is absolutely right.

This chapter has shown which key elements and developments form the basis of e-health and the tools for patient empowerment. But it has also tried to make clear the enormous challenges that go with these new developments. If applied correctly, these developments can be of help in creating patient empowerment, however, the state of mind is one of the essential elements. Not only that of the patient but also from the care-provider.

The internet will be an important tool in diminishing digital and literacy divides, however creating a new divide at the same time. The acceptance of these new technologies is a generational thing. Children currently grow up with the presence of the internet and all the tools that come with it. For them there is no existence without their cellphones, their social networks (Ärzte-Zeitung 2010). They do have a different view of what privacy is due to their growing up with networks like Facebook and living with computers with camcorders. They will be more open about sharing experiences.

The generation of their parents and grandparents are the big social challenge for patient empowerment. They will have to learn to deal with these new "technical" developments. We have seen that the elderly increasingly use cellphones. They use Facebook, Skype to contact their grandchildren. The generations of the parents are great adopters of cellphones and increasingly of smartphones. Work is becoming dependent on connectivity, availability of internet. That's also the case of the health professional. New toys/tools like iPhone and iPad and their applications are rapidly becoming very popular in medical circles (Blankenhorn 2010) and medical education (White 2010).

However, there is more to patient empowerment than embracing technological innovation. To achieve true patient empowerment we will have to change attitudes. The ease of access to information has caused a major shift in the way we want to have access to our own. When we start sharing our experiences, reading about our conditions we want to base ourselves on the only data that really are important; our own data. Patient empowerment got an enormous boost in the United States with the

---

[5] http://reginaholliday.blogspot.com/.

heartfelt outcry by that other patient empowerment advocate Dave deBronkart (e-patient Dave)[6]: "Gimme my damn data!" (deBronkart 2009).

The paradigm shift that access to data will cause is enormous. We will have to train health professionals how to deal with (seemingly) knowledgeable patients. Discussions about ownership of data are already in full swing.

We will have to make patients realize that the information they search might come from not so reliable sources. We will have to develop new ethical standards, patients are no consumers, even if we promote choice by creating rating sites (doctors, hospitals). How are we going to deal with the fact that we know where we can get the best treatment (both cure and care) but will not be able to pay or be financially covered for it?

We will have to take a different perspective on technology. The amount of data we will have to deal with in the future will grow exponentially, also (especially?) in health. Monitoring devices, blogs, tweets, networks, all creators of data considered "ours" and possibly influential in the way we deal with our cure and care path and definitely important in changing our lifestyles in a preventative way. How to handle these data will become a growing concern for those dealing with (bio)statistics and knowledge management.

To be able to exchange the data and the information/knowledge derived from it we will have to agree on standards, global standards (global as in cross-border). It will be impossible to create "risk-free" information but we can at least make an effort. Simply Googling "obesity" does certainly not bring a guaranteed high quality result. Properly standardizing and coding elements contained in Electronic Health Records (SNOMED CT, ICD10, etc.) are essential. Recent developments indicate decisive moves in that direction (Monegain 2010; Ingram 2010). Semantic and ontological standards will be another necessary step that is getting more attention (Bos et al. 2010). By doing so we could and should be able to use our EHR as input for information search (Bos et al. 2008).

Patient empowerment will change. For the next three to four decades we will have to deal with making those who did not grow up with internet technology aware of its possibilities, realizing that many of them do not want to deal with the consequences. Many, in the beginning even the majority of patients will not want to live according to these new concepts. They still want their doctors to be in charge, they will not want to be "in the driver's seat" or be responsible for their health data. At the same time as our society will become more internet-based patient empowerment might need to focus on changing views on privacy (Manning and Benton 2010).

In 2004 ICMCC created the term compunetics, the social, societal and ethical consequences of the use of computing and networking[7]. It might become the scientific base of patient empowerment.

---

[6] http://epatientdave.com/.

[7] www.icmcc.org.

References

[Online] Available from http://twitter.com/ReginaHolliday/status/24337346433. Accessed September 8, 2010.

9th "Health on the net survey of health and medical online use" [Online] Available from http://www.hon.ch/Survey/Survey2005/res.html. Accessed September 3, 2010.

Adams, S. A. (Jun 2010). Revisiting the online health information reliability debate in the wake of "web 2.0": An inter-disciplinary literature and website review. *International Journal of Medical Informatics, 79*(6), 391–400.

Ahern, D. K., Kreslake, J. M., & Phalen, J. M. (Mar 2006). What is eHealth (6): Perspectives on the evolution of eHealth research. *Journal of Medical Internet Research, 8*(1), e4. Available from http://www.jmir.org/2006/1/e4/. Accessed August 29, 2010.

Anderson, C., & Wolff, M. (Sep 2010). *Wired Magazine.* [Online] Available from http://www.wired.com/magazine/2010/08/ff_webrip/all/1. Accessed September 5, 2010.

Ärzte-Zeitung. (Sep 2010). Studie: Online ist für Jugendliche wichtigstes Leitmedium. [Online] Available from http://www.aerztezeitung.de/panorama/default.aspx?sid=618646. Accessed September 10, 2010.

Bächlin, M., Plotnik, M., Roggen, D., Giladi, N., Hausdorff, J. M., & Tröster, G. (2010). A wearable system to assist walking of Parkinson's disease patients. *Methods of Information in Medicine, 49*(1), 88–95.

Blanch, D., Sciamanna, C., Lawless, H., & Diaz, J. (2005). *The Journal on Information Technology in Healthcare, 3*(3), 179–201. Available from http://www.hl7.org.tw/jith/pdf/JITH_Volume_3,_Issue_3.pdf#page=43. Accessed September 1, 2010.

Blankenhorn, D. (Aug 2010). The iPad makes its first hospital rounds. *ZDNet healthcare.* [Online] Available from http://www.zdnet.com/blog/healthcare/the-ipad-makes-its-first-hospital-rounds/3880. Accessed August 2, 2010.

Born, K., Rizo, C., & Seeman, N. (2009). Participatory storytelling online: A complementary model of patient satisfaction. *Electronic Healthcare, 8*(2), e3–e8.

Bos, L. (2007). Medical and care compunetics the future of patient-related ICT. In L. Bos & B. Blobel (Eds.), *Medical and care compunetics 4* (pp. 3–17). Amsterdam: IOS Press. Available from http://www.icmcc.org/pdf/bosios2007.pdf

Bos, L., Blobel, B., Benton, S., & Carroll, D. (Eds.), *Medical and care compunetics 6.* See section Knowledge representation and Ontologies. Amsterdam: IOS Press.

Bos, L. (Apr 2010). *Europe's Health 2.0.* ICMCC Blog. [Online] Available from http://blog.icmcc.org/2010/04/10/europes-health-2-0/. Accessed September 2, 2010.

Bos, L., Marsh, A., Carroll, D., Gupta, S., & Rees, M. (2008). Patient 2.0 empowerment. In H. R. Arabnia & A. Marsh (Eds.), *Proceedings of the 2008 international conference on semantic web & web services SWWS08* (pp. 164–167), Las Vegas.

Bruce, S. (Aug 2007). Pill that texts trialled in UK. *eHealth insider.* [Online] Available from http://www.e-health-insider.com/news/6165/pill_that_texts_trialled_in_uk. Accessed August 17, 2010.

Capstrat. (2010). *Health care information – Where do you go? Who do you trust?* [Online] Available from http://www.capstrat.com/elements/downloads/files/health-care-information-where-do-you-go-who-do-you-trust.pdf. Accessed September 3, 2010.

CBI. (Oct 2009). Doing more with less. Available from http://www.cbi.org.uk/ndbs/Press.nsf/38e2a44440c22db6802567300067301b/f2aa76202344d1a880257650005a50e7/$FILE/CBI-Doing%20More%20With%20Less.pdf. Accessed September 8, 2010.

Centola, D. (2010). The spread of behavior in an online social network experiment. *Science, 329*(5996), 1194–1197.

Chen, P. W. (Jun 2009). Medicine in the age of Twitter. *The New York Times.* [Online] Available from http://www.nytimes.com/2009/06/11/health/11chen.html. Accessed September 3, 2010.

Cheng, M. (Aug 2010). Africans text message to check if drugs are real. *Associated press.* [Online] Available from http://m.apnews.com/ap/db_15901/contentdetail.htm?contentguid=ADMQe1QJ. Accessed August 20, 2010.

Coberly, E., Boren, S. A., Davis, J. W., McConnell, A. L., Chitima-Matsiga, R., Ge, B., Logan, R. A., Steinmann, W. C., & Hodge, R. H. (2010). Linking clinic patients to Online-based, condition-specific information prescriptions. *Journal of the Medical Library Association, 98*(2), 160–164. Available from http://www.ncbi.nlm.nih.gov/pmc/articles/PMC2859275/. Accessed September 4, 2010.

Coombes, R. (Sep 2007). Who are the doctor bloggers and what do they want? *British Medical Journal, 335*, 644. Available from http://www.bmj.com/content/335/7621/644.long. Accessed September 5, 2010.

deBronkart, D. (Sep 2009). Give patients (that's you) access to all their (your) data – so they can help. *E-patient Dave*. [Online] Available from http://epatientdave.com/2009/09/20/give-us-our-data/. Accessed September 8, 2010.

Eng, T. (2001). The e-Health landscape – a terrain map of emerging information and communication technologies. In *Health and health care*. Princeton: The Robert Wood Johnson Foundation. Available from http://www.informatics-review.com/thoughts/rwjf.html. Accessed September 1, 2010.

ESDIS. (Apr 2006). Health and ageing in the knowledge society: employment, social cohesion and e-health potential. Working document of the high level group on employment and social dimension of the information society (ESDIS). [Online] Available from http://www.umic.pt/images/stories/publicacoes/healthinks_20060429_esdis.pdf. Accessed September 1, 2010.

Eysenbach, G. (Jun 2001). What is e-health? *Journal of Medical Internet Research, 3*(2), e20. Available from http://www.jmir.org/2001/2/e20/. Accessed August 29, 2010.

Friedlin, J., & McDonald, C. J. (May 2010). An evaluation of medical knowledge contained in Wikipedia and its use in the LOINC database. *Journal of the American Medical Informatics Association, 17*(3), 283–287.

García-Lizana, F., & Muñoz-Mayorga, I. (2010). What about telepsychiatry? A systematic review. *Primary Care Companion to the Journal of Clinical Psychiatry, 12*(2), e1–e5.

Garner, J., & O'Sullivan, H. (Jun 2010). Facebook and the professional behaviours of undergraduate medical students. *The Clinical Teacher, 7*(2), 112–115. Available from http://onlinelibrary.wiley.com/doi/10.1111/j.1743-498X.2010.00356.x/full. Accessed September 10, 2010.

Gaßner, K., & Conrad, M. (Mar 2010). *ICT enabled independent living for elderly*. VDI/VDE/IT. Available from http://www.vdivde-it.de/publikationen/dokumente/ICT_for_Elderly.pdf. Accessed September 8, 2010.

Gerber, B. S., & Eiser, A. R. (2001). The patient–physician relationship in the online. *Journal of Medical Online Research, 3*(2), e15. [Online] Available from http://www.jmir.org/2001/2/e15/

Giansanti, D., Morelli, S., Maccioni, G., & Costantini, G. (Apr 2009). Toward the design of a wearable system for fall-risk detection in telerehabilitation. *Telemedicine Journal and E-Health, 15*(3), 296–299.

Gibbons, M. C. (Apr 2005). A historical overview of health disparities and the potential of eHealth solutions. *Journal of Medical Internet Research, 7*(5), e50. Available from http://www.jmir.org/2005/5/e50/. Accessed August 29, 2010.

Giustini, D. (2006). How Web 2.0 is changing medicine. *British Medical Journal, 333*, 1283–1284.

Gliddon, J. (Sep 2010). *Danish portal chief warns of ehealth delays*. eHealthSpace.org. [Online] Available from http://ehealthspace.org/news/danish-portal-chief-warns-ehealth-delays. Accessed September 9, 2010.

Google Scholar. (2010). [Online] http://scholar.google.com/scholar?cites=3220290637136728330&as_sdt=2005&sciodt=2000&hl=en. Accessed August 29, 2010.

Gravitz, L. (Jul 2010). Biosensors comfortable enough to wear 24–7. *MIT Technology Review*. [Online] Available from http://www.technologyreview.com/biomedicine/25701/?a=f. Accessed July 7, 2010.

Greenhalgh, T., Stramer, K., Bratan, T., Byrne, E., Russell, J., & Potts, H. W. W. (Jun 2010). Adoption and non-adoption of a shared electronic summary record in England: A mixed-method case study. *British Medical Journal, 340*(jun16_4), c3111.

Halpern, S. M. (2010). Does teledermoscopy validate teledermatology for triage of skin lesions? *British Journal of Dermatology, 162*, 709–710. Available from http://www.molesafe.com/bjd1.pdf. Accessed September 1, 2010.

Hannan, A., & Webber, F. (2007). Towards a partnership of trust. In L. Bos & B. Blobel (Eds.), *Medical and care compunetics 4* (pp. 108–16). Amsterdam: IOS Press. Available from http:// www.icmcc.org/pdf/recordaccess/hannan.pdf

Ingram, D. (Aug 2010). openEHR/IHTSDO explore IP integration, governance, SNOMED archetypes. *openEHR*. [Online] Available from http://www.openehr.org/302-OE.html?branch= 1&language=1. Accessed September 3, 2010.

Iskowitz, M. (Aug 2010). Avandia warning signs seen online as early as '04. *Medical Marketing & Media*. [Online] available from http://www.mmm-online.com/avandia-warning-signs-seen-online-as-early-as-04/article/177982/. Accessed September 3, 2010.

Jain, S. H. (Aug 2009). Practicing medicine in the age of Facebook. *The New England Journal of Medicine, 361*(7), 649–651. Available from http://www.nejm.org/doi/full/10.1056/ NEJMp0901277. Accessed September 4, 2010.

Johansson, T., & Wild, C. (Apr 2010). Telemedicine in acute stroke management: Systematic review. *International Journal of Technology Assessment in Health Care, 26*(2), 149–155.

Kamel Boulos, M. N., & Wheeler, S. (2006). Wikis, blogs and podcasts: A new generation of Web-based tools for virtual collaborative clinical practice and education. *BMC Medical Education, 6*, 41. Available from http://www.biomedcentral.com/1472-6920/6/41. Accessed August 31, 2010.

Kaplan, A. M., & Haenlein, M. (2010). Users of the world, unite! The challenges and opportunities of social media. *Business Horizons, 53*(1), 59–68.

Karkalis, G. I., & Koutsouris, D. D. (Oct 2006). E-health and the Web 2.0. In *Proceedings of ITAB 2006*, Ioannina, Greece. IEEE EMBS, 2006. [Online] Available from http://medlab.cs.uoi.gr/ itab2006/proceedings/eHealth/124.pdf. Accessed September 2, 2010.

Kemper, D. W., Del Fiol, G., Hall, L. K., Myers S., & Gutierrez, J. (Jan 2010). Getting patients to meaningful use using the HL7 "Infobutton" standard for information prescriptions. *Healthwise*. [Online] Available from http://hwinfo.healthwise.org/docs/DOCUMENT/8325.pdf. Accessed September 3, 2010.

Kroes, N. (2010). Telemedicine and infrastructures in Europe. In *The European files: The telemedicine challenge in Europe*. [Online] Available from http://ec.europa.eu/information_society/activities/health/docs/publications/2010/2010europ-files-telemedicine_en.pdf. Accessed July 23, 2010.

Landro, L. (Aug 2010). *The Wall Street Journal*. [Online] Available from http://online.wsj.com/ article/SB10001424052748703960004575427531544486778.html. Accessed August 17, 2010.

Leithner, A., Maurer-Ertl, W., Glehr, M., Friesenbichler, J., Leithner, K., & Windhager, R. (Jul 2010). Wikipedia and osteosarcoma: A trustworthy patients' information? *Journal of the American Medical Informatics Association, 17*(4), 373–374.

Lenhart, A. (Sep 2010). *Cell phones and American adults* (Report Pew Online). [Online] Available from http://www.pewOnline.org/Reports/2010/Cell-Phones-and-American-Adults. aspx. Accessed September 3, 2010.

Lintonen, T. P., Konu, A. I., & Seedhouse, D. (Jun 2008). Information technology in health promotion. *Health Education Research, 23*(3), 560–566. Available from http://her.oxfordjournals. org/cgi/content/full/23/3/560. Accessed August 29, 2010.

Lupiáñez-Villanueva, F., Mayer, M. Á., & Torrent, J. (Sep 2009). Opportunities and challenges of Web 2.0 within the health care systems: An empirical exploration. *Informatics for Health and Social Care, 34*(3), 117.

Manning, B., & Benton, S. (2010). Setting core standards: Privacy, identity & interoperability. In L. Bos, B. Blobel, S. Benton, & D. Carroll (Eds.), *Medical and care compunetics 6* (pp. 32–39). Amsterdam: IOS Press.

Manning, B., & Kun, L. (2009). Information highway to the home and back: A smart systems review. In K. Yogesan, L. Bos, P. Brett, & M. C. Gibbons (Eds.), *Handbook of digital homecare* (pp. 5–31). Heidelberg: Springer.

McMullen, M. (Oct 2006). Patients using the Online to obtain health information: How this affects the patient–health professional relationship. *Patient Education and Counseling, 63*(1–2), 24–28.

Meijer, W. J. (2009). Standards for digital homecare. In K. Yogesan, L. Bos, P. Brett, & M. C. Gibbons (Eds.), *Handbook of digital homecare* (pp. 53–74). Heidelberg: Springer.

Meijer, W. J., & Ragetlie, P. L. (2007). Empowering the patient with ICT-tools: The unfulfilled promise. In L. Bos & B. Blobel (Eds.), *Medical and care compunetics (Vol 4)* (pp. 199–218). Amsterdam: IOS Press.

Merrill, M. (Aug 2010). Study: Texting improves medication adherence in teens with diabetes. *Healthcare IT news*. [Online] Available from http://www.healthcareitnews.com/news/study-texting-improves-medication-adherence-teens-diabetes-0. Accessed August 10, 2010.

mHealth Initiative. [Online] Available from http://www.mobih.org/. Accessed September 8, 2010.

Monegain, B. (Jul 2010). Standards group to bolster interoperability worldwide. *HealthcareITNews*. [Online] Available from http://www.healthcareitnews.com/news/standards-group-bolster-interoperability-worldwide. Accessed September 3, 2010.

Monteagudo, J. L., & Moreno, O. (Mar 2007). *Patient empowerment opportunities with eHealth, eHealth ERA Report on Priority Topic Cluster Two and recommendations*. Available from http://ec.europa.eu/information_society/newsroom/cf/document.cfm?action=display&doc_id=320. Accessed September 3, 2010.

Nissen, S. E., & Wolski, K. (2007). Effect of rosiglitazone on the risk of myocardial infarction and death from cardiovascular causes. *The New England Journal of Medicine, 356*(24), 2457–2471.

O'Reilly, T. (Sep 2005). *What is Web 2.0 – Design patterns and business models for the next generation of software*. [Online] Available from http://www.oreillynet.com/pub/a/oreilly/tim/news/2005/09/30/what-is-web-20.html. Accessed September 3, 2010.

Oh, H., Rizo, C., Enkin, M., & Jadad, A. (Feb 2005). What is eHealth (3): A systematic review of published definitions. *Journal of Medical Internet Research, 7*(1), e1. Available from http://www.jmir.org/2005/1/e1/. Accessed August 29, 2010.

Pagliari, C., Sloan, D., Gregor, P., Sullivan, F., Detmer, D., Kahan, J. P., et al. (Mar 2005). What is eHealth (4): A scoping exercise to map the field. *Journal of Medical Internet Research, 7*(1), e9. Available from http://www.jmir.org/2005/1/e9/. Accessed August 29, 2010.

PatientsLikeMe (2010). [Online] Available from http://www.patientslikeme.com/

PatientsLikeMe Facebook. (2010). *Success is putting patients first*. [Online] Available from http://www.facebook.com/notes/patientslikeme/success-is-putting-patients-first/470378470860. Accessed September 10, 2010.

Pho, K. (Aug 2010). Should doctors friend their patients on Facebook? *KevinMD.com*. [Online] Available from http://www.kevinmd.com/blog/2009/08/should-doctors-friend-their-patients-on-facebook.html. Accessed August 14, 2009.

Pho, K. (Jul 2009). USA Today. [Online] Available from http://www.kevinmd.com/blog/2009/08/op-ed-wikipedia-isnt-really-the-patients-friend.html. Accessed September 10, 2010.

Pisani, E., & AbouZahr, C. (2010). Sharing health data: Good intentions are not enough. *Bulletin of the World Health Organization, 88*(6), 401–480.

Prabhakaran, L., Chee, W. Y., Chua, K. C., Abisheganaden, J., & Wong, W. M. (Jul 2010). The use of text messaging to improve asthma control: A pilot study using the mobile phone short messaging service (SMS). *Journal of Telemedicine and Telecare, 16*(5), 286–290.

Prado-Velasco, M., Fernández-Peruchena, C., & Rubio-Hernández, D. (2009). Model-based methodology for the analysis of e-health systems diffusion: case study of a knowledge-centered telehealthcare system based on a mixed license. In K. Yogesan, L. Bos, P. Brett, & M. C. Gibbons (Eds.), *Handbook of digital homecare* (pp. 75–94). Heidelberg: Springer.

Project HealthDesign. (2009). Rethinking the power and potential of personal health records. Available from http://www.projecthealthdesign.org/media/file/Round%20One%20PHD%20Final%20Report6.17.09.pdf. Accessed September 8, 2010.

Pubmed. [Online] Available from http://www.ncbi.nlm.nih.gov/pubmed/. Accessed September 8, 2010.

Rahme, E., Kahn, S. R., Dasgupta, K., Burman, M., Bernatsky, S., Habel, Y., & Berry, G. (Aug 2010). Short-term mortality associated with failure to receive home care after hemi-arthroplasty. *Canadian Medical Association Journal, 182*(13), 1421–1426.

Rajagopalan, M. S., Khanna, V., Stott, M., Leiter, Y., Showalter, T. N., Dicker, A., et al. (2010). Accuracy of cancer information on the Online: A comparison of a Wiki with a professionally maintained database. *Journal of Clinical Oncology.* ASCO, 2010, abstract 6058. [Online]Available from http://www.asco.org/ASCOv2/Meetings/Abstracts?&vmview= abst_detail_view&confID=74&abstractID=41625

Reuters. (Sep 2010). *People are quicker to change when they hear the message from more than one source.* [Online] Available from http://www.vancouversun.com/news/Groups±friends±changi ng±health±behaviours/3499383/story.html. Accessed September 8, 2010.

Rutherford, J. J. (Jun 2010). Wearable technology. *IEEE Engineering in Medicine and Biology Magazine, 29*(3), 19–24.

Salmon, P., & Hall, G. M. (Feb 2004). Patient empowerment or the emperor's new clothes. *Journal of the Royal Society of Medicine, 97*(2), 53–56. Available from http://www.pubmedcentral.nih. gov/picrender.fcgi?artid=1079288&blobtype=pdf. Accessed September 3, 2010.

Saltman, R. B. (1994). Patient choice and patient empowerment in northern European health systems: A conceptual framework. *International Journal of Health Services, 24*(2), 201–229.

Scanfeld, D., Scanfeld, V., & Larson, E. L. (Apr 2010). Dissemination of health information through social networks: Twitter and antibiotics. *American Journal of Infection Control, 38*(3), 182–188.

Schieppati, A., Jan-Henter, I., Daina, E., & Aperia, A. (2008). Why rare diseases are an important medical and social issue. *Lancet, 371,* 2039–2041. [Online] Available from URL:http://www. sbgm.org.br/artigos/art_rare_diseases.pdf. Accessed September 3, 2010.

Sermo (2010). [Online] Available from http://www.sermo.com/. Accessed September 3, 2010.

Sevillano, E. (Sep 2010). *Salud en la Red, no todo es mentira.* El País. [Online] Available from http:// www.elpais.com/articulo/sociedad/Salud/Red/todo/mentira/elpepusoc/20100911elpepusoc_1/Tes. Accessed September 11, 2010.

Society for Participatory Medicine. [Online] Available from http://participatorymedicine.org/. Accessed September 8, 2010.

Sommerhalder, K., Abraham, A., Zufferey, M. C., Barth, J., & Abel, T. (2009). Online information and medical consultations: Experiences from patients' and physicians' perspectives. *Patient Education and Counseling, 77,* 266–271.

Spallek, H., O'Donnell, J., Clayton, M., Anderson, P., & Krueger, A. (Apr 2010). Paradigm shift or annoying distraction. *Applied Clinical Informatics, 1*(2), 96–115.

Sweet, M. (2010) What could Web 2.0 do for the health sector? In: N. Gruen (Ed.), *Croakey the Crikey Healthblog.* [Online] Available from http://blogs.crikey.com.au/croakey/2010/09/02/ what-could-web-2-0-do-for-the-health-sector-nicholas-gruen/. Accessed September 2, 2010.

Tamura, L. (Aug 2010). Physicians use photos from patients' cellphones to deliver 'mobile health'. *The Washington post.* [Online] Available from http://www.washingtonpost.com/wp-dyn/con-tent/article/2010/08/30/AR2010083003939.html. Accessed September 1, 2010.

The Harris Poll #95. (Aug 2010)."Cyberchondriacs" on the Rise? [Online] Available from http:// www.harrisinteractive.com/vault/HI-Harris-Poll-Cyberchondriacs-2010-08-04.pdf. Accessed August 31, 2010.

van der Heijden, J. P., Spuls, P. I., Voorbraak, F. P., de Keizer, N., Witkamp, L., & Bos, J. D. (2010). Tertiary teledermatology: A systematic review. *Telemedicine Journal and E-Health, 16*(1), 56–62.

Vesely, R. (Sep 2008). *Data privacy concerns remain as Google PHR grows.* ModernHealthcare. com. [Online] Available from http://www.modernhealthcare.com/article/20080929/ REG/309299997/. Accessed September 9, 2010.

Via PrNewswire. (2010). comScore/ImpactRx Physician Behavioral Measurement™ solution. [Online] Available from http://www.prnewswire.com/news-releases/4-out-of-5-physicians-online-visited-health-care-professional-sites-in-q1-2010-101570778.html. Accessed September 3, 2010.

Warshaw, E. M., Lederle, F. A., Grill, J. P., Gravely, A. A., Bangerter, A. K., et al. (2009). Accuracy of teledermatology for pigmented neoplasms. *Journal of the American Academy of Dermatology, 61*(5), 753–765.

White, T. (Sep 2010). Will iPad transform med school? *Stanford Medical School.* [Online] Available from http://med.stanford.edu/ism/2010/september/ipads-0913.html. Accessed September 10, 2010.

Whitten, P., Holtz, B., & LaPlante, C. (2010). Telemedicine what have we learned? *Applied Clinical Informatics, 1*(2), 132–141.

Wickramasinghe, N. S., Fadlalla, A. M. A., Geisler, E., & Schaffer, J. L. (2005). A framework for assessing e-health preparedness. *International Journal of Electronic Healthcare, 1*(3), 316–334. Available from http://citeseerx.ist.psu.edu/viewdoc/download?doi=10.1.1.88.4973&rep=rep1 &type=pdf. Accessed August 29, 2010.

Wiki. (2010). Wikipedia. [Online] Available from http://en.wikipedia.org/wiki/Wiki. Accessed September 8, 2010.

Wiljer, D., Leonard, K., Urowitz, S., Apatu, E., Massey, C., Quartey, N. K. et al. (2010). The anxious wait: Assessing the impact of patient accessible EHRs for breast cancer patients. *BMC Medical Informatics and Decision Making, 10*(1), 46. [Online] Available from http://www.biomedcentral.com/content/pdf/1472-6947-10-46.pdf. Accessed September 2, 2010.

Yogesan, K., Bos, L., Brett, P., & Gibbons, M. C. (Eds.). (2009). *Handbook of digital homecare* (p. 1). Berlin: Springer.

Zanaboni, P., Scalvini, S., Bernocchi, P., Borghi, G., Tridico, C., & Masella, C. (Dec 2009). Teleconsultation service to improve healthcare in rural areas: Acceptance, organizational impact and appropriateness. *BMC Health Services Research, 9*, 238. Available from http://www.biomedcentral.com/1472-6963/9/238. Accessed September 8, 2010.

Chapter 15
Citizen eMPOWERment

Amir Hannan

Abstract This chapter outlines the need for full patient access to their healthcare records and reports on hypothetical and real-life UK-based scenarios. These serve to illustrate the importance of supporting patients, clinicians and managers to understand how personal health information can be shared across a health and social care setting and to promote best practice by combining local expertise with national and international experience and knowledge.

Keywords Patient empowerment • IT in health care • Patient • Partnership

15.1 Introduction

The current trend towards electronic healthcare overwhelmingly appears to put forward information and communication technologies (ICTs) as the panacea for the contemporary shortcomings in medical delivery to the patient. However, working in closer partnership with patients should reap exponential rewards in the form of more accurate diagnosis and prognosis, trust, encouraging patients to learn more about their own health and result in better health outcomes for individuals and society as a whole. This chapter will illustrate the efforts of the author, a full-time UK-based general practitioner (GP), an advocate of patient empowerment (Hannan and Webber 2007), to bring greater transparency to electronic patient records.

A. Hannan (✉)
Haughton Thornley Medical Centres, Hyde, Cheshire, UK
e-mail: amir.hannan@nhs.net

N. Wickramasinghe et al. (eds.), *Critical Issues for the Development
of Sustainable E-health Solutions*, Healthcare Delivery in the Information Age,
DOI 10.1007/978-1-4614-1536-7_15, © Springer Science+Business Media, LLC 2012

15.2   A Typical Patient Vignette

The following scenario serves as a useful vignette which illustrates some of the challenges of contemporary healthcare. The chapter will finish with a revised vignette once our hypothetical patient has become suitably empowered.

15.2.1   Before Empowerment

An obese diabetic smoker in his mid 50s is sat on the chair watching TV, eating crisps and chocolates. He has missed lots of appointments at the surgery because he was too busy and "they would only tell him off for doing the wrong things". He suddenly develops chest pains in the middle of his chest, making him feel breathless, nauseous and clammy lasting for about an hour. He had been getting them recently when he walked but thought it was indigestion and had not bothered about them.

He stays still fearing for his life. "Maybe it isn't indigestion". Unsure what the cause is, he rings the surgery, finds the phone is engaged and is asked to try again. So he keeps trying and after the fifth occasion, finally gets through to the receptionist. He asks for an urgent appointment for his chest pains. She immediately advises him to call an ambulance but he disagrees and would like his general practitioner (family physician) to see him first. She tells him that this is not appropriate and that he must call an ambulance because that is all the doctor will do anyway when he sees him. He refuses and so she has to disturb the annoyed doctor who tells him what he MUST do.

Reluctantly, he agrees and calls an ambulance. The ambulance comes within 5 min, asks him questions about his health such as when he was diagnosed with diabetes and whether he has ever had chest pains before. They ask him what tablets he is taking but he cannot remember. It's a frightening experience and he is unable to answer. He has never felt like that before. So they pick up his medication from the cupboard, noting that there seem to be a lot of packets of simvastatin and aspirin that he has not been taking. They forget to collect his byetta injection for his diabetes, which he keeps in the fridge "for safe keeping". He gets to the hospital, is swiftly seen by the A&E doctors who take a quick history, examine him, arrange for some blood tests and a series of ECGs. They then inform him that he is having a "heart attack", confirming his worst fears, and that they will be transferring him urgently to the catheter lab for an urgent coronary angiogram. They mutter something about a 1–2% risk of death but explain this is what they tell everybody "because they have to".

The patient doesn't really listen – he feels a hypoglycaemic attack is coming on and has a sudden urge to eat something and wonders if anybody would notice if he puts a sweet in his mouth. "It won't matter and anyway a hypo would be much more worrying". He gets the angiogram done and it confirms he has two vessel disease. He is advised to have an angioplasty and two coronary stents inserted because "that is the best advice for this type of condition" and is asked to sign the consent form.

Following surgery, he is transferred to the main ward, has an uneventful few days and then is discharged back home. He feels he has been in a prison and unable to smoke. They keep telling him he must stop but it's not that easy. He has always smoked since he was 12 years old and what could a young 30 something year old teach him! He's heard about terrible rashes people get with nicotine patches – much worse than the cigarettes!

The doctor scribbles something down on a piece of paper and asks him to hand it into the surgery. He congratulates him on how well he has done (because he has not had any further chest pains). But he can't wait to get home, light a cigarette and eat his chocolates and crisps. He has been denied his creature comforts for the past week and is looking forward to being at home once again. He briefly remembers that he never told them about his byetta injection that he should also have taken. "It probably won't matter", he thinks to himself as his wife drives him out of the hospital. He will start it from tomorrow once things are "back to normal". But for now he lights up a cigarette. "You won't believe how much I craved for this cigarette and they just wanted to give me patches or see a smoking advisor! Who are they kiddin'? I'm cured!"

15.2.1.1   The Case for Patient Empowerment

Established research has advocated the importance of patient empowerment (Anderson et al. 1995; Salmon and Hall 2003; Segal 1998; Roberts 2001; Munir and Boaden 2001; Falcão-Reis and Correia 2010). Traditionally the patient was expected to come to the doctor or latterly the nurse for "pearls of wisdom" as somebody who is there to "fix" or "cure" the patient of their disease. Whilst this may have been what doctors did in the early/mid part of the twentieth century, our role has changed with the advances in medicine such that people often no longer die of a "heart attack" or "diabetes" but are left with the burden of chronic disease that they then need to continue to manage.

The challenge is that the clinician, with a few notable exceptions, can no longer tell patients that they are cured. Instead they have to inform them about a new treatment regimen that they will need to adopt for their own with regular checkups, possibly tests and investigations and ever more powerful treatments with side effects and interactions that may or may not suit the patient. These necessitate regular interval reviews with the hope of identifying problems early and hence prevent further deterioration in their health.

Another challenge is the incessant rise in the proportion of people leading sedentary lifestyles. Technological advancements such as the motor car, entertainment in the home such as television and latterly video games and easy access to "junk food", high in calories, have led to the obesity epidemic and alongside it increasing numbers of people diagnosed with diabetes as well as associated conditions such as depression, back pain, hypertension and ischaemic heart disease. Although there is often a genetic component to these conditions, the sedentary lifestyle makes the likelihood of these conditions manifesting themselves more likely.

Patient empowerment means "to promote autonomous self-regulation so that the individual's potential for health and wellness is maximized" (Funnell et al. 1991). Patient empowerment is about giving back control to patients so they feel they are in charge of their health destiny instead of being controlled by the disease or by the healthcare system around them. Much controversy still exists on whether this is possible when doctors and nurses still decide to give patients a label and order them on what they should do or not do, what treatments they should take and when and get upset with them when patients do not follow "their" advice (Salmon and Hall 2004). But the increased access to the internet for the population at large does give them the opportunity to learn more for themselves instead of being reliant on the clinician. Health 2.0 defines the combination of health data and health information with (patient) experience through the use of ICT, enabling the citizen to become an active and responsible partner in his/her own health and care pathway. Combining these two concepts together, patient 2.0 empowerment is the active participation of the citizen in his or her health and care pathway with the interactive use of Information and Communication Technologies.

15.3   The Best Patient is One that is Enabled, Informed, and Empowered

The patient scenario at the start of this chapter describes a disempowered patient who does as he pleases without realizing the consequences, suddenly develops a life-threatening condition and is thrust into a difficult series of encounters feeling out of control throughout and unable to make informed decisions for himself. How does such a patient become empowered?

The first step is to *enable* the patient to feel they can make decisions about themselves. This may be dependent on their own "locus of control". People who have a strong internal locus of control need to have self belief in themselves to be able to make a difference in their life. People with a strong external locus of control are reliant on external factors to help them achieve enablement such as an authoritarian figure as a doctor or society itself informing them that they should do this. People with an external locus of control still go to work, get food for themselves and live in a home they choose. Whatever the locus of control a patient has, they must become enabled to take the first steps towards patient empowerment. They must feel that they can and must take a more active role in their own care and not simply be recipients of care handed down to them.

Having become enabled, the next step is to become *informed*. This requires patients to be able to view different trustworthy information in a variety of different formats that suit their needs. The information may well be contradictory (as is often the case in medicine) but they need to be able to see different perspectives and hence different choices they could enact for themselves and learn to weigh up what is right for them given their particular circumstances. The more information they gather from different trustworthy sources, the more informed they will become. Sources may include their doctor or nurse, articles they read from newspapers, the internet, programs they watch on TV or listen to the radio or discussions they have with friends, family, work colleagues and their peers. Whilst the trustworthiness of these sources may vary considerably, they will influence the patient's thinking and help them to become better (or worse) informed. We will see later how patients can become better informed.

Once informed, patients must then be *empowered* to make decisions for themselves based on the choices they feel are right for them. This is an important prerequisite. The choice needs to be made by the patient and not made for them. This should take into account the patient's own ideas, concerns and expectations. Even those with a high degree of external locus of control still need to be encouraged to determine their own choice even if this is what the external authority is telling them to do so! But empowered patients cannot just act on their own based on "generic information". They need to have an understanding of their own health condition as well before determining how best to proceed. I have adapted the word empowerment to stand for:

e
Medical
Patient and the Public
c**O**mmunication
World wide web
Record
ed

So an eMPOWERed patient (Medical, Patient and the Public, cOmmunication, World wide web, Record) is one who is empowered and also has access to their own electronic health record (Fisher et al. 2007; Hannan 2007; Hannan 2010) which they can use as a reference, as a reminder and help to drive the choices they have to get the best outcomes.

eMPOWERed patients are able to read about their own health, understand the context of their own health in relation to medical knowledge as well as the services available locally to them and also what is available afar, use this information to work out how best to use the resources available to them (their time, the service provider they go to, for example: general practitioner or dietician and information sources they trust) to determine the next steps that could help prevent problems, manage ongoing problems and be prepared for an emergency in the future should it arise.

But why should it matter that we have eMPOWERed patients? Throughout the world, healthcare costs are rising at an exponential rate far out-stripping the money available for an increasingly aging population. Costs need to be contained but this is not at the expense of quality of care delivered. Innovation and delivering higher quality care should help to deliver more care to more people with a corresponding increase in cost. This is extremely hard to deliver sustainably in the current financial climate. But eMPOWERed patients may hold a key to achieving this. If patients are able to take more responsibility for their own care needs then they are less reliant on the healthcare system and are more likely to take the treatments offered, particularly those that have strong evidence behind them and hence more convinced by them to help them with their own healthy outcomes they wish to achieve. That in turn should mean less out of hours urgent care and better managed patients that ultimately cost the health system less. Another further benefit is that a healthier patient population is more able to work longer creating more wealth for the nation (through taxes but also by spending more of what they earn) so that there is more opportunity for others to benefit too. Patient eMPOWERment is therefore not just for patients but also a benefit to clinicians (who want patients to get better and are able to return to work instead of remaining in an illness state) as well as to organizations (that are struggling to see ever more patients within a given time span) and more broadly to businesses so that their workforce is in work for longer.

But why is this sustainable? The explosion of knowledge coupled with the advent of the internet to help easily share information means that more and more patients are likely to learn more about the benefits of them taking an active role, choosing to share their experience with others. This will encourage others to do the same until a new happy medium is reached where patients are spontaneously becoming more eMPOWERed to make decisions in conjunction with their clinician without necessarily needing a consultation to do so. Patients will choose to come to the clinician when they really need to. Clinicians will inform patients (either directly or via information sources such as an organization's website) what care patients should expect to receive. The clinicians' role will be to help patients to become enabled, better informed, help to guide them through the choices they need to make and how access to their medical records can help them to make better decisions about their health. As the population ages and more sophisticated IT systems are developed with adequate access controls, carers of patients may also be able to take a more active role too – further lessening the burden on strained healthcare services. Organizations will change the way they deliver care from simply being a place where patients attend to receive care to ones that encourage patients and clinicians to act in a way that supports patient eMPOWERment.

All this however presumes the patient is able to make choices for themselves. There are some patients who will not be able to make choices for themselves. There are some patients who cannot give consent. Perhaps they are very young children or suffer with severe learning difficulties, dementia or severe mental health problems. Sometimes patients may be acutely unwell, for example when they are having a heart attack and need/expect a clinician to act in their best interests when they are unable to do so. Advanced Directives (which determine what a patient would be happy to have if confronted by a certain eventuality, for example, Jehovah Witness not wanting blood products if they have a catastrophic bleed) and Advanced Care Planning (where a patient who may be in the terminal stage of their life and describes how he or she wishes to be cared for) help to ensure the patient's desires are enacted if they are no longer able to communicate. Another legal entity is where the family of the patient apply for lasting Power of Attorney which also gives them access to their medical records too. Where there is a difference of opinion between the patient and the clinician and it is deemed appropriate, then either party can apply to the courts for further clarification.

There will however be some patients who refuse to become eMPOWERed, preferring to keep this function with the clinician or the organization or society. They are capable of making decisions for themselves but do not feel willing to do so. Rather than ostracizing such patients, we will need to understand their needs better, how to work with them and find out how to best support them. They may not be ready to do everything all at once but may be happy to be enabled or simply to gather information from sources, which they present to the clinician. Healthcare systems may need to develop sophisticated ways of enabling the rest of the information to be made available at the point of care, for example the patient's electronic health record. But there is a fine balance between the need to have access to the information and the patient's right to privacy and confidentiality. Some patients may not want to present information to clinicians and we need to respect their wishes but continue to strive to deliver high quality care.

Finally there are a third group who may wish to be empowered but do not wish their medical records to be electronically stored in a way that provides other clinicians access to their medical information for justifiable reasons (www.thebigoptout.org 2010). More research is needed to understand this better and how best to support such patients.

What about those people that are not patients? Wikipedia defines a patient as somebody who receives medical attention, care or treatment (Wikipaedia 2010). What about those that do not consider themselves to be patients? If healthcare was about treating those that are ill then this would not matter. However there is an increased realisation that people need to learn to change their behaviour/lifestyle to help reduce their risk of developing certain conditions, for example obesity or diabetes. Gene therapy may offer further options for people that thought they will almost certainly develop certain conditions. Such citizens can become eMPOWERed to look after themselves better and prevent disease from occurring. More and more effort and resources are being applied to encourage all people to look after themselves better and so citizen empowerment may be a better all encompassing term which includes everybody else as well. Everybody that has the ability needs to become eMPOWERed – they will help to get better quality care for themselves and reduce their dependency on others to look after them.

15.4   How Can we Enable Patient eMPOWERment?

People already have the propensity to "self care". Our instincts are to look after ourselves. Self care means "looking after (ourselves) in a healthy way, whether it's brushing (our) teeth, taking medicine when (we) have a cold or doing some exercise" (What is self care? 2010). This is a commonly used term but how does this relate to patients increasingly presenting at their general practice, urgent care centre or casualty?

Patients usually do not want to waste time, money and their energy trying to get seen by a clinician unless they have good reason to. Usually this is because their ability to cope with the symptoms they have, have been exhausted or they feel they need something that they can only get from the clinician, for example advice, medication or perhaps a note that confirms their illness. Sometimes they may have forgotten to do something and then need to present as an emergency in order to get a treatment that they could have got without having to ask for an urgent appointment. Telling patients to simply "self care more" is not enough. We need to understand each of these scenarios and others better and consider how an eMPOWERed patient may approach these problems. Contrary to what one might think, patients may not be aware of solutions that exist or other strategies that patients use which could help them. So the clinician/organization begin to understand why the patient has presented when they do, what information they provide on what matters and what are they hoping to achieve by the encounter. The clinician then arms the patient with further information to help them self care better, where else they could get information from to help them besides asking for an appointment, other services that may be available to support the patient and perhaps a series of actions the patient needs to take this time but which they could refer to in the future if the same problem arose again. They need clear instructions on when to return back to the clinician rather than continuing to self care. When a patient is having a heart attack, it is essential that they seek urgent help rather than trying to self manage.

But how can patients learn such skills? This may be answered by asking how one learns to get a job, choose which bank account to open and with which institution, find a partner to get married to, get a mortgage, choose a school for their child or choose a holiday. The first step is to recognize that this is an action that should be the patient's responsibility and not devolved to others. But the patient is not alone. There is ample advice available for all the actions described above such as speaking to family and friends that have had different experiences or knowledge, learning the skills in school, visiting different banks, collecting their information brochures about the services they offer, school tables which inform us about how schools are doing, and speaking to travel agents about different holidays and which would suit us best based on our preferences. There are articles in newspapers and magazines and often programs on television and the radio that also inform the viewer on how to choose. Increasingly there are now a large number of websites that offer advice too. Sometimes it may be appropriate to go directly to the provider's own website, for example the bank or the school one is thinking about joining. Other times, it may be better to go to a trusted website which gives general information about how to compare one institution with another, for example a mortgage comparison website or even Which? Finally sometimes it may be worth looking at actual comments posted by individuals on blogs. Each of these methods have advantages and disadvantages associated with them. We will have our own preference of the type of information and how we receive such information to determine a course of action.

Healthcare is different though because generally in the UK we do not pay for specific treatments at the point of care and often patients would prefer to go to the local services close to where they live rather than having to travel further afield. But none-the-less there is other information that may be more relevant, for example the types of treatments that are available such as anti-depressant medication or counselling or both. But this means it is essential patients are even clearer about what they are getting and what they hope to achieve. Is the goal cure or to control symptoms? In the future, other services may develop such as health trainers used by employers to keep employees healthy or other health 2.0 websites may open that encourage further sharing of information between patients and citizens in a responsible manner so that everybody can benefit from this. www.patientslikeme.com is an example of such a website.

eMPOWERed patients may challenge clinicians and establishments to prove the value of the service being offered. This may be quite challenging for clinicians who are used to giving advice to patients. They may feel the patients are challenging their authority, wasting their time or being neurotic, focusing on things that may not be considered important for the clinician. Alternatively clinicians may devolve their responsibility to the patient and not help the patient through their healthcare journey as long as the clinician does what they are paid to do. Clinicians have a responsibility to take an adequate history, examination, arrange appropriate investigations and determine a plan of action. However they should also take account of the patient's ideas, concerns and expectations so that a joined plan of action can be agreed with shared understanding and shared goals so that there is joined clinical and patient ownership. Benefits may be accrued for both by this joined way of working so that there is win/win for both parties. Patients who understand their health better will make life easier for clinicians because they are more likely to understand the condition, the importance of taking treatment, being able to explain better what treatments suit them, the importance of taking their treatment and to come back if they have problems with their treatment.

15.5   Changes in Healthcare and IT

If eMPOWERed patients are really to benefit from the information stored about them, it will be essential for their records to be easily accessible at a time of their convenience. This really means that their record must be stored in an electronic format which can be accessed over the internet via a variety of different internet-enabled devices including desktop computers, laptops, tablet PCs, smartphones and other devices that have yet to come. Most healthcare institutions besides General Practice are still based on paper records although some institutions have began to move towards installing electronic health record systems. This is a pre-requisite for the change to happen. Once a record is in an electronic form, it can be made available for access via the internet through a suitable adequately secure patient identification system.

There are many benefits of having an IT-based system including clearly legible notes that contain coded data as well as free text and easily accessible from multiple locations with the data re-usable for other secondary purposes too besides describing patient care. If the notes are coded using a universal language such as SNOMED-CT then the data can be understood by other clinical systems throughout the world that also read SNOMED-CT and in theory at least they could write back into the original electronic health record even if it was written in a different language too so that the record remains complete. Decision support tools can also be added to help the clinician and the patient to understand and manage the patient better. This will help to improve the quality of care by helping the patient and clinician to see what could happen next and what choices there may be. The patient can also see any errors and omissions that may exist in the record and help to correct them before they may cause further harm. This helps to build a "Partnership of Trust" between patient and clinician with the electronic health record helping to support both.

However simply being able to view data is not enough. Patients need to be placed on a patient pathway that describes where they are and ideally what should happen next. Clinicians often have imaginary pathways in their head for patient pathways. There are many guidelines that describe how patients should be managed. But these can often be quite different and conflict with one another especially where there is less evidence. Consequently patients get a variable experience even when different clinicians from the same institution are presented with the same information. To help improve quality and reduce costs further, it has become essential to develop agreed evidence-based care pathways for a variety of conditions that cross organizational boundaries and are agreed between commissioners and providers for use at the point of care by clinicians and patients too. One such tool widely deployed in the NHS is the "Map of Medicine". In areas where it has been deployed, there has been a significant increase in improved quality of care and significant reduction in costs.

eMPOWERed patients need access to trusted information from a variety of different sources that they can use to help manage their care. NHS Choices provides national healthcare information about a variety conditions as well as information about providers and the quality of services they provide. Some practices are now beginning to offer information specific to their own patient population how care is managed. We have developed a practice web portal www.htmc.co.uk as an example too. It provides information, videos and links to trusted websites that eMPOWERed patients can use to help them manage their care.

How can patients assimilate different information to help them to determine the best course of action? Different patients will have different ways of doing this. Some patients may present different evidences they have seen or read with their trusted doctor or nurse asking for their advice. Decision Aids have also been produced to help patients weigh up the different choices including their own personal preferences too. Patients are being encouraged to check their own blood pressures as the costs of the machines have dropped. Patients can record their blood pressure, weight, blood glucose readings and other parameters in www.healthspace.nhs.uk, Google Health or even Microsoft HealthVault. They can then share this information with others including their health professional if they so wish. Instead of determining how well controlled a patient's blood pressure is based on 1 or 2 readings, they can now show a wide variety of readings taken at different times of the day or night and during work days as well as weekends.

Telehealth also provides patients with the ability to monitor their own health more regularly so that they can see how their control is and be monitored by another health professional who can intervene before their health deteriorates significantly. This allows patients to be managed without having to come to the health care establishment as often. The data could be used to see how well the treatment is working and whether further changes are necessary or not.

These developments could come together so that an eMPOWERed patient could look at the practice web portal to learn about blood pressure or they could see their practice nurse who advises them to get a blood pressure machine to check their blood pressure a few times a week at a time and place convenient to them. The patient gets a suitable blood pressure machine which they monitor their blood pressure with using advice from the Map of Medicine. This also informs them about lifestyle changes that have shown proven benefit. If their blood pressure starts to rise above the normal threshold then they may choose to share it with the nurse or doctor for advice on what to do next. If the patient is considered at high risk as advised by a localized Map of Medicine pathway and unable to come to the surgery then they may be given a telemonitoring machine too which automatically checks the blood pressures and sends them back to a monitoring service. A nurse or doctor could then regularly check the results and call the patient if they go outside the normal range. An advanced care plan drawn up by the practice may be kept in the patient's record describing what care the patient wishes to receive. This could be provided to the out-of-hours service or the casualty department if the need arises so that the patient's wishes along with the doctor's are enacted. Patient Reported Outcome Measures could ensure that there is an overall improvement for the patient as perceived by the patient and not just some abstract blood pressure reading that is within a normal range but leaves the patient feeling miserable because of the side effects of treatment. As patients see for themselves the positive outcomes, it will encourage them to continue to follow the treatment without needing to regularly see their doctor or nurse. If on the other hand the outcomes are not what they are expecting then they may wish to see their clinician sooner. The clinician would also be able to see the PROMS too so that there is a further opportunity for the clinician to intervene too if the patient does not. Patients, clinicians and information come together to help deliver a higher level of care.

15.6   What is Needed from the System to Enable Citizen eMPOWERment?

All the elements are now available for patients, clinicians and organizations to benefit from eMPOWERed citizens. Citizens need to come together with clinicians whom they trust to help build partnerships to discuss how the change may come about. To a large extent, the changing relationship has already started from a father-child relationship to an adult-to-adult relationship where both partners bring equal expertise to the table – the patient brings their personal experience, what they know and what they want to happen. The clinician brings their experience of the local health service as well as their expertise of the condition. The computer system provides information for both patient and clinician on the patient's medical history (the electronic health record) as well as advice on local services (NHS Choices) and guidance on evidence based patient pathways (Map of Medicine). Patients are encouraged to think about their own condition or what they may be at risk of and are invited to learn more about what they need to know, what skills they may need to acquire (for example computing skills as well as how to check their own blood pressure or how to read the Map of Medicine pathway). At subsequent consultations, their attitudes may be assessed to see how committed they are to becoming eMPOWERed. This may include checking what they have learned previously but also what they would like to do over the coming months. The clinician with the patient try to determine what outcomes they are trying to achieve and how they will know if they have succeeded. The clinician becomes the personal trainer for the patient to learn for himself or herself. The patient is advised to practice what they have learned and to continually describe that experience to ensure it remains positive. If problems arise then the patient with the clinician attempt to look at why things have not happened as they might have done and what could be done differently.

Of course the patient has the right not to do this but then the patient may not get a better service as a result. The clinician is continually trying to explain why patient empowerment helps the patient to get where they want to be but that this comes with responsibilities that the patient has to fulfill.

As much of healthcare is inextricably linked with social care too, eMPOWERed patients may also need guidance on social care needs that could help them too. Such guidance does not readily exist at present but will be necessary to unlock the full potential that patients have to self care and stay away from institutionalized care such as residential/nursing homes. As patients understand these better, they will begin to understand where significant choices in their patient pathway are to be made and to try to plan ahead for the next one involving other third parties where necessary to support them, for example daughter and the family doctor along with the health trainer and their employer. Looking at outcome data as well as monitored date, patients may be able to look at how they compare with other similar patients locally, identify aspects of their care that differ from the ideal evidence based care pathways and work with their trusted clinician to see how such variability may be reduced to help improve outcomes for both the patient, the clinician as well as the organization. Large groups of eMPOWERed citizens could then come together to support wider healthcare reform by ensuring all health and social care organizations are locally accountable to help deliver the best care possible with available resources and the citizen is at the centre of their care.

15.7 Returning to Our Vignette

15.7.1 After Empowerment

The obese diabetic ex-smoker in his mid 50s has returned from a "weight matters" class on his bicycle where he has won an achievement award for losing 3 kg on average per week over the past 3 months. He has changed his diet considerably and now rarely eats snacks. He only watches television for a maximum of an hour a day as he realized this was a big culprit for causing him to gain weight. Nowadays he would much rather go for gentle walks or cycle to the local shops. He has rekindled an old interest in spotting birds and noticing the flowers in people's gardens as he walks past them which he never did when he drove everywhere before.

He uses the *Nintendo Wii* to play some active games when he wants to have a little fun with his teenage children – something he never had time to do before. He goes online to check if his test results are back and then adds the latest weight, blood pressure and how many steps he has walked this week. He has an application on his computer which shows how far he is walking compared with a colleague at work. This week he has walked 2 km more than him and so decides to celebrate with a banana. He has noticed his potassium is a little on the low side and so can afford to take a banana which is high in potassium.

He has a quick look at the practice website and sees a talk on chest pains and know what to do if is having a suspected heart attack. He looks at what medications he should be on and compares it with what the *Map of Medicine* says. He checks his own records and wonders whether he should be on an ACE inhibitor. He makes a note in *HealthSpace* to remind himself to raise it with the doctor or nurse when he next meets them. He is pleased that he is doing everything as it should be. Over the next week, he develops some increased frequency of chest pains when walking and decides he ought to make an urgent appointment with his doctor.

He brings his wife with him and also his diary as he thinks he will need further investigations and be referred to the hospital. He knows that diabetic patients are more likely to suffer with ischaemic heart disease and just wants to make sure everything is as it should be. He sees his GP who confirms that it may possibly be angina and that he will refer him to the 2 week chest pain clinic to be assessed by a cardiologist. He takes a printout of his summary record including all his repeat medication as well as any over-the-counter medication and herbal remedies he is taking and his personal localized *Map of Medicine* pathway. He knows they can sometimes affect his medication or condition too. He arrives at his appointment early and reads through the *Map of Medicine* pathway to see what next steps will be.

He presents this to the doctor who also has a copy of the same pathway in front of him. This is very reassuring for both – they are both using the same guidelines. Following the consultation, his doctor arranges a coronary angiogram for him. He confirms that he needs to continue to take all his medication and not stop any. He also checks on the hospital website for what to do the night before an angiogram. It advises not to eat anything or drink anything from 10 p.m. the night before besides a drop of water with his tablets in the morning. It also says he should not smoke either.

He's glad he stopped smoking many years ago when his doctor advised him to change his ways and become an eMPOWERed citizen by taking control of his own health. The angiogram confirms he has developed two vessel disease and so has angioplasty done at the same time. He knows that the angioplasty will not in itself enable him to live longer. But it will improve his symptoms. Although he is now

pain free, he resolves to try to reduce his weight even more and do more walking
and cycling. He also wants to take his family with him on walks and cycles too – he
really does not want them to have to go through what he has had to. And there is so
much to enjoy and get satisfaction from. Why not? Life is to enjoy and not throw
away. He feels very positive about himself and wonders what would have happened
to him and his family had he not changed his ways!

References

Anderson, R. M., Funnell, M. M., Butler, P. M., Arnold, M. S., Fitzgerald, J. T., & Feste, C. C.
(1995). Patient empowerment. Results of a randomized controlled trial. *Diabetes Care, 18*(7),
943–949.

Falcão-Reis, F., & Correia, M. E. (2010). Patient empowerment by the means of citizen-managed
electronic health records: Web 2.0 health digital identity scenarios. *Studies in Health Technology
and Informatics, 156*, 214–228.

Fisher, B., Fitton, R., Poirier, C., & Sables, D. (2007). Patient record access – The time has come.
British Journal of General Practice, 57, 507–511.

Funnell, M. M., Anderson, R. M., Arnold, M. S., Barr, P. A., Donnelly, M. B., Johnson, P. D., et al.
(1991). Empowerment: An idea whose time has come in diabetes patient education. *Diabetes
Education, 17*, 37–41.

Hannan, A. (2007). The paradigm shift in healthcare – Overcoming challenges in giving patients
access to their records. *Journal of Communication in Healthcare, 1*(1), 7–19.

Hannan, A. (2010). Providing patients online access to their primary care computerised medical
records: A case study of sharing and caring. *Informatics in Primary Care, 18*, 41–49.

Hannan, A., & Webber, F. (2007). Towards a partnership of trust. *Studies in Health Technology and
Informatics, 127*, 108–116.

Munir, S., & Boaden, R. (2001). Patient empowerment and the electronic health record. *Studies in
Health Technology and Informatics, 84*, 663–665.

Roberts, K. J. (2001). Patient empowerment in the United States: A critical commentary. *Health
Expectations, 2*(2), 82–92.

Salmon, P., & Hall, G. M. (2003). Patient empowerment and control: A psychological discourse in
the service of medicine. *Social Science & Medicine, 57*(10), 1969–1980.

Salmon, P., & Hall, G. M. (2004). Patient empowerment or the emporor's new clothes. *Journal of
the Royal Society of Medicine, 97*(2), 53–56.

Segal, L. (1998). The importance of patient empowerment in health system reform. *Health Policy,
44*(1), 31–44.

What is self care? (2010). Retrieved August 29, 2010, from NHS Choices: www.nhs.uk/Planners/
Yourhealth/Pages/Whatisselfcare.aspx.

Wikipedia. (2010). Retrieved August 29, 2010, from Wikipedia: http://en.wikipedia.org/wiki/
Patient.

www.thebigoptout.org (2010). Retrieved August 29, 2010, from www.thebigoptout.org.

Chapter 16
E-Health: Focusing on People-Centric Dimensions

Rajeev K. Bali, Michael C. Gibbons, Vikraman Baskaran, Caroline De Brún, and Raouf N. G. Naguib

Abstract This chapter highlights the essential issue of people skills and knowledge for E-Health based initiatives. People-based issues have Knowledge Management (KM) at their core and the best KM implementations rely heavily on skilfully integrating technology with human requirements. The chapter features three short E-Health cases and discusses the human dimensions of each of these. Finally, we call for increased use of Populomics (a comprehensive way of studying health issues and providing focused solutions) when implementing E-Health as this produces a powerful solution taking into account multiple factors.

Keywords Knowledge Management • Populomics • Organisational Development • Healthcare information system • Breast screening • Crohn's disease • Maternity services

16.1 E-Health

The multidisciplinary nature of E-Health has resulted in a plethora of definitions focussing on one or more of the following themes: information and technology technologies (ICTs), process-driven activities and people-focussed dimensions.

R.K.Bali (✉) • C. De Brún • R.N.G. Naguib
Biomedical Computing and Engineering Technologies (BIOCORE) Applied Research Group,
Health Design and Technology Institute (HDTI), Coventry University, Coventry, UK
e-mail: r.bali@ieee.org; debrunc@uni.coventry.ac.uk; r.naguib@coventry.ac.uk

M.C. Gibbons, MD, MPH
Public Health and Medicine, Center for Community Health,
Johns Hopkins Urban Health Institute, Johns Hopkins Medical Institutions, Baltimore, MD, USA
e-mail: mgibbons@jhsph.edu

V. Baskaran
Ted Rogers School of Information Technology Management,
Ryerson University, Toronto, Ontario, Canada
e-mail: vikraman@ryerson.ca

N. Wickramasinghe et al. (eds.), *Critical Issues for the Development of Sustainable E-health Solutions*, Healthcare Delivery in the Information Age, DOI 10.1007/978-1-4614-1536-7_16, © Springer Science+Business Media, LLC 2012

These three aspects are also the essential components of contemporary Knowledge Management (KM) which results from the intersection of people, process and technology (Bali et al. 2009; Wickramasinghe et al. 2009). As with KM, when discussing people-centric issues, there is inevitable cross-over with process and technology issues as all three of these concepts are inextricably linked.

In essence, E-Health has at its core the intent to effectively share health information by way of technology. The term E-Health "…characterizes not only a technical development, but also a state-of-mind, a way of thinking, an attitude, and a commitment for networked, global thinking, to improve health care locally, regionally, and worldwide by using information and communication technology" (Eysenbach 2001). Due to the potentially wide definitions of the term, the NHS Service Delivery and Organisation (SDO) Programme has funded mapping projects to understand the field. Literature review articles have identified the range of E-Health definitions used worldwide (Pagliari et al. 2005; Oh et al. 2005). Even though these definitions address a wide array of areas within healthcare, the benefits of E-Health are universally accepted and include:

- Supporting the delivery of care tailored to individual patients
- Improving transparency and accountability of care processes
- Facilitating shared care across boundaries
- Patient-centric care delivery
- Aiding evidence-based practice and error reduction
- Improving diagnostic accuracy and treatment appropriateness
- Improving access to effective healthcare by reducing barriers created (physical location or disability)
- Facilitating patient empowerment for self-care and health decision making
- Improving cost-efficiency by streamlining processes, reducing waiting times and waste (OpenClinical.org 2005).

Much of the current E-Health literature focusses on the role of technology. Whilst technology is integral to the success of E-Health initiatives, we must also understand the importance of process and people. This paper will focus on the people issue and will provide an overview of key concepts. Brief case studies will be presented which illustrate how people-centric activities are central to E-Health success.

16.2   Examples of People-Based Issues in E-Health

16.2.1   Social Networks

In its simplest form, a social network is a structure comprised of several nodes (entities which could be companies, institutions or people) which are interconnected according to varying dependencies and interdependencies. These could include common interest, value, linkages and so forth. Given the myriad of different possibilities, the resulting visualization can often be very complex. Social Network Analysis (SNA) examines these relationships as linkages (ties) between nodes (the actors within the network). The social networks (and contacts) combine to form social capital, considered to be of vital importance for communities and individuals (Putnam et al. 2000).

The fact that relationships matter is a key concept within social capital theory (Field 2003). As interactions allow people to create communities and a sense of belonging, the rich experience of a trustworthy social network can produce great advantages to the individuals within the social network. The "trustworthiness" of the network is essential as trust between individuals (known persons within the network) has broader implications for people outside the network (strangers) with whom interactions (face-to-face) would eventually take place (Beem 1999). Without this essential interaction, trust breaks down causing major social problems. The NHS Faculty of Health Informatics has conducted special training sessions for its staff on social networking tools (NHS Faculty of Health Informatics 2008). These training sessions were aimed at educating their staff on the various facets of social networking and to apply them for effective collaboration within NHS. Such networking tools increase the efficacy of delivering healthcare and also ensure that the people delivering them can actually enjoy doing their jobs (NHS Faculty of Health Informatics 2008).

The proliferation of web-based social networking includes recent phenomena such as wikis, blogging, chat, instant messaging, file sharing, file exchange, video and contact management. The "social" aspect (the ability for individual users within the trustworthy environment to "tag" important documents and items – thus saving valuable time for other interested users) has key advantages for contemporary organizations. When this is combined with opinion and fact-finding from individuals, these comment-based contributions can combine to provide the basis for a useful Community of Practice (CoP).

16.2.2   Community of Practice

The term "Communities of Practice" (CoP) refers to a network of people, working on the same or similar areas, coming together (either physically or virtually) to share and develop their collective knowledge (Wenger 1998). The intention is that this would benefit themselves as individuals as well as the organization. Engagement in CoPs may be viewed as a way in which the individual helps establish his or her own identity and this identity relates to processes of change. CoPs may be within a subject discipline, or they may be within an application area that involves people from a variety of subject disciplines. Wenger explains practice as meaning – an experience which is of interest located in a process referred to as the negotiation of meaning. This negotiation requires active participation defined as "…the social experience of living in the world in terms of membership in social communities and active involvement in social enterprises … it can involve all kinds of relations, conflictual as well as harmonious, intimate as well as political, competitive as well as cooperative" (Wenger 1998).

A Community of Practice created and facilitated by the Knowledge Management for Healthcare (KARMAH) research subgroup (working under BIOCORE) at Coventry University in the UK is exemplified by the "KARMAH Starwheel". Essentially, as the group's interests match those of KM within the healthcare environ, the span of knowledge is widespread, depicted by five distinct avenues: OB (Organizational Behaviour, including change management, strategy, ICTs, clinical governance), CI (Clinical Informatics and Engineering, including AI, cybernetics, expert systems), ET (Education and Training, including HRM, work study, industry-academic interfaces), PS (Privacy and Security, including technical, legal, ethical and organizational aspects), DM (Data Mining, including algorithms, knowledge discovery, genomic mining).

Having recognized that the nature of Healthcare KM is such that a blend of key skills is required to achieve true progress in this rapidly evolving area, the "Starwheel" depicts the group's strategy for efficient sharing and debate of current knowledge in the field. The schematic shows how participants, with expertise and competencies in the given areas (e.g. OB, CI etc) can bring key ideas to a central repository (the centre of the star) from which other members can draw/amend/add before returning back to the centre for final refinement. At the same time, members are free to interact by moving directly across the wheel. In this manner, it is envisaged that this will lead to an increased and rapid level of publication and/or collaborative projects for all active participants. This is a useful example of a multidisciplinary Community of Practice.

16.2.3 Organisational Development and Mess Management

Organisation Development (OD) refers to long term programme, led and supported by top management, to improve an organisation's visioning, empowerment, learning, and problem-solving processes, through an ongoing, collaborative management of the organisation's culture. There is special emphasis on the culture of intact work teams and other team configurations, particularly on the consultant-facilitator role and the theory and technology of applied behavioural science, including action research (French and Bell 1995). The approach: (1) emphasises goals and processes with emphasis on processes, (2) deals with change over medium and long-term, (3) is about people and recognises their worth, (4) involves the organisation as a whole as well as its parts and (5) emphasises the concept of a change agent/facilitator.

Some organisational scenarios, by the nature of their complexity and particular characteristics – such as E-Health, require a soft rather than a hard systems approach to change. The philosophy, value orientation and theoretical underpinnings of Organisation Development (OD) as a generalised example of soft systems models for change are ideally suited to E-Health initiatives. Factors such as power bases, organisational culture, leadership styles and changes in the organisation's environment can make organisational change a lot more complex and emotionally charged (or "messy") than traditional models of change can adequately deal with.

The traditional (hard systems) model of change is not likely to be effective for E-Health scenarios as the nature of the presented (and multidisciplinary) problems are defined differently by different stakeholders. E-Health systems are therefore inherently complex and quantitative criteria cannot always readily be agreed upon. Work by Ackoff (1993) on "Mess Management" concludes that the issues involved with such complex scenarios should be "dissolved" (or "idealised"). This would involve three broad stages: (1) changing the nature of the problem context (or system) so as to remove the problem, (2) development-orientation (and therefore keen to improve the quality of organisational life for self and others), (3) redesign of the systems at various levels of the organisation in order to dissolve the problem.

16.3 Populomics

The healthcare domain not only provides challenging opportunities for managing knowledge but also is one of the areas where it is often most poorly understood and deployed. This predicament is slowly being addressed as more and more KM-focussed projects are initiated and healthcare professionals (and other stakeholders) with better understanding of KM are being involved. More family and community residents are becoming "caregivers" and "care providers". This shift is enhancing the impact of social, behavioural, community and economic realities on their therapeutic regimens and provider relationships. In short, the social and behavioural sciences, which traditionally had not been considered within the domain of healthcare, are increasingly recognized as fundamentally linked to illness, health and healthcare outcomes (Galea and Vlahov 2005) while the need for an integrated approach to health research and healthcare is gaining appreciation, thinking across disciplinary lines can be challenging.

The growing realization of healthcare disparities is forcing clinical researchers to think about disease causation not only among individual patients, but also across entire groups or populations of people. Among patients who have vastly differing cultural beliefs and practices, diets, educational or literacy levels and socioeconomic resources, clinical practitioners and researchers developing interventions that ignore these sociocultural realities may struggle to demonstrate or maintain therapeutic efficacy across increasingly multicultural populations of patients. Focussing on electronic health care records, a growing number of patients want both access and control of their own information, large employers are exploring new methods to improve employee (and beneficiary) health while reducing healthcare costs and leading technology companies are anxious to offer an effective technology solution.

Increasingly, scientific evidence suggests that disease causation results from complex interactions of social, environmental, behavioural and biologic factors which simultaneously and often cooperatively act across more than one level of existence over time (Gibbons et al. 2007). Thus a comprehensive understanding of health and disease requires the integration of knowledge derived from the bench, sociobehavioral and population sciences. Most historic and contemporary conceptual models of health though, have often been derived either from the socio-behavioural sciences or the biomolecular sciences. With the exception of those pathways based on stress (neuro-immunological) mechanisms, the published frameworks in the behavioural sciences and epidemiological literature largely lack clearly stated, causal biologic connections to observed health outcomes (Macintyre 1997; Acheson 1998; Williams 1999; LaLonde 1981; Evans and Stoddart 1990). On the other hand, most biologically oriented formulations poorly account for socio-environmental and behavioural effect modifiers that may profoundly influence the pathogenesis of disease and the development of health disparities (Burger and Gimelfarb 1999; Phillips and Belknap 2002; Sharma 1998; Meyer and Breitner 1998).

Populomics represents a new comprehensive way of studying health problems and crafting health solutions. It is being advocated by some officials at the National Institutes of Health as a new science that should be supported as the population level equivalent of genomics, which may lead to quantum leaps forward in understanding health challenges and developing new effective therapies and treatments (Office of Behavioral and Social Sciences Research (OBSSR) 2010). The three case studies illustrate how KM and knowledge-based initiatives such as Populomics can be used to create powerful health outcomes.

Both Populomics and the people-centric theories described earlier can be applied to E-Health cases as they embody organisational processes that seek a synergistic combination of data and information processing capacity of information technologies, and the creative and innovative capacity of human beings. We now present three case studies which illustrate the importance of human expertise as part of their E-Health focus.

16.3.1 Case Exemplar #1: Breast Screening

Breast cancer is the most common cancer in women with over forty thousand women being diagnosed with the disease each year in the UK (Cancer Research 2005). Any information related to the breast can largely affect a women's consciousness and a threat of breast cancer will have varying impacts on women psychology. Typically breast cancerous cells originate in the mammary glands (lobules) or in the ducts connected to these glands or in other tissues around these glands (American Cancer Society Inc. 2005). When in close proximity to the lymphatic system, these cells can result in being carried to other organs of the body. This subsequently results in cancerous growth in that organ and is described as metastatic breast cancer (American Cancer Society Inc. 2005). Although many causes had been identified for breast cancer, the knowledge of finding a cure is still not within the reach of modern medicine.

Breast cancer should ideally be diagnosed at the earlier stages of its development. Possible treatments include removing or destroying the cancer cells to avoid the spread of the affected cells. Breast Self Examination (BSE) is an effective and non-intrusive type of self diagnosis exercise for checking any abnormalities/lumps in the breast tissue. Unfortunately this greatly depends on the size of the lump, technique and experience in carrying out a self examination by the woman. An ultrasound test using sound waves can be used to detect lumps but this is usually suited for women aged below thirty-five owing to the higher density of breast tissue (American Cancer Society Inc. 2005). Having a tissue biopsy via a fine needle aspiration or an excision is often used to test the cells for cancer. These tests are mostly employed in treatments or post-treatment examination and as second rung diagnostic confirmation methods. Performing a Computed Tomography (CT) or a Magnetic Resonance Imaging (MRI) scan would result in a thorough examination of the breast tissue but this technique is not favoured due to reasons including that it may not be economical, needs preparation, noisy, time consuming and images may not be clear.

16.3.1.1   Breast Screening Programme

Mammography is a technique for detecting breast tissue lumps using a low dosage of x-ray. This technique can even detect a three millimetre sized lump. The x-ray image of the breast tissue is captured and the image is thoroughly read by experienced radiologists and specialist mammogram readers. Preliminary research suggests that women aged 55 and above are more susceptible to breast cancer; mammography is more suited to the women aged 55 and above (due to the lower density of breast tissue) (Blanks et al. 2000). Even though mammography has its critics – mainly due to its high rate of false positives and false negatives (Burton 1997) – it has still become the standard procedure for screening women by the National Health Service (NHS) National Breast Screening Programme UK (Forrest 1986). Mammography is the best and most viable tool for mass screening to detect cancer in the breast at an early stage (Medicine net 2002); however, the effectiveness of diagnosis through screening is directly dependent on the percentage of women attending the screening programme. The NHS Breast Screening Programme, catering to the entire eligible women population is funded by the Department of Health in the UK and is the first of its kind in the world. It covers nearly four million women and detected more than 13,000 cancers in the screened population for the year 2005 (NHS Review 2005). Currently the screening programme routinely screens women between the ages of 50 and 70, and employs two views of the breast, medio-lateral and cranio-caudal. The lack of breakthroughs in finding a definitive cure means that preventive medicine is the only viable alternative to reduce deaths due to breast cancer.

The UK National Health Service (NHS) National Breast Screening Programme (NBSP) is unique as it provides free breast screening for the female population aged between 50 and 70 at a national level (Forrest 1986; Cancer Research 2004). The recent increase of the upper age limit from 63 to 70 for screening and making a two-view mammogram mandatory has greatly increased the efficiency of benign or malignant tumour detection. The NBSP currently runs a massive screening programme catering to almost two million eligible women across the UK (Cancer Research 2004). This programme runs on a call/recall cycle which screens all eligible women in a 3 year interval. The information published by the UK Government Statistical Service (NHS Health and Social Care Information Centre) in its Community Health Statistics report for the year 2006 agrees that, for the past 10 years since 1995, the uptake has remained constant at around 75%. The number of non-attendees has been significantly increasing and has reached half a million. Simple projection of this data submits that nearly 4,000 cancer incidences would not have been diagnosed. Even if a small percentage of these non-attendees could be made to attend, it would result in the saving of significant lives. Indirectly we can also infer that, despite focussed efforts on these non-attendees for the past 10 years, there was no real effect on their attendance. Moreover, early stage cancer detection would have a huge impact in reducing cancer related deaths. From these facts and data, we see that the primary concern is to reduce non-attendance (Bankhead et al. 2001). These challenges can be addressed by a resource saving strategy which has better healthcare at its core. The technical details involved mean that it is beyond the remit of this paper.

16.3.1.2 Human Dimensions of this Case

The objective of this work was to identify the challenges which are being faced by the UK NHS' national breast screening programme and find approaches to alleviate these impediments and eventually reduce mortality due to breast cancer. When the algorithm is executed, the resulting knowledge can be shared with the GPs (with whom the women are registered) can initiate personally interventions. Such interventions can educate the non-attending women and clarify their attitudes and beliefs – this can only occur by way of human interaction (i.e. doctor and patient). The expected outcome is that the women commits to a positive informed decision, which would culminate in attending the screening appointment. This work not only confirms that breast screening attendance can be predicted through an automated software solution, but also can be leveraged to increase screening attendance by employing emerging KM tools and techniques. This research work draws its strength from such KM tools and techniques. This work is also one such initiative addressing the NHS' breast screening attendance through efficient KM methodologies. A 25% success in GP interventions will result in saving more than 350 women's lives per year.

16.3.2   Case Exemplar #2: Maternity Services

At its conception in 1948, the UK's National Health Service (NHS) held three core principles: (a) to meet the health care needs of everyone, (b) free at the point of delivery and (c) based on clinical need, and not the ability to pay. The aim was to create an uniform service combining all hospitals under one central system with the ideal that healthcare should be available to all regardless of wealth status. Sixty years on, the NHS is relatively uniform but with significant inequalities in service and quality of care with access to treatment. This case will examine some of the various KM issues induced by the introduction of ICTs into the NHS with a particular focus on Maternity Services.

Maternity Services were not particularly affected by various changes in policy and NHS maternity care is given without charge at the point of delivery. However, in comparison to other European countries, the UK Government has contributed approximately 1–1.5% less to healthcare on an annual basis. This has been a contributory factor in the inadequacies of healthcare provided by the NHS today (Bankhead et al. 2001). The NHS organization consists of multiple layers of health service providers each responsible for the procurement of their own IT systems. This has led to a vast amount of systems that have not been introduced in a coherent approach, therefore integration and sharing of information between providers and across the services has not been efficient or effective. In order to increase efficiency, effectiveness, equity and reduce risk, particularly at the point of care, The National Programme for Information and Technology (NPfIT) was introduced in 2002. Connecting for Health (CfH) is the Government agency responsible for the implementation of NPfIT. It is the largest civil technology program undertaken and is intended to unite separate NHS organizations. This is a centrally driven mandate.

The aim is to electronically connect all 50 million plus patient records, allowing access by patients and health professionals in over 30,000 General Practitioners (GP) Practices and 300 hospitals. It was envisaged that during an incremental period of 10 years, NPfIT will bring modern computer systems into the NHS changing the way the NHS works to improve patient care and services. However, the formation of a single demographic database gives rise to many concerns. In particular, how this information will be used, by whom and how patient confidentiality and security will be maintained are common themes amongst those resistant to a national database. Many patients and clinicians are concerned that the system is not secure (Wanless 2002; Carvel 2006). A number of clinicians are sceptical of the need for integrated records via a national database, as systems already exist for locality data sharing between relevant GP's and hospitals 'without the need to leave a copy of the information on the nationally accessible database' (Leigh 2006). In order to satisfy patient concerns and control access, the consequence of illegal misuse of data from the databases may require greater legal penalties than the current financial ones.

16.3.2.1 Proposed Changes Within Maternity Services

Current NHS reforms aim 'to develop a patient led NHS that uses available resources as effectively and fairly as possible to promote health, reduce health inequalities and deliver the best and safest healthcare' (Department of Health 2006). Maternity organizations must therefore supply accessible, efficient, quality care. Services should provide care that is women focused considering individual needs of health status, culture, religion, social needs and disabilities. High quality, efficient Maternity Services are essential in contributing the attainment of the Department of Health's Public Service Agreement (PSA) targets (Treasury 2004). In relation to Maternity Services, the PSA targets include: (a) reduction by 10% of health inequalities, measurable by infant mortality and life expectancy at birth, (b) a substantial reduction of mortality rates, (c) reduce by 1% per annum women who smoke in pregnancy, (d) reducing the under 18 year old conception rate and (e) increase breastfeeding rates by 2% per annum.

In addition, the Department of Health produced the *Maternity Standard, National Service Framework (NSF) for Children Young People and Maternity Services* (2004) identified as best practice guidance. The NSF is based on a care pathway approach which place value on women-focused care rather than meeting the needs of the service. In doing so, an emphasis is placed on evidenced-based procedures and guidelines representing a method for continuous quality improvement. Maternity care pathways will provide a system through which services will be integrated between primary, secondary and social services to provide comparable high quality effective clinical care.

The large scale and constituents of the work force will have a major impact of change within the NHS. In comparison to other countries the UK has a lower number of health care professional per population (Wanless 2002). Recruitment and retention of staff in some services, particularly midwifery, create significant difficulties and can seriously effect patient care. The NHS Plan proposes new ways of working to reduce professional barriers resulting in a more flexible workforce between staff groups. In addition, it aims to increase the amount of skilled workforce. Nurse Practitioners/ Midwives could assume 20% of doctor's work, whilst Health Care Assistants (HCAs) could perform duties of the Nurse/Midwife workload. This skill mix change would increase the workforce capacity. However significant investment in IT would reduce administration time allowing increased time providing patient care.

16.3.2.2 Human Dimensions of this Case: Patient Expectations

Patients today are better informed with access to better information regarding treatment, management and prevention of illness and diseases. Patients have rights to informed consent but also demand informed choice of type and place of their care. Healthcare does not meet patient expectations particularly regarding access of care and waiting times for treatment. In addition, the health service is not yet sufficiently patient-centred; the Wanless Report included survey evidence showing that patients commonly feel that they have insufficient involvement in decisions, there is not one to talk to about anxieties and concerns, tests and treatment are not clearly explained with insufficient written information provided. A survey by the Department of Health in 2005 observed that women using NHS Maternity Services would have preferred more choice in type of care and place of delivery. Certain geographical locations have experienced an increase in European migrants which has had an impact on Maternity Services, particularly with language difficulties. For local Trusts there are cost implications involving translators and written forms of communications that are not met centrally. With widening access to current maternity health care information, for example via the internet, the general public are more assertive and better informed to demand change within Maternity Services.

16.3.3   Case Exemplar #3: Crohn's Disease – Availability of Internet Based Information and Person-to-Person Support

Crohn's disease is an inflammatory bowel disease, affecting about one in 700 people, both male and female, but mainly adults. It is not contagious, but there is a higher risk if a family member already suffers from the condition. It is a chronic condition, and can affect people for the rest of their lives. The condition flares up causing excruciating pain and discomfort, and then goes into remission. The quality of life of sufferers is greatly affected as there is often no obvious trigger for a relapse (Bupa's Health Information Team 2008). For this reason, it is essential that sufferers have access to good quality information and support, available online, as sometimes they may not be able to leave the house.

This case study acted as a critical review to search for online patient information and support, and assess the quality of the resources. Assessment was based on whether the sites are supported by adverts or sponsorship, whether they have the HONCode symbol, and whether they adhere to Silberg's criteria (Silberg et al. 1997), namely:

1. Authorship – identifiable author with no conflict of interest
2. Attribution – copyright information relating to material on the website
3. Disclosure – ownership of the site accurately determinable
4. Currency – clearly visible date showing when the information was updated
5. Content – appropriate for patient population.

A search on PubMed (www.pubmed.gov) was carried out, searching for "*Crohn disease*" (this is how it is classified on PubMed) combined with "*Patient Education*" or "*Patient Education Handout*" or "*Self-Help Groups*", all as MeSH (Medical Subject Headings or Thesaurus terms). Seventy-five papers were identified, the majority of which were aimed at clinicians rather than patients. The remaining 22 discussed Crohn's disease from the point of view of the patient (Torpy et al. 2008; Zutshi et al. 2007;

American Family Physician 2003), and some assessed the quality of patient information and support (Moody et al. 1993; Verma et al. 2001; Probert et al. 1991), again, from a patient-point-of-view. The reason for this search was to identify if a previous critical review existed, and to get some general background information on the availability of online patient information and support for this condition.

The next step of this review was to search the Internet for appropriate results. "crohn's disease" was searched on Google, with no restrictions. 2,730,000 results were received. A free text search on PubMed found 20,026 results, of which 16,524 were in English. When restricted to a MeSH or thesaurus search, there were 17,686 papers in English, specifically about "Crohn disease". An amended search on Google for "crohn's disease" "support groups" produced 96,700 results. The search was amended to first include "NHS", which improved the results, and then changing "support" to "patient", which did not improve the results. Having reviewed the results from Google, it was decided to restrict the search to "UK", for reasons which will be discussed in the results section. This restriction produced 381,000 results. A final search was performed via a subject gateway. *Intute Health and Life Sciences* (www.intute.ac.uk/healthandlifesciences) is a search engine that applies filters to its search so that only good quality information is found. A search was carried out which retrieved only 21 results only 10 of which were patient-related.

For the purpose of this critical review, the results of the Google searches will be restricted to the first ten results. In 2005, Google carried out an eye tracking study (PRWeb 2005) to verify the importance of page position. It seems to show that people look at the top, left-hand side of the page, (for example, the first five results), the most. The author cannot prove that this is the method that everyone uses when searching, but to review more results would not be possible within the word limitations of this review. Five searches were carried out, producing 50 websites to be reviewed. A summary was produced of the web-sites with an assessment of the sites, based on Silberg's criteria, whether they have the HONCode symbol, and whether or not they are supported by adverts or sponsorship.

The first search found only one web-site from the UK. The rest were from the US. Two (*MedicineNet* and *WebMD*) looked as though there were different organisations with different URLs, but they were produced by the same organisation. Both sites had the HONcode symbol on their screens, yet they did not meet Silberg's criteria for quality (Silberg et al. 1997). Both sites promoted drugs, which is inappropriate and confusing for patients, particularly as different drugs are available in the US, compared to the UK. Neither site contained links to the original research, only further resources on each other's web-sites. Wikipedia was slightly better, as it produced a long list of original research that was used to produce the content. However, there was no information about the authors. The Crohn's Disease Web Site was the worst one for meeting the criteria. There were lots of adverts and pop-ups, and no evidence of ownership or attribution. The Crohn's and Colitis Foundation of America is a non-profit organisation, but it does have corporate sponsors, including pharmaceutical companies, so there may be some bias. Furthermore, they say that their content is reviewed by members of their National Scientific Advisory Committee, but no further details were available. Two of the best sites were the

National Institute for Health and Medline Plus. However, both of these are aimed at the US population. As Crohn's disease can be affected by diet, there may be differences in treatment, between UK and US populations. For this reason, the search was re-run, adding "UK" to the search terms, and the results of this search will be discussed further on. The best result that was retrieved was from NHS Choices, which had a review date, and no sponsorship, and is aimed towards UK patients.

The next search looked at ""crohn's disease" uk". These were much more relevant to the UK patient. However, the first result was the *National Association for Colitis and Crohn's Disease*, which although it is a charity, has corporate sponsorship from pharmaceutical companies. The best resource was again, the NHS Choices page on Crohn's disease. But, again, this was last in the Google ranking, which means that if their eye tracking study is to be believed, it may not be picked up by the patient. The search using the Subject Gateway wasn't really helpful as it only retrieved 21 results, and only 10 of these were for the patient. It retrieved items such as the *National Association for Colitis and Crohn's Disease*, *MEDLINEplus*, *MayoClinic*, and *Crohn's and Colitis Foundation of America*, all of which had been picked up via Google. It did not, however, pick up anything from NHS Choices, which is surprising as Intute is a UK-based resource. It did retrieve a patient leaflet from the Clinical Knowledge Summaries service (CKS) however, which is also UK-based, but predominantly for clinicians.

The final searches, built "support groups" into the equation. Again, unless specifically limited to the UK, only American support groups were displayed, which is not helpful to UK-based patients. When "UK" was added to the search, results were displayed, some for physical support groups, and some providing online support in the form of discussion lists and chatrooms. Google Directory was one of the results and linked to a list of 14 online support groups. These results seemed most useful as they linked to other people suffering from the same complaint. Some of the sites did have adverts, which is how they are able to offer the service freely, but on the whole, they looked user-friendly and there was a fair selection for patients to choose from, all based in the UK.

It is clearly very difficult to find appropriate patient information on "Crohn's disease" unless the searcher is familiar with methods for limiting searches. In reality, if they are researching a condition for themselves or for someone close to them, the last thing they will probably think of will be to apply good searching skills or to use a tool like Discern (www.discern.org.uk), a questionnaire to help patients assess the quality of a web-site. It is also unlikely that they will be familiar with symbols such as the HONcode (www.hon.ch), which could help them make judgements.

16.3.3.1   Human Dimensions of this Case

Out of all of the sites reviewed, the patient information produced by BUPA, a commercial organisation, appears to tick the most boxes, with NHS Choices coming second for UK patient information. The reason that NHS Choices comes second is because it is unclear where the evidence supporting the patient information comes from. Ideally, patients in the UK should be aware of, and rely on NHS Choices as their first port-of-call for finding the best available information on their conditions. However, although it contains patient information on 750 conditions, not all illnesses are recognised on NHS Choices. Rarer conditions will require more in-depth searching, and this is where a public librarian can help, although perhaps if the condition is sensitive, this might not be the most favoured option for the patient.

16.4 Conclusion

Our current work includes additional research continuing to investigate the human dimensions of the three cases. For all of the given case studies, the knowledge created is useful for contemporary E-Health. The outcomes leverage the health knowledge created in order to share it with the healthcare deliverers to alleviate the particular predicaments faced, be they increasing uptake of breast screening, fostering better access to maternity services or aiding the gathering of patient-focused information. Such work has direct synergies with the central component of Populomics, one of the key aims of which is to reduce disparities and inequalities. Although the role and importance of E-Health for the three provided case scenarios are central to their success, their focus on large patient communities empowers Populomics to add its inherent value to the case studies. Socio-behavioural factors and community-wide risk profiles can be integrated into the existing knowledge-based initiatives as, in combination, Populomics and E-Health can come together to produce a powerful focus for current and future, patient-focussed, practice. We encourage researchers in similar fields to include Populomics into relevant E-Health studies.

References

Acheson, D. (1998). *Independant inquiry into inequalities in health*. London: UK Department of Health.

Ackoff, R. (1993). *From mechanistic to social systematic thinking, systems thinking in action conference*. Pegasus: Pegasus Communications, Inc.

American Cancer Society Inc. (2005). Cancer reference information. www.cancer.org/docroot/CRI/content/CRI_2_4_1X_What_is_ breast _cancer_5.asp. Accessed 10 Aug 2005.

American Family Physician. (2003). Information from your family doctor: Crohn's disease. *American Family Physician, 68*(4), 17–18.

Bali, R. K., Wickramasinghe, N., & Lehaney, B. (2009). *Knowledge management primer*. New York: Routledge.

Bankhead, C., Austoker, J., Sharp, D., Peters, T., et al. (2001). A practice based randomized controlled trial of two simple interventions aimed to increase uptake of breast cancer screening. *Journal of Medical Screening, 8*(2), 91–98.

Beem, C. (1999). *The necessity of politics: Reclaiming American public life*. Chicago: University of Chicago Press.

Blanks, R. G., Moss, S. M., McGahan, C. E., Quinn, M. J., et al. (2000). Effect of NHS breast screening programme on mortality from breast cancer in England and Wales, 1990–8: Comparison of observed with predicted mortality. *British Medical Journal, 321*(7262), 665–669.

Bupa's Health Information Team. (2008). Crohn's disease Bupa. http://hcd2.bupa.co.uk/fact_sheets/html/crohns_disease.html. Accessed 2 Jan 09.

Burger, R., & Gimelfarb, A. (1999). Genetic variation maintained in multilocus models of additive quantitative traits under stabilizing selection. *Genetics, 152*(2), 807–820.

Burton, G. (1997). *Alternative medicine*. Washington: Future Medicine Publishing.

Cancer Research UK. (2004). Breast cancer factsheet. http://publications.cancerresearchuk.org/epages/crukstore.sf/en_GB/?ObjectPath=/Shops/crukstore/Categories/BrowseBySubject/BreastCancer. Accessed 18 Sept 2004.

Cancer Research UK. (2005). CancerStats incidence-UK. http://www.cancerresearchuk.org/about-cancer/statistics/statsmisc/pdfs/cancerstats_incidence_apr05.pdf. Accessed 10 Aug 2005.

Carvel, J. (2006). NHS plan for central patient database alarms doctors. The Guardian. 21 Nov 2006, http://society.guardian.co.uk/e-public/story/0,,195318500.html. Accessed 1 July 2011.

Department of Health. (2006). *Health reform in England: Update and commissioning framework*. London: HMSO.

Evans, R. G., & Stoddart, G. L. (1990). Producing health, consuming health care. *Social Science & Medicine, 31*(12), 1347–1363.

Eysenbach, G. (2001). Editorial. *Journal of Medical Internet Research, 3*(2), e20.

Field, J. (2003). *Social capital*. London: Routledge.

Forrest, P. (1986). *Breast cancer screening – A report to the health ministers of England, Scotland, Wales and Northern Ireland*. London: HMSO.

French, W. L., & Bell, C. H. (1995). *Organisation development: Behavioural science interventions for organisation improvement*. Englewood Cliffs: Prentice-Hall.

Galea, S., & Vlahov, D. (2005). Urban health: Evidence, challenges and directions. *Annual Review of Public Health, 26*, 341–365.

Gibbons, M. C., Brock, M., Alberg, A. J., Glass, T., LaVeist, T. A., Baylin, S. B., et al. (2007). The Socio-biologic integrative model: Enhancing the integration of socio-behavioural, environmental and bio-molecular knowledge in urban health and disparities research. *Journal of Urban Health, 84*(2), 198–211.

LaLonde, M. (1981). *A new perspective on the health of Canadians*. Ottawa: Government of Canada.

Leigh, D. (2006). What health professionals say about the new NHS database. The Guardian. 1 Nov 2006, http://society.guardian.co.uk/health/news/0,1936174,00.html. Accessed 1 July 2011.

Macintyre, S. (1997). The Black report and beyond: What are the issues? *Social Science & Medicine, 44*(6), 723–745.

Medicine net. (2002). Breast cancer. http://www.medicinenet.com/breast_cancer/page3.htm. Accessed 10 Aug 2005.

Meyer, J. M., & Breitner, J. C. (1998). Multiple threshold model for the onset of Alzheimer's disease in the NAS-NRC twin panel. *American Journal of Medical Genetics, 81*(1), 92–97.

Moody, G. A., Bhakta, P., & Mayberry, J. F. (1993). Disinterest in local self-help groups amongst patients with inflammatory bowel disease in Leicester. *International Journal of Colorectal Disease, 8*(4), 181–183.

NHS Faculty of Health Informatics. (2008). The power and the perils of using social networking tools in the NHS. http://kingsfundlibrary.co.uk/commissioning/Social-networking-tools-in-the-NHS-FINAL%5B1%5D%5B1%5D.pdf. Accessed 13 Mar 2010.

NHS Review. (2005). The breast screening programme annual review 2005. http://www.cancer-screening.nhs.uk/breastscreen//publications/2005review.html. Accessed 14 July 2007.

Office of Behavioral and Social Sciences Research (OBSSR). (2010). Strategic plan. http://obssr.od.nih.gov/about_obssr/strategic_planning/strategicPlanning.aspx. Accessed 3 May 2010.

Oh, H., Rizo, C., Enkin, M., & Jadad, A. (2005). What is eHealth: A systematic review of published definitions. *Journal of Medical Internet Research, 7*(1), e1.

OpenClinical.org. (2005). E-Health. http://www.openclinical.org/e-Health.html. Accessed 24 April 2010.

Pagliari, C., Sloan, D., Gregor, P., et al. (2005). What is eHealth?: A scoping exercise to map the field. *Journal of Medical Internet Research, 7*(1), e9.

Phillips, T. J., & Belknap, J. K. (2002). Complex-trait genetics: Emergence of multivariate strategies. *Nature Reviews Neuroscience, 3*(6), 478–485.

Probert, C. S., Godber, D., Calcraft, B., & Mayberr, J. F. (1991). Patient's assessment of an information booklet on Crohn's disease written by a patient. *Italian Journal of Gastroenterology, 23*(5), 9–43.

PRWeb. (2005). Did-it, Enquiro, and Eyetools uncover Google's golden triangle. http://www.prweb.com/releases/2005/03/prweb213516.htm. Accessed 3 Jan 2009.

Putnam, R. D., Feldstein, L. M., & Cohen, D. (2000). *Bowling alone: The collapse and revival of American community*. New York: Simon & Schuster.

Sharma, A. M. (1998). The thrifty-genotype hypothesis and its implications for the study of complex genetic disorders in man. *Journal of Molecular Medicine, 76*(8), 568–571.

Silberg, W. M., Lundberg, G. D., & Musacchio, R. A. (1997). Assessing, controlling, and assuring the quality of medical information on the viewor – Let the reader and viewer beware. *Journal of the American Medical Association, 277*(15), 1244–1245.

Torpy, J. M., Lynm, C., & Glass, R. M. (2008). JAMA patient page: Crohn disease. *Journal of the American Medical Association, 299*(14), 1738.

Treasury, H. M. (2004). *Spending review: Public service agreements 2005–2008*. London: HMSO.

Verma, S., Tsai, H. H., & Giaffer, M. H. (2001). Does better disease-related education improve quality of life? A survey of IBD patients. *Digestive Diseases and Science, 46*(4), 865–869.

Wanless, D. (2002). *Securing our future health: Taking a long-term view*. London: HMSO.

Wenger, E. (1998). *Communities of practice: Learning, meaning, and identity*. Cambridge: Cambridge University Press.

Wickramasinghe, N., Bali, R. K., Lehaney, B., Schaffer, J., & Gibbons, M. C. (2009). *Healthcare knowledge management primer*. New York: Routledge.

Williams, D. R. (1999). Race, socioeconomic status, and health: The added effects of racism and discrimination. *Annals of the New York Academy of Sciences, 896*, 173–188.

Zutshi, M., Hull, T. L., & Hammel, J. (2007). Crohn's disease: A patient's perspective. *International Journal of Colorectal Disease, 22*(12), 1437–1444.

Chapter 17
A Model of Estimating the Direct Benefits of Implementing Electronic Data Exchange of EMRs and State Immunization Information Systems

Michael L. Popovich and Xiaohui Zhang

Abstract In the U.S. significant investments in health information technology are being made to ensure a patient's health data is sharable between providers. Incentive programs exist to facilitate the implementation of electronic health/medical record systems. State and regional health information authorities are challenged to facilitate the exchange of patient clinical data to improve quality of care and the management of limited resources. Interoperable health information technology is the new interstate highway system for health data flow. The exchange of timely and accurate information and its use to support decisions among patients, providers, clinicians, researchers, and public health professionals is the payoff.

Investment in new health information systems will mount to hundreds of billions of dollars in the next few years alone. The unanswered question is what is the return on this investment? The assumed answer is improved patient quality of care which improves the health and economic impact on families and communities. In time, cost benefit studies will produce improved business case models for information technology investments. However, today there is an opportunity to illustrate a return on such technology investments by considering the current health information national objectives and measurement of these objectives through metric driven outcomes as specified by new meaningful use regulations.

This paper summarizes an example case study that modeled the exchange of immunization records between provider-based electronic health records and state immunization registries, demonstrating the potential for increased provider revenue. The national movement to electronic health/medical record and health information exchange is underway. The return on investment for individual providers is being accelerated through new incentive programs for qualified clinicians. However, the

M.L. Popovich, MSSE(✉) • X. Zhang, PhD
Scientific Technologies Corporation,
Tucson, AZ, USA
e-mail: Michael_Popovich@stchome.com; Xiaohui_Zhang@stchome.com

N. Wickramasinghe et al. (eds.), *Critical Issues for the Development*
of Sustainable E-health Solutions, Healthcare Delivery in the Information Age,
DOI 10.1007/978-1-4614-1536-7_17, © Springer Science+Business Media, LLC 2012

true effectiveness of this effort will be measured over time by monitoring health outcomes in provider-based populations.

Keywords EHR • Electronic date exchange • Electronic health record • Electronic medical record • EMR • Health information exchange • Health information technology • HIE • HITECH • Immunization • Immunization information system • Meaningful use • Public health • Return on investment

17.1 Background

The rapid expansion of electronic health records in the United States is a direct response to federal initiatives in support of the Health Information Technology for Economic and Clinical Health Act (HITECH) (U.S. Department of Health and Human Services 2009). This Act includes incentives and penalties for clinical practices and hospitals that serve Medicare and Medicaid eligible populations. As a result of the HITECH initiative, a qualified provider who implements Electronic Health Record (EHR) systems may receive up to $ 44,000 (through Medicare), and up to $ 63,750 (though Medicaid). These incentives are intended to "jump start" the clinical community to move to implementing interoperable electronic health/medical record systems.

HITECH emphasizes demonstrating a return on the provider incentive payments by linking the payments to specific functionality and outcomes of the implemented electronic systems. Specifically, Meaningful Use (MU) objectives have been defined in support of HITECH which can be used to demonstrate compliance and thus receipt of incentive payments.

The recent MU regulations that have been approved for the first stage of EHRs have been established to include 35 measurable objectives ranging from maintaining active medication lists and reporting of quality measures to electronic exchange of information to public health. Of these 35, an eligible provider's EHR must achieve 25 core objectives and five of the ten additional criteria (Blumenthal and Travenner 2010) in order to qualify for incentive payments.

HITECH and the accelerated national efforts to move toward electronic exchange of patient information between providers and other healthcare stakeholders are targeting approximately 72% of the U.S. physicians who currently do not have electronic medical records (The Information Technology and Innovation Foundation 2009). This initiative has significantly short timelines associated with it. Over the course of the next 2 years providers wishing to receive funding must move to implement EHRs and validate their implementation through meaningful use reporting. This is not a small task and for providers this will be challenging and disruptive to current workflow. It is understood however that the eventual outcome will be improved patient care and more efficient medical business practice resulting in added benefits for the provider, their paying partners, and most important, the patient.

It is a given that EHRs will continue to expand within the clinical community. It is a given that their functionality will impact provider operations and that costs will only partially be off-set by incentive payments and that the on-going sustainability of these systems must be supported through the clinical business model. It is a given some clinicians will embrace this effort while others will be less than enthusiastic. But in time EHRs will be standard within all medical practices. The more important and significant challenges of sharing and using the information to improve patient health and provider-based population outcomes will be centermost.

This paper illustrates through a case example how compliance with just one Meaningful Use objective, the electronic exchange of immunization records of EHRs with a public health state registry, will create value-added benefits for the provider. The benefits will increase their return on this investment and accelerate movement toward electronic sharing of patient health information.

17.2 EHR Public Health Meaningful Use Objectives

The final MU regulations that have recently been accepted include three objectives that specifically support public health (PH):

- Submit electronic immunization data to immunization registries or immunization information systems.
- Submit electronic syndromic surveillance data to public health agencies.
- Submit electronic data on reportable laboratory results to public health agencies.

In addition, there are a number of other meaningful use criteria which require the reporting of quality measures and the ability to generate lists of patient subpopulations by condition to improve their quality of care, reduce disparities, and increase outreach. These objectives begin to establish measurable values for the use of the data within an EHR to support provider-based population health outcomes.

Given the investment required to implement and sustain an electronic record system, a case can be made in support of increasing the value of this investment to the provider if they support the public health meaningful use objectives and actively implement data exchange. The question becomes: is it possible to measure the value of ensuring that the EHR is interoperable with public health, and how this can increase or impact the provider's patient care, their business operations, or impact their cost and revenue. In short, is there an EHR-PH ROI? If so, how can we quantitatively estimate it?

17.3 EHR Return on Investment

Implementation of electronic health/medical record systems consists of ensuring a clinical practice has the correct hardware, operating software, telecommunication, and staff to support vendor requirements, train users, and migrate data in order to validate and operate the optimal EHR for the physician's practice. Each is a cost element to the business. Each has an impact on operations and patient services through this process, and each has associated risks.

Consultants, vendors, blogs, and peer-based anecdotal evidence provide information on costs, risks and benefits, as well as best practices for options and alternative EHR solutions. The American Academy of Family Physicians (Valancy 2002) has provided guidance to assist in calculating the implementation and annual support costs of an EHR. Typical initial costs vary by practice type, number of providers and concurrent users, functionality of the solution, and the vendor business model. Nowadays, in the U.S., for a small office of fewer than ten physicians with a primary care practice, the EMR pricing ranges from under $10,000 for low-end options, up to approximately $80,000 for a comprehensive EMR system. In addition, the hardware, telecommunication, and application support expenses need to be added on top of these option estimates.

The ability for a provider to qualify for new federal incentive money means EHR vendors will articulate the value of their systems to support the meaningful use objectives to facilitate qualifying for the funds and in turn to support the basic return on investment model. The current ROI model includes:

- Revenue increases through increased patient volume, increased reimbursement, and improved cash flow.
- Cost reductions through more efficient operations, fewer errors, and supply savings (i.e., vaccines) once the systems are fully operational and integrated with other systems.
- Improved services for patients and third party insurers through more accurate data, data exchanges, and reporting (including to public health).

Detailed cost benefit studies illustrate EHR hard dollar savings in the $60,000–$80,000 per year range, simply by eliminating chart pulls and transcriptions (Zaroukian 2004). As a result, an investment in a new medical record system can be recovered in just a few years.

The ROI of implementing an EHR can be significantly expanded by examining specific clinical work flows and calculating the quantifiable impacts at each step. For example, Fig. 17.1 illustrates a typical work flow process that traces the activities associated with a patient receiving an immunization. Within each step of the process an effective EHR will add value as illustrated by the accumulation of patient benefits. Cost benefit analysis at each step would support the ROI calculations that will augment the above hard dollar numbers through reduced labor of chart pulls and transcription.

Under HITECH a provider's EHR system is no longer expected to be an isolated island of patient data. Rather it will become a health data resource within a clinical care community that extends beyond the primary physician. The EHR is expected to be a "data node" within a Health Information Exchange (HIE) in which patient medical information is available electronically to the appropriate clinician at the appropriate time. Moreover, it is expected that this information is now also available to the patient to encourage patient empowerment.

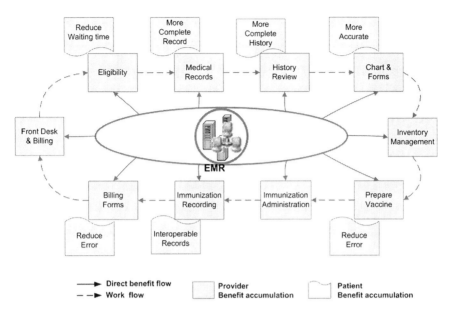

Fig. 17.1 Value-added benefits of an EHR within immunization workflow

Figure 17.2 illustrates the comprehensive benefits of an EMR with an HIE network aligned with the HITECH vision. The HIE framework includes the basic clinical care settings (clinics, hospitals, laboratories and pharmacies), health care management organizations, and the public health community. As a result the value-added benefit by considering the EHR within a larger system perspective can be expanded.

The ability to share information in this larger framework has "payoffs" not commonly measured or included in an ROI calculation. The fact that HITECH will accelerate information sharing increases the benefit to a larger stakeholder community and as such increases the opportunity to demonstrate ROI. This is examined through an example case study.

17.4   EHR Extends the Return on Investment:
A Case Example in Immunization

In 2005 during the aftermath of Hurricane Katrina, Louisiana's statewide immunization registry remained on-line. Through electronic exchanges with providers and other state health departments across the U.S., Louisiana's Electronic Health immunization Record (EHiR) exchange provided an estimated $4.6 million in savings in revaccination costs (Urquhart et al. 2007). This was determined by

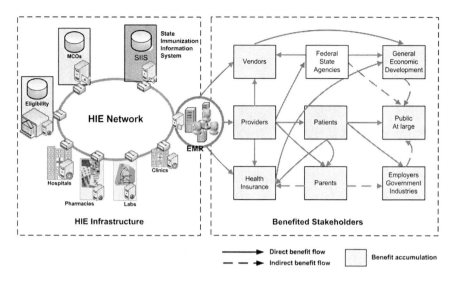

Fig. 17.2 Extended stakeholders to benefit from EHR investments

calculating the cost impact of not revaccinating for the following eight childhood immunizations:

- DTaP – Diphtheria and tetanus, toxoids and acellular pertussis
- IPV – Polio
- MMR – Measles, Mumps and Rubella
- Hib
- HepB
- Varicella
- PCV – Pneumococcal conjugate vaccine
- Meningococcal

This event demonstrated a ROI for a public health information system that exchanged patient immunization records. It did not illustrate the value to the individual providers that benefited from having this information available as families moved throughout the country.

However, it established best practices for EHR exchange within a national HIE. It provided a specific hard dollar value for the sharing of patient health data, immunization records, thus establishing the value for inclusion of immunization exchange as a meaningful use objective within the 2010 regulations. Determining the potential benefit to an individual provider that implements an EHR that is interoperable with a state immunization registry is a derivative expansion of the Hurricane Katrina/Louisiana EHiR concept.

To demonstrate how this objective adds value to the provider and increases their ROI for implementation of an EHR, a case study was undertaken that used data from two other existing state-based immunization registries. The first registry has been in operation for over ten years and the second for over five. Each is fully operational and fully deployed within their respective states. Combined they include over 7 million patient records and 60 million immunization histories. Combined they support over 1,600 providers, and as of mid 2010 they included over 140 electronic immunization exchanges with provider-based EHRs.

Each registry supports both private and public immunization providers and each registry includes decision tools to forecast past, current, and next due vaccinations. Each includes functionality to support generations of subpopulations at risk to vaccine preventable disease, all of which is available to the clinicians within each state. Given this baseline data, a model was developed to estimate revenue value for exchanging immunization records and increasing the EHR-PH ROI. For consistency with the 2005 Katrina study, only childhood immunization data was used. This model was built using the variables listed in Table 17.1.

The intent of this case study was not to provide the exact benefit to an individual provider in each of the two states but to illustrate across all providers the potential impact of immunization record exchange to the required access of patient data within the state HIE. A scenario was used to calculate the costs and revenue. While the exact numbers in each state could not be determined, this illustrative scenario assumes 50% of the childhood immunizations were given to privately insured patients and 50% were given to VFC qualified patients. The scenario also assumes provider reimbursement rates that allow for a 10% profit on their vaccine and administration costs and uses averages for the number of immunizations given on each visit.

Table 17.2 provides the total immunizations within each state by type and the number of providers reporting. It includes the cost and reimbursement numbers used and calculates expected provider costs and revenues to provide childhood patient immunizations. It does not include the addition of adult immunization and normalizes the information across all providers. The net revenue increase is $ 60,000 for "State A" and $ 24,000 for "State B" as a result of implementing the meaningful use immunization data exchange.

The exact potential for revenue increase can only be measured by individual providers knowing the numbers and types of immunizations they provide, their cost and reimbursement rates, and their business approach to immunization of their patients. This model illustrates that there is the potential to increase revenue which further contributes to the ROI by including public health data exchange as one of the key implementation features of a medical record system and pro-actively implementing a provider-based immunization program. As a result this HITECH meaningful use objective improves a provider's revenue stream and offers an opportunity to accelerate the payback period for a new EHR.

17.5 Conclusion

Over the next few years health care providers will be faced with their own perfect storm. The bright spot however is the opportunity to add or improve their health information technology while participating in a meaningful exchange of data with other health care stakeholders. This undoubtedly will result in improved patient

Table 17.1 EHR-PH ROI cost and revenue model variables

Variable	Data	Notes
Vaccine types	8 Childhood vaccines as above	Two sources for Vaccine, the Vaccine for Children (VFC) Program and Private Purchase
Vaccine purchase costs	Government supplied	$ 0 – Govt. supplied VFC vaccine is provided at no cost to eligible providers
	Private purchase	CDC published vaccine price tables (non-negotiated) (Vaccine Price List 2010)
Vaccine reimbursement costs	Government	$ 0 – No reimbursement payments are made to VFC supplied vaccine
	Private sector examples	$ Varies – Reimbursement varies though negotiated rates by state, insurance companies, location, area and provider (Freed et al. 2009). For example these rates are for two separate locations and illustrate the inconstancy:

Vaccine	(1)	(2)
DTaP	$ 14.56	$ 25.76
IPV	$ 26.32	$ 26.53
MMR	$ 44.70	$ 46.48
Hib	$ 21.69	$ 25.25
HepB	$ 23.01	$ 25.04
Varicella	$ 77.55	$ 78.78
PCV	$ 90.71	$ 79.89
MCV	$ 79.46	$ 95.68

Variable	Data	Notes
Vaccine administration costs	Government VFC program	$ 10 – Current VFC reimbursement if Medicaid eligible, capped at $ 15 if not Medicaid eligible.
	Private sector negotiated rates	$ Varies – reimbursement from $ 10–$ 20+ are paid. Factors include age of the child and if counseling was included at that time of administration and the number of immunizations given at one time. For example reimbursement rates in two different locations are illustrated below:

	< age 8 with counseling	< age 8 each additional
(1)	$ 20.29	$ 10.22
(2)	$ 16.39	$ 11.17

Variable	Data	Notes
Numbers of vaccines by type	Annual immunizations given	Data from two state based immunization registries
Number of providers	Total providers reporting	Same as above

Table 17.2 Potential increased revenue from implementation of a meaningful use immunization data exchange

Costs

Pediatric vaccine	VFC cost/dose	Private sector cost/dose	VFC administration costs/dose	Private administration costs/dose	State A total immunizations	State B total immunizations	State A total costs 50% VFC 50% private	State B total costs 50% VFC 50% private
Notes	CDC price list		(1)		2009 totals		Assumed ½ in each sector	
DTaP	$ 13.98	$ 22.30	$ 11.51	$ 11.51	108,900	525,554	$ 2,467,674	$ 11,909,054
Polio	$ 18.77	$ 25.70	$ 11.51	$ 11.51	67,289	284,190	$ 1,639,160	$ 6,922,868
MMR	$ 18.64	$ 48.31	$ 11.51	$ 11.51	73,360	307,734	$ 2,616,384	$ 10,975,333
Hib	$ 9.67	$ 23.07	$ 11.51	$ 11.51	11,843	105,197	$ 272,922	$ 2,424,265
HepB	$ 10.25	$ 21.98	$ 11.51	$ 11.51	38,455	171,876	$ 865,238	$ 3,867,210
Varicella	$ 67.08	$ 80.58	$ 11.51	$ 11.51	76,673	321,008	$ 3,971,661	$ 16,628,214
PCV	$ 91.75	$ 108.75	$ 11.51	$ 11.51	80,763	346,963	$ 5,321,070	$ 22,859,657
Meningococcal	$ 79.75	$ 103.41	$ 11.51	$ 11.51	43,958	258,439	$ 2,778,849	$ 16,337,480
				Totals	501,241	2,320,961	$ 19,932,958	$ 91,924,081

Revenue

Pediatric vaccine	VFC reimbursement/dose	Private sector reimbursement/dose	VFC administer reimbursement	Private payer administer reimbursement	State A total immunizations	State B total immunizations	State A total costs 50% VFC 50% private	State B total costs 50% VFC 50% private
Notes		Used a 10% profit on cost		Average				
DTaP	$ –	$ 24.53	$ 12.66	$ 15.00	108,900	525,554	$ 2,841,800	$ 13,714,594
IPV (Polio)	$ –	$ 28.27	$ 12.66	$ 15.00	67,289	284,190	$ 1,881,771	$ 7,947,515
MMR	$ –	$ 53.14	$ 12.66	$ 15.00	73,360	307,734	$ 2,963,817	$ 12,432,761
Hib	$ –	$ 25.38	$ 12.66	$ 15.00	11,843	105,197	$ 314,065	$ 2,789,719
HepB	$ –	$ 24.18	$ 12.66	$ 15.00	38,455	171,876	$ 996,734	$ 4,454,940
Varicella	$ –	$ 88.64	$ 12.66	$ 15.00	76,673	321,008	$ 4,458,497	$ 18,666,455
PCV	$ –	$ 119.63	$ 12.66	$ 15.00	80,763	346,963	$ 5,947,630	$ 25,551,396
Meningococcal	$ –	$ 113.75	$ 12.66	$ 15.00	43,958	258,439	$ 3,108,143	$ 18,273,472
				Totals	501,241	2,320,961	$ 22,512,456	$ 103,830,854
					Net		$ 2,579,497	$ 11,906,772
					Providers reporting		43	490
					Net income per provider		$ 60,339	$ 24,287

care, operational efficiencies, and increased revenue (or the offset of lost revenues). The business side of a provider's operation has always benefited from improved technology and new information systems. Under the new HITECH law, a federally driven emphasis is placed on improved technology to improve patient care and over-all disease prevention.

The meaningful use objectives of the HITECH law ensure accountability for federal expenditures supporting EHR incentive plans which in turn improve the provider ROI. The case study of immunization record exchange after Katrina illustrated one real example of value-added benefits in revaccination savings. Detailed case studies of provider exchanges with state immunization systems are emerging. Early modeling analysis reveals tangible indicators that public health data exchange adds significant value to both patient care and provider business operations.

References

Blumenthal, D., & Travenner, M. (2010). The "meaningful use" regulation for electronic health records. *The New England Journal of Medicine, 363*(6), 501–504.

CDC Vaccine Price List. (2010). http://www.cdc.gov/vaccines/program/vfc/cdc-vac-price-list. htm. Accessed 3 Sept 2010.

Freed, G., et al. (2009). Variation in provider vaccine purchase prices and payer reimbursement. *Pediatrics, 124*(6), S459–S465.

The Information Technology & Innovation Foundation. (2009). *Health IT report*. Accessed Sept 2009.

U.S. Department of Health & Human Services. (2009). Health information technology for eco-nomic and clinical health (HITECH) act. .http://www.hhs.gov/ocr/privacy/hipaa/administra-tive/enforcementrule/hitechenforcementifr.html. Accessed 18 Feb 2009.

Urquhart, G., Williams, W., Tobias, J., & Welch, F. (2007). Immunization information systems use during a public health emergency in the United States. *Journal of Public Health Management and Practice, 13*(5), 481–485.

Valancy, J. (2002). Computers: how much will that EMR system really cost? *Family Practice Management, 9*, 57–58.

Zaroukian, M. (2004). EMR cost-benefit analysis: Managing ROI into reality. *Centricity healthcare user group slide set presentation*. http://www.himss.org/content/files/EMRCost-BenefitReality. pdf.

Section IV
Innovation in eHealth

ICT is attributed with making healthcare more effective and efficient by, e.g., improving the accuracy of diagnosis, optimizing clinical pathways, avoiding doubled examinations or treatments, and fostering collaboration of healthcare stakeholders by means of loosely coupled, adaptive healthcare services. As such, ICT holds high promises. The history of eHealth tells that these promises must be analyzed and assessed carefully. The bottom line is that ICT provides an ever-growing plethora of *inventions* thus novel ideas, whereas only their successful application to a domain transforms them into *innovations* which deliver benefits to a group respectively wealth to the society. Therefore, eHealth innovation research studies the adoption, usage, and effects of ICT as well as their key success factors. It provides theories, models, methods, and tools for describing, explaining, and ultimately predicting the level of innovation of specific ICT inventions. This section contains chapters that are devoted to eHealth innovation research and study ICT inventions from different perspectives.

The chapter "Smart Objects in Healthcare – Impact on Clinical Logistics" by M. Sedlmayr and U. Münch is concerned with automatic identification and data capture (AIDC) technologies. Hospitals are confronted with a great variety of respective solutions and have implemented them for various scenarios. The problem is that these solutions are not adequately integrated into hospital information systems and healthcare processes. Solution providers and early adopters paid little attention to the specific setting of the healthcare environment. The authors propose a holistic view on the entire hospital value system and introduce the concept of smart object. The key idea is to separate the physical implementation (hardware, communication software) from the functions which are then made available by software services. The usefulness and efficiency of this new approach is demonstrated by a case study and an assessment of effects on time, quality, and costs.

The chapter "Business Models for Electronic Healthcare Services in Germany" by S. Dünnebeil, J.M. Leimeister, and H. Krcmar explores the business opportunities that a new nationwide telematics infrastructure may offer to IT service providers. Being a case study from Germany, this chapter addresses the general problem of developing sustainable, ICT-based business models in the healthcare sector.

The analysis reveals several barriers of the underlying infrastructure as well as the key success factors for service providers. The proposed business model is evaluated by using the e3value methodology. A major finding is that a lack of financial incentives hinders the development of value-added services on top of the telematics infrastructure.

The chapter "Cost Accounting and Decision Support for Healthcare Institutions" by L. Waehlert, A. Wagner, and H. Czap studies the new role of accounting in networked healthcare. In such healthcare, patients are guided via patient pathways through a system of healthcare services, both from internal and external providers. ICT provides tremendous opportunities for collaboration and has already reshaped healthcare delivery. These changes require new means for accounting and decision making; in particular, for assessing the performance of services and deciding about service providers. This chapter proposes an accounting model based on standardized cross-organizational clinical pathways and reports about a prototype system.

Networked healthcare is also subject of the chapter "Agency Theory in E-Healthcare and Telemedicine: A Literature Study" by J. Leukel, J. Fernandes, A. Heidebrecht, and S. Schillings. In networked healthcare, diverse bilateral relationships exist between participants. A particular type of relationship is that between a principal and an agent, e.g., patient and physician, or hospital management and physician. Introducing ICT affects necessarily these relationships. Agency theory can provide useful insights into ICT effects. This chapter analysis to which extent agency relationships have been considered in eHealth research, and to which extent eHealth research makes use of the insights, and results of agency theory. The comprehensive literature review of IS and eHealth outlets suggests that an important factor of the organizational setting has not been considered in studying ICT adoption, which is the existence and nature of agency relationships.

Finally, the chapter "A Comprehensive Approach to the IT-Clinical Practice Interface" by D. Zakim and M.D. Alscher argues that ICT adoption has to acknowledge essential defects of medical practice instead of just aiming at "tweaking around the edges". These defects are due to finite human cognitive capacity and memory, which both put a burden on physicians and any medical professional. This fact gets even more important because of the exponential growth of medical knowledge. The authors deduce that the only feasible approach is to making this knowledge explicit and understandable to computers. From this perspective, the chapter revisits the seminal idea of medical expert systems, proposes a new approach to knowledge acquisition from various data sources and decision support for physicians, and reports about a commercial implementation. The authors relate the ICT approach closely to the self-conception of physicians.

Chapter 18
Business Models for Electronic Healthcare Services in Germany

Telemonitoring of Chronic Heart Failure: A Case Study

S. Duennebeil, J. Leimeister, and H. Krcmar

Abstract Health information systems have the potential to improve healthcare quality. Accordingly, German health authorities are currently building a nationwide telematics infrastructure (TI) to connect care providers' information systems via a common network. Telemedicine services based on this TI will offer communication cooperation documentation and analysis features such as web services to ensure pervasive availability and integrity of medical data in the German public health system. Fields of applications involve pharmaceutical drug safety, insurance data maintenance, electronic healthcare records (EHR) and emergency records. These services are specified by the German public health authorities for all caregivers. Value added applications that use the infrastructure and its services to support treatment and administration, can be deployed by software vendors thus supplying innovative services in the field of e-health.

In order to enable a vital competition for value adding services, it is essential to provide sustainable business models for medical service providers to foster development and adoption of innovations deployed via the TI. This chapter uses a case study to illustrate the situation of a services provider that wants to offer a solution for telemonitoring via the TI. The analysis of the current state of the German public health system and the TI reveals several barriers hindering the progress of the proposed system. Pointing out critical issues for the development of sustainable e-health solutions, the work elaborates key success factors of past e-health projects. The most significant findings, such as privacy, controlling structures and incentive mechanisms, are addressed and analyzed in depth. A corresponding business model for the service provider is developed, using an integrative business model approach to address external factors, such as legal conditions, competitors and strategy development. The result is an actor, revenue and services model for the provider of the telemonitoring solutions.

S. Duennebeil (✉) • H. Krcmar
Department of Informatics, Technical University of Munich (TUM) , München, Germany
e-mail: duennebe@in.tum.de

J. Leimeister
Research Center for IT Design (ITeG), University of Kassel, Kassel, Germany

N. Wickramasinghe et al. (eds.), *Critical Issues for the Development of Sustainable E-health Solutions*, Healthcare Delivery in the Information Age, DOI 10.1007/978-1-4614-1536-7_18, © Springer Science+Business Media, LLC 2012

For verification of the revenue model, the article uses the e3 value methodology to assess the financial profitability of the approach. The discussion includes the adjustment of financial incentives for the developers of sustainable e-health innovations that boost the improvement of information technology utilization in healthcare.

Keywords Telemonitoring • Business models • E-health • Telemedicine • Chronic heart failure • Healthcare telematics • Germany • Ambulatory care

18.1   Introduction

18.1.1   Motivation

Health systems around the world have seen multiple innovations in the field of electronic health (e-health). The benefits of these applications are proven in many cases (European 2007; Shekelle et al. 2006). Telemonitoring – remote computer aided patient observations – has strong evidence of being beneficial in many aspects of healthcare. Hospitalization, mortality rate, disablement, and the overall treatment costs can be reduced tremendously by this e-health application (Helms et al. 2007; Kempf and Schulz 2008). Further, medical errors, which are called adverse events and cause more casualties than breast cancer, traffic accidents and AIDS combined, can be limited by the usage of e-health application. Compared to the traditional medication handling, applications managing the ac-curate discharge of prescriptions show significant advantages. These are able to decrease the unadjusted absolute death rate by 27% for cardio-vascular patients after one year (Lappé et al. 2004). Considering the fact that wrong medication in the United States in 2006 cost $4.4 billion (IOM 2006) and that 37.4% of all adverse events were caused by wrong medication (Aranaz-Andrés et al. 2008), the diffusion of such technologies should be subject of major efforts. Hence, utilization of supporting information systems (IS) is urgently recommended by European health authorities (European 2007). However, the diffusion speed of such applications is currently very low (DesRoches et al. 2008; European 2010), despite the enormous potential for fund saving. The low adoption rate of e-health indicates a lack of sustainable business models. As the technology is theoretically available and the benefits have been proven, a working market to organize and accelerate distribution and adoption is an important factor. The intention of this chapter is the development of a sustainable business model for providers of e-health. The overall goal is to enable the utilization of information technology (IT) in healthcare to improve the overall treatment quality. For this purpose German health authorities are currently building a nationwide telematics infrastructure (TI) to connect care providers' IS via a common network (Fraunhofer 2005). On the basis of the proposed TI, telemedicine services will offer communication, cooperation, and documentation features implemented as web services to ensure pervasive availability and integrity of medical data among the German public health system. In the case of the proposed infrastructure, medical patient data is either stored on central servers or portable smart cards. The secure infrastructure is considered as a major enabler of electronic health services, e.g., for telemonitoring.

18.1.2 The Public Health System in Germany

In 2008 the German public health system was the biggest national service industry, responsible for total revenue of €263.2 billion, of which healthcare spending accounted for 10.5% of the German gross domestic product (GDP) (KVB 2008). According to estimates, the spending will rise to €453 billion in 2020, which will represent approximately 15.5% of the national GDP at that time (Karette et al. 2005). Healthcare spending can be divided into public and private funds. The public spending represents the major proportion, about 75% of all funds, amounting to €3,210 per citizen. Annual private spending for healthcare in Germany does not exceed the sum of €800 per capita and is mostly expended for medication, wellness or medical appliances that are not covered by health insurances (OECD 2010). In Germany employees and employers pay solidary contributions to public and private health insurances via a public health fund. The fund was established by health authorities and is equally financed by employees and employers, and receives a tax money subvention in case of insufficient coverage. The fund pays a standard amount for each insured citizen to health insurances. The financial resources are distributed quarterly by physicians associations to registered caregivers, according to the recorded treatment of the last quarter. All allowable treatments are fixed in a treatment or medication catalogue ex ante in order to be refundable (Lisac et al. 2010). As a result, treatments and medication are part of a fixed service portfolio, which has to be reimbursed by all health insurances. The distribution is based on a common weighting point value, called "Einheitlicher Bewertungsmaßstab" (EBM) that distributes the overall fund to caregivers. The more services are claimed by caregivers, the lower the point value becomes (Fig. 18.1).

Currently, IT services are not part of the treatment catalogue, and can therefore not be billed by caregivers in the regular allowance process. There are some direct contracts between health insurances and caregivers that allow the funding of additional health services and treatments. The health insurance can collect an extra amount of money from their insurants and distribute financial surpluses in order to achieve competitive advantage and diversification (Lisac et al. 2010).

Normal markets generally organize the flow of materials and services between individuals and institutions according to demand, supply and external mechanisms. Market forces determine design, price, quality and delivery time of products and services. The buyers demand goods and services according to these parameters and their personal requirements, thereby implicitly regulating markets (Malone et al. 1987). Health systems, in contrast, are characterized by an organized flow of funds from citizens and companies to caregivers (Lisac et al. 2010). The flow is regulated by various public mechanisms and institutions. Public health systems thus differ from normal markets, as: (1) they normally offer unlimited access to the services offered in the

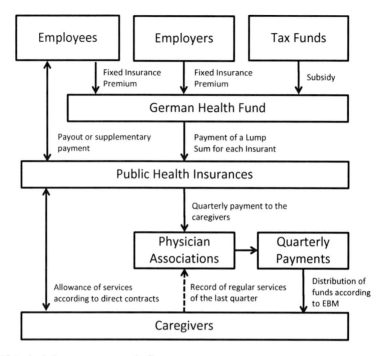

Fig. 18.1 Ambulatory care system in Germany

public health system, (2) they show information asymmetries between the suppliers (caregivers) and consumer (patients) of health services, and (3) the future personal health status of their customers is uncertain and subject to random fluctuations. These characteristics, in sum, lead to market failure (Smith et al. 1997) and explain why the demand for e-health solutions is low, despite the positive effects. Therefore, business models in healthcare – if they involve public funds – must be designed differently from business models in the free market. Despite the special characteristics within public health system, business models are considered to be the most important success factor for the adoption of information technology in healthcare (European 2010).

18.1.3   Research Method

We conducted a case study, based on a region in southern Germany with 452,000 inhabitants on 2,847 km^2. The region is geographically well definable because of its heterogeneous structure, which makes the region suitable for field testing since it represents the structure of Germany very accurately (ZTG 2009). The caregivers of the region, their physician network, as well as two health insurances are willing to establish telemonitoring. Therefore, the health insurances want to allocate funds to enable business models for telemonitoring in order to encourage companies to supply solutions. The telemonitoring solution should be embedded in the rollout process of the national electronic health card (eHC) system, which will be piloted in the region. The exploratory nature of

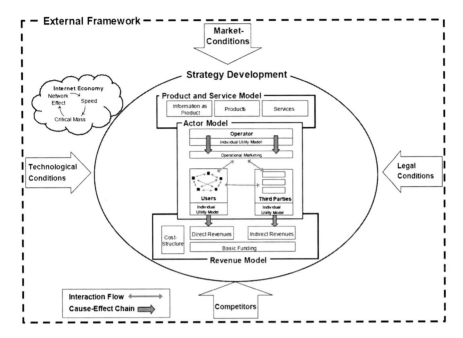

Fig. 18.2 Research framework according to Leimeister and Krcmar (2004)

this research within the context of a physician network that was related to the IT project of the eHC guided the authors to adopt a qualitative and interpretive approach to the inquiry. The empirical part of this research follows an exploratory research design with the intention of generating an empirically motivated business model; it is not with the intention to test a given research model. Methodological aspects of explorative research designs can be found in Bortz and Döring (2002) or Becker (1993). Case study research itself is widely used in IS research. For an approach on how to build theories from case study research see Eisenhardt (1989). Four semi standardized oral interviews were conducted: two with board members of the physician network (the business manager and the chairman who additionally works as a general practitioner) and further two board members of a health insurance, which insures 80,000 people in the region. Additionally, data from two general practitioners' health information systems was analyzed. The literature on previously conducted research was (where available) also included. The study is still ongoing but the main interviews were conducted in a 2 month period in 2010 as part of the introductory project of the eHC.

According to Timmers (1998), a business model describes architecture for the services and information flows, including a description of the various business actors and their roles, a description of the potential benefits for the various business actors and their roles, as well as a description of the sources of revenues. This definition does not include external factors such as legal or technological issues. The work employs an integrative business model approach (Leimeister and Krcmar 2004), which adds external perspectives as the technological, legal and technical conditions to the approach of Timmers (Fig. 18.2).

18.2   The German Telematics Infrastructure

18.2.1   Architecture of the Telematics Infrastructure

In Germany the Telematics Infrastructure (TI) is the technical base for new e-health applications and used as the backbone for the mandatory eHC system. The infrastructure connects the existing IS of care providers via a common network (Marschollek and Demirbilek 2006). Within the service-oriented architecture (SOA) of the TI, centralized servers or decentralized components provide web services, e.g., the encryption, digital signature and authorization of medical data. The primary systems of the TI, i.e., information systems of medical institutions, can utilize these services to communicate or collaborate with other care providers to maintain, review or share medical data objects (Fig. 18.3). A local connector component encapsulates all local services as encryption or card access and establishes a secure virtual private network (VPN) connection to the central servers if needed (gematik 2008a). The connector is connected to smart card readers that allow access to the eHC. All individually related medical and administrative data uploaded to central servers have to be encrypted using a hybrid encryption method (gematik 2008b). The private keys are located on the smart card chip of the eHC and cannot be extracted; hence, they can be used for digital signatures and the encryption of medical data. Decryption of the access key happens within the microchip of the smart card after authorization with a Personal Identity Number (PIN). Patients can use public keys of health care institutions to encrypt the data for the receiver in order to grant them access to their personal medical data. Given that the receiver of the medical data is a specific physician, the patient needs to access the physician's certificate, either located on the so-called health professional card (HPC) or via a public key infrastructure.

To encrypt the medical data for larger groups of caregivers, e.g., for emergency physicians, the institutional smart cards, called Secure Module Card (SMC), hold private keys of institutions (gematik 2008a).

18.2.2   Taxonomy of Value-Added Applications

The TI is specified by a government controlled institution called gematik. In addition to the infrastructure, some services, such as a service for patient master data, a prescription service, or an emergency data service, are specified by this institution. These services are either medical or administrative services and complement the infrastructure services, as encryption or digital signature, and are available to all stakeholders with access to the TI. Value-added services in the context of the TI are web services, which provide an additional value that is not delivered by any service, specified by the gematik. All services can be used in various applications running on caregivers' primary systems. To extend amount and variety of value-added services, the TI can be enriched in several ways. There are four alternatives, depending on the level of security required within for the service (gematik 2008c) An application that utilizes

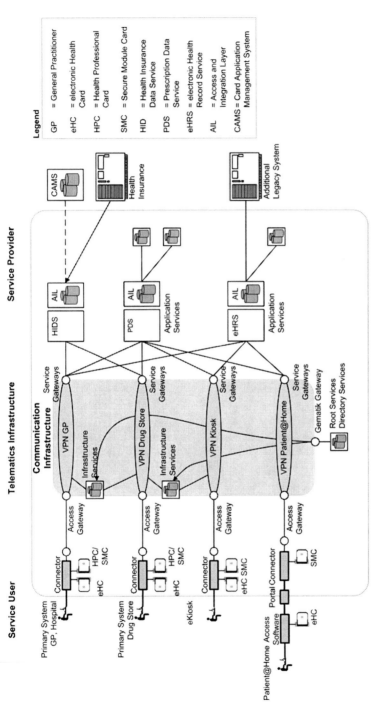

Fig. 18.3 The architecture of the German TI in Fraunhofer (2005)

any value added service, apart from the medical, administrative and infrastructural services of the TI, is considered a value added application. These applications are supposed to contribute billions of Euros of added value to the TI (Bernnat 2006). Such applications are the subject of the business model developed in this work.

18.2.3 Telemonitoring as Value Added Service

Telemonitoring is a telemedicine application that transfers medical data through interactive audiovisual channels to a physician for the purpose of monitoring patients with various diseases, such as diabetes or heart failure. The addressed physician can observe the disease permanently, without the necessity of daily visits. Telemonitoring applications can be deployed via the TI as a value-added application. To realize telemonitoring within such a distributed SOA, services can offer the exchange of encrypted medical data via a centralized server. The analysis of the data cannot be performed on a centralized server, as only encrypted patient data can be stored there (Gesundheit 2005). Calculations on encrypted data could be proven for all arithmetic operations (Gentry 2009); however, current IT is not yet feasible to realize encrypted computing. Local components are therefore necessary on the patients' and caregivers' side in order to perform the logical operations on raw data. The patient has to maintain an application which can obtain the vital parameters and deliver them to the caregiver. Medical devices, as a scale or a blood pressure meter can offer the functionality as web service. The value-added application on the patient's computer will call the service in order to obtain vital parameters. Afterwards, the local signature service will be employed to verify the patient's identity. The local encryption service will encrypt the set of vital parameters in order to secure the data for later transfer to the telematics server. All services must be integrated within a value added application on the patient's and caregiver's side. The service integration on the caregiver's side will retrieve the data at first, use the decryption service to extract the raw data, after which the information can be analyzed for medically relevant patterns. This action can be either done manually or semi-automatic. Such an application for telemonitoring will automatically implement the security and authorization standards of the German TI and provide additional services for medical purposes (Fig. 18.4).

18.3 Case Study

18.3.1 Telemonitoring of Chronic Heart Failure (CHF)

Heart failure is one of the most widespread chronic diseases in Germany (Neumann et al. 2009). The patients' hearts are not able to supply the organism with sufficient blood flow and oxygen, to ensure that the human metabolism is working well during

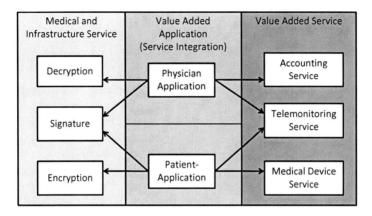

Fig. 18.4 Value-added applications and services

exposure or rest. During chronic heart failure (CHF) the metabolism compensates the low oxygen supply by higher heart rate, vascular stenosis, thickening the myo-cardial muscle or an increase in blood volume. This can temporarily compensate the low oxygen delivery to the end organs. Patients with chronic stable heart failure temporarily do not show any symptoms of CHF (Krum and Abraham 2009). Decompensation of CHF, caused e.g., by heart attack or pneumonia, leads to fluid retention and uncontrolled hypertension, during rest or light exposure. Medical guidelines provided by the German Medical Association therefore advise daily monitoring of patients' blood pressure, heart frequency and weight (Ärztliches Zentrum für Qualität in der Medizin 2009). A significant increase in a patient's weight during a short period is a strong indicator of a fluid retention caused by a decompensation in the case of a heart attack. Also, low hypotension (systolic blood pressure) indicates a decompensation.

Early identification of a decompensation allows caregivers to take counteractive measures as early as possible – before the patient's hospitalization – because of dyspnea (breathlessness), pulmonary edema or acroedema (water retention in lungs or legs) is inevitable. The application for telemonitoring should support this moni-toring action in the best possible manner. Sensors record the vital parameters and transmit them to physicians for monitoring (Helms et al. 2007). In 2006, there were 317,000 patients with a diagnosis of chronic heart failure (CHF) in Germany. The treatment cost in the same year summed up to €2.9 billion, representing about 1.1% of all national health expenses (KVB 2008). CHF furthermore caused the highest number of hospitalizations, reportedly due to a single disease. 60% of all CHF related costs were caused by hospital stays. In 2008, CHF caused 48,918 cases of death, representing a share of 5.8% of the annual German death rate (Neumann et al. 2009).

18.3.2 External Framework Model

18.3.2.1 Market Condition

The region in southern Germany counts 450,000 inhabitants. More than 550 of the 600 ambulatory physicians treating the patients of the region are organized in a physician network (ZTG 2009). The physician network has the organizational setup of a GmbH: a private company limited by shares (the German equivalent to a Limited Company). The network is thereby able to generate revenue, which can then be distributed to the shareholders. All physicians have equal shares in the physician network, and the earnings of the network are either distributed equally or according to dedicated contracts. The physician network can negotiate treatment contracts with the health insurances of the region directly. This enables physicians to earn money beyond the fixed allowance catalogue of the German ambulatory health system. Two health insurances were contacted by the physician network and asked whether they were willing to set up a market for telemonitoring. Each of the two health insurances has approximately 80,000 insurants. Including the co-insured family members, about half of the inhabitants of the region are insured by either of the two health insurances. Both health insurances – one a dominant German health insurance and the other the health insurance of a globally operating company with headquarters in the region – are willing to allocate funds in order to enable the business model for telemonitoring. The market conditions for telemonitoring depend on the health insurances. If a pilot program in the region is successful, further applications are possible, as both health insurances have a larger number of insurants. Of the 317,000 patients with CHF in Germany, the region has 1,700 patients suffering CHF, which is representative. Hence, the physician network is responsible for the treatment of about 1,500 patients. 750 of these patients are insured by one of the two insurers that want to donate funds for telemonitoring. The case study employs estimations, as no detailed data were available during the research. The physician network has 250 general practitioners responsible for monitoring of CHF (Ärztliches Zentrum für Qualität in der Medizin 2009): hence, each physician treats approximately three patients with CHF. The numbers taken from the IS of two caregivers indicated a higher number of clients. Over a period of five years 53 respectively 45 patients with the corresponding diagnosis were recorded in the health information system. Despite the variation, the calculation is based on the estimation that three patients with CHF are monitored by one physician.

18.3.2.2 Legal Model

The patient related requirements for the development of the TI are derived from legal conditions in the German code of social law (Bundesrepublik 1988). Following the political goals of achieving high patient involvement in medical processes, patients are required to be in full control of their data. They have to agree on collection, usage and processing of their medical data for each service and care provider ex ante. In order to warrant this requirement, the medical data need to be encrypted with the public key of the source patient and is therefore solely accessible with the private key stored on the patient's smart card (gematik 2008b). It is thus a mandatory requirement for the TI that patients can view all their data and the record of its usage.

18.3.2.3   Technical Model

To ensure that patients could exercise these legally granted rights, patient interfaces were suggested. An internet-based front end for home usage was announced in the initial architecture (Fraunhofer 2005). A citizen front end for the new German ID-Cards that is compatible with the eHC was already released. This software can be employed to transfer data from patients' locations to caregivers. Available are also sensors that can transmit data of weight, blood pressure and heart rate to caregivers. The implementation of the TI is based on the SOA paradigm, with two centralized web services. These are hosted by the physician network due to caregivers' distrust to private institutions and health insurances concerning storage of health related data (Dünnebeil et al. 2010). The health service allows saving of communication between patients and physicians, while the accounting service supports the communication between the service provider and the caregivers. Service-oriented device integration of sensors is possible (Mauro et al. 2009), as the data is encrypted by the eHC and decrypted with the physicians' HPC, according to the description in Sect. 2.1.

18.3.3   Business Model Development

18.3.3.1   Development of an Actor Model

The actor model is derived from a typical use case, worked out during the interviews. Afterwards the use case is transferred into a high level model, illustrating the stakeholders' interactions within the use case. Due to the introduction of the eHC in Germany and the region's character as a testbed, the implementation of the application is based on the German TI. The following use case was the suggested interaction model for the telemonitoring solution. Figure 18.5 shows its integration into the TI. (1) The patient monitors the daily weight, heart rate, and blood pressure. (2) The sensors transfer the vital parameters to the patient's computer. (3) The patient encrypts the data for his/her caregiver and transfers it to the medical server. (4) The medical service flags the data for the caregiver and sends a notification. (5) The physician checks the medical service and downloads the monitoring record. (6) The physician

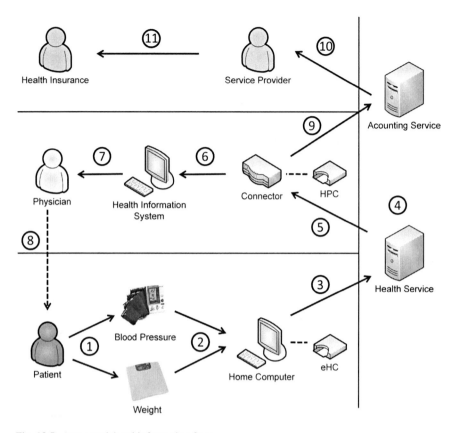

Fig. 18.5 Actor model and information flow

decrypts the data each working day and transfers them to his IS. (7) The physician validates the data within his IS and judges the patient's health status. (8) The physician consults the patient personally, as required from the monitoring data. (9) The physician compiles a report and submits it to the accounting service each quarter. (10) The service provider downloads all reports and inserts measures in the overall monitoring sheet. (11) The service provider compiles a report and transfers it to the health insurance company.

18.3.3.2 Development of a Service Model

The main service provided by the telemonitoring supplier is the processing of information objects for the purpose of remote monitoring. Medical information is highly confidential data, which must not, according to regulations in the German law, be processed without the patient's agreement. Furthermore, health insurance companies must not be in control of all transaction objects, even though they finance the information objects (Gesundheit 2005). The interviewers therefore recommend splitting the information object into three different objects, each processed by two of the major stakeholders. The first transaction object is derived from the medical recommendation settled in medical guidelines in order to achieve the best possible monitoring of patients with CHF (Ärztliches Zentrum für Qualität in der Medizin 2009). It is processed from the patient to his/her general practitioner for pure medical purposes. The transaction object directly follows a paper based recommendation developed by the Heart Failure Association of the European Society of Cardiology (HFA 2010). It consists of a daily recording of weight, heart rate, and blood pressure (diastolic and systolic). The patient measures this data, either manually or automated and transmits them to the general practitioner. Precondition is the patient's registration to the program, which is not mandatory. Patients agree on the financial benefits and the processing of anonymous measures to the health insurance and the service provider. Caregivers receive the monitoring record once a day. The caregivers compile the data continuously into a diagram that helps to supervise patients' status of health. At the end of each quarter, caregivers create a report for each patient. Lack of work, monitoring compliance, hospitalization and the CHF related treatments are added to the report, which is the second transaction object and processed to the service provider (Fig. 18.6). The data enables providers to organize the accounting and integrate global measures. The global measures contain overall data of all patients with CHF and enable the health insurance to monitor the success of the market and adjust the incentive structures accordingly.

18.3.3.3   Development of a Revenue Model

According to a study on telemonitoring (Helms et al. 2007), the average annual financial benefit of telemonitoring for one patient with CHF is at least 3,000 Euros. Considering the total cost of approximately 9,000 Euros per year, a treatment cost reduction of one third can be achieved. Hence, the health insurances try to save money by the avoidance of hospital treatment, which involves partially redirecting funds from hospitalization to prevention, by construction of a market for telemonitoring solutions If the underlying studies prove to be accurate – the assumption of this paper – utilization of telemonitoring is more efficient for health insurances than is hospitalization, that is, the savings achieved by telemonitoring are sufficient to cover the additional treatment cost of the physician and the market price of a telemonitoring solution, and thus the health insurances will save money. Initially, a share of one third of the estimated total cost reduction was the saving target of the market initiators. Two thirds should be set up as funds for the provider of the telemonitoring solution. This represents the total market volume

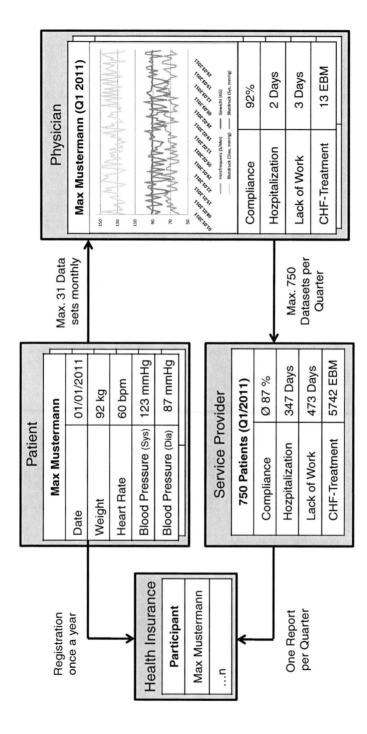

Fig. 18.6 Information flow and architecture

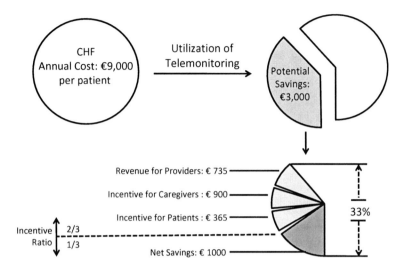

Fig. 18.7 Financial environment

for the region. The solution provider will need to partly use the funds as an incentive for patients and caregivers to regularly participate in the monitoring. The payment should depend on the compliance of patients and caregivers. An incentive of one Euro per transaction per patient is suggested here and an incentive of maximal 225 Euros for a caregiver per quarter. This was reported in an interview to be a sufficient amount for a monthly time effort of one hour. As Fig. 18.7 indicates, when monitoring at least three patients with CHI, the additional annual income totals 2,700 Euros.

Figure 18.7 illustrates the financial flow and names the most important stakeholders apart from the health insurances: service providers, patients and caregivers. For health insurances even a zero saving is considered a success, as the treatment quality can be increased when reducing the hospitalization. Further, the current calculation considers only the actual treatment costs; however, the adjusted expenses for CHF are much higher. Including the indirect costs, caused by lack of work, the adjusted annual advantage of telemonitoring totals 6.300 Euros per patient (Helms et al. 2007). The distribution of the funds to the stakeholders aims to maximize the savings of the annual treatment costs. The total market volume for CHF-telemonitoring in Germany adds up to approximately €230 million per year. In the region the market volume is only 500,000 Euros; however, the character of a pilot project can justify higher investments.

The financial flow is the adverse flow of the transaction objects, developed in the previous chapter. The health insurance wants to redirect funds of CHF treatment in hospitals to prevention by telemonitoring. A contract between the service providers and the health insurance should be concluded and extended on an annual base. In the first year (period t_1) the health insurance is not able to quantify the savings achieved by telemonitoring, but can estimate the cost of CHF for the last year (period t_0). To distribute the funds in the first year (t_1), the savings measured in the studies are taken as the initial calculation base. The initial fund in t_1 will allocate two thirds of all CHF-related costs of t_0. The funds should be adjusted afterwards, reflecting the actual savings achieved after t_1. In general, savings in the later periods are as following:

$$\text{Saving } t_n = \text{CostCHF}_{t0} - \text{CostCHF}_{tn}$$

$$= \left(\sum \text{EBM}_{t0} - \sum \text{EBM}_{tn}\right) + \left(\sum \text{Hospital Cases}_{t0} - \sum \text{Hospital Cases}_{tn}\right)$$

In Germany health insurances pay allowances for hospital cases based on a diagnosis. CHF has three different hospital cases, priced between €2,382 and €4,242 (Hellmann and Eble 2009) covering all hospital expenses with little exceptions (Lisac et al. 2010). Further, certain treatments and medication in ambulatory care can be associated with CHF and quantified in an EBM-value (Helms et al. 2007). Lack of work could also be included into the savings gained by the telemonitoring business model; it is neglected for now, since an inclusion of employers would be necessary.

Service providers will pay parts of the total fund to caregivers and patients. In our example, the physicians will receive the sum of all patients, where each patient consists of the product of gain sharing, compliance factor and savings, divided by the payment division, which is agreed. This is the allowance for the second information. In our case, the allowance in t_1 will be paid four times (each quarter) and will be 30% of the saving, which was estimated to be €3,000. In case of full compliance (>80%), the compliance factor is agreed to be 1. This would lead to a quarterly amount of €225 per patient and €900 over the whole year. With the estimated treatment of three patients, a total amount of €2,700 could be earned, if patients of the region subscribed to telemonitoring and participated with high compliance.

$$\sum_{i=1}^{n} \frac{\text{gain sharing i} \times \text{compliancefactor i} \times \text{saving}}{\text{payment division i}} = \sum_{i=1}^{3} \frac{0{,}3 \times 3000 \times \text{compliance i}}{4}$$

Formula 2 – Allowance caregivers in t_1

The allowance for the first transaction object, the vital parameters, is paid on a monthly basis to the patients, by deducting it from the monthly insurance premium or the extra premium. Patients are paid 12% of initial savings in t_1, if they reach a compliance factor of one.

$$\frac{\text{gain sharing} \times \text{compliancefactor} \times \text{saving}}{\text{payment division}} = \frac{0{,}12 \times 3000 \times \text{compliancefactor}}{12}$$

Formula 3 – Allowance patients in t_1

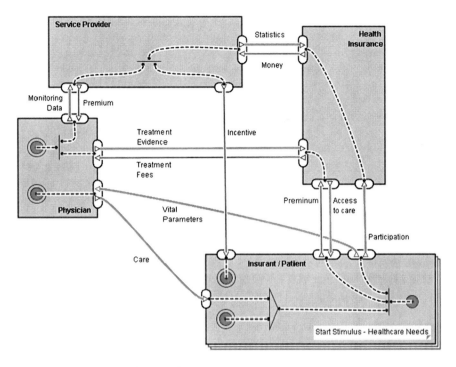

Fig. 18.8 Value network of telemonitoring

In period t₂ the whole process should be adjusted according to market results. The market result is determined by the behavior of the market participants (Weinhardt et al. 2003). Currently the business model expects that the saving potential is high enough to ensure a sustainable telemonitoring without extra funds from the health insurance. Other cased might require extra funds, but the medical use could justify the allocation also in such cases.

Figure 18.8 illustrates all value exchanges of between the actors in an e3value network according to healthcare patterns described in Kartseva et al. (2010). Patients' insurance payments are the initial stimulus for the business model. The health insurances redirect some financial flow via service provides to patients and caregivers, which in exchange deliver data. The data delivery is the record of medical monitoring that saves the funds to finance the business model. Financial flows in Fig. 18.8 are marked blue, services and information brown.

18.4   Discussion and Outlook

Unlike treatment, medication or medical appliances, the German health system currently has no regular business model for e-health. This chapter has illustrated how health insurances and physician networks can enable business models for electronic health services in order to harvest the benefits identified in clinical studies.

Allocating funds for e-health solutions can create a well-defined market, including secure transaction objects and a predefined service model for applications as telemonitoring. Medical studies can be employed at first to identify potential business models, estimate the initial efforts and long term saving potentials that can be achieved by e-health applications. In the case of CHF, the potential fund savings seem to be sufficient to finance a market by the increase in treatment efficiency.

The case study has a facilitating environment for a regional business model, as a big physician network could encourage the caregivers of a region to participate in a pilot project. Further, they could sign contracts for multiple caregivers, which is difficult to achieve for single physicians or small physician networks. Since close contact already existed between health insurances and the physician network, this was an advantage for case study. The approach is not necessarily limited to telemonitoring, as business modeling needs to consider several specific aspects, and it is therefore difficult to generalize. In any case, business models, as, for example, the one developed for telemonitoring, seem to be an approach to create sustainable business models for e-health applications, and thus overcome the low adoption of information technology in healthcare. It must be further ensured that necessary treatments, medications or hospitalizations are not neglected due to the financial incentive. Lack of work could not be included into the business model, as companies were not yet asked to support the utilization of e-health solutions. It is also currently legally difficult to pay allowance directly to patients with chronic diseases, a benefit which healthy patients do not receive.

18.4.1   Implications for the TI

The current state of the German TI does not allow for a setup according to the actor model suggested in this paper. The rollout of local components is not yet completed, nor have the smart cards been distributed to caregivers and patients. The TI must develop a feasible approach to enable both – the deployment of value-added services and applications. The infrastructure can provide a common security standard, as well as a common process for signature and data exchange. Utilization of the TI can ease business models, as data security and authentication do not need to be implemented by the provider of e-health application. Currently, value added applications must be integrated into the local IS of the caregiver as well, as no patient data can be obtained from an EHR. The TI should encourage developers of local software to extend the SOA approach to the local software components, as value-added applications can utilize local services as patient data, as well as device services and telematics services. Common software architectures ease the goal of achieving seamless healthcare support.

18.4.2   Implications for Service Providers

As long as there is no regular allowance for e-health applications funded by health insurances, there are only two possible alternatives to find financiers of e-health applications. Either physicians or the patients finance the application. As physicians have no chance to bill telemonitoring as a regular service, they do not receive any funds for their treatment. This issue will probably occur for most new and innovative e-heath applications, as they are unlikely to be part of the well-established treatment catalogue. Therefore, no financial incentives are currently fostering the adoption of e-health. Patients could finance the service by themselves; however, the annual costs for the treatment by caregivers are already near the amount that patients spend in one year on the private health market in total. The overall costs will likely lay beyond the financial scope of patients with chronic diseases, especially as they are often in high age groups.

Service providers should be in contact with health insurances and physician networks to develop of innovative business models. Business model developments could originate in e-health studies for first financial estimation. Contact with physician networks could reduce the marketing approach for the e-health providers, as the marketing efforts are limited to the physician network. Also, the technological architecture should be driven towards a SOA approach, which allows combining various services and achieving major functionalities of value added applications by combining the web services, offered by different institutions already. The availability of encryption, authentication, signature services, as well as a secure centralized infrastructure, can enable a rapid development approach. This can, in the case of telemonitoring, be combined with services provided by medical devices to create a working solution.

References

Aranaz-Andrés, J. M., Aibar-Remón, C., & Vitaller-Murillo, J. (2008). Incidence of adverse events related to health care in Spain: Results of the Spanish National Study of Adverse Events. *Journal of Epidemiology and Community Health, 62,* 1022–1029.

Ärztliches Zentrum für Qualität in der Medizin. (2009). Nationale VersorgungsLeitlinie Chronische Herzinsuffizienz. Bundesärztekammer, Kassenärztliche Bundesvereinigung, Arbeitsgemeinschaft der Wissenschaftlichen Medizinischen Fachgesellschaften, Berlin.

Becker, F. (1993). Explorative Forschung mittels Bezugsrahmen – ein Beitrag zur Methodologie des Entdeckungszusammenhangs. In *Empirische Personalforschung: Methoden und Beispiele* (pp. 111–127).

Bernnat, R. (2006). Kosten-Nutzen-Analyse der Einrichtung einer Telematik-Infrastruktur im deutschen Gesundheitswesen. Booz Allen Hamilton GmbH.

Bortz, J., & Döring, N. (2002). *Forschungsmethoden und Evaluation für Human- und Sozialwissenschaftler* (Vol. 3). Berlin: Springer.

Bundesministerium für Gesundheit. (2005). The German eHealth Strategy (Target and strategy, concept, legal framework, activities/roll-out plan, costs and return of investment, European perspective). Berlin/Bonn.

Bundesrepublik Deutschland. (1988). Sozialgesetzbuch (SGB) Fünftes Buch, Gesetzliche Krankenversicherung.

DesRoches, C., Campbell, E., Rao, S., Donelan, K., Ferris, T., Jha, A., Kaushal, R., Levy, D., Rosenbaum, S., Shields, A., & Blumenthal, D. (2008). Electronic health records in ambulatory care – A national survey of physicians. *The New England Journal of Medicine, 359*(1), 50.

Dünnebeil, S., Sunyaev, A., Leimeister, J. M., & Krcmar, H. (2010). Strategies for development and adoption of EHR in German ambulatory care. In *4th international conference on pervasive computing technologies for healthcare (PervasiveHealth)* (pp. 1–8), Munich: IEEE.

Eisenhardt, K. M. (1989). Building theories from case study research. *Academy of Management Research, 14*, 532–550.

European Commission. (2007). EuropäischeUnion (2007). *eHealth for safety report*. Luxembourg.

European Commission. (2010). *Business models for ehealth. European commission DGINFSO ICT for health*, Luxembourg.

Fraunhofer Institut. (2005). Spezifikation der Lösungsarchitektur zur Umsetzung der Awendungen der elektronischen Gesundheitskarte. Fraunhofer, Projektgruppe FuE-Projekt.

gematik. (2008). Einführung der Gesundheitskarte – Gesamtarchitektur. vol 1.5.0. Gesellschaft für Telematikanwendungen der Gesundheitskarte mbH.

gematik. (2008). Übergreifendes Sicherheitskonzept der Telematikinfrastruktur. Specification. Gesellschaft für Telematikanwendungen der Gesundheitskarte mbH.

gematik. (2008). Facharchitektur Mehrwertanwendungen Typ 4 vol 1.0.0. Gesellschaft für Telematikanwendungen der Gesundheitskarte mbH, Berlin.

Gentry, C. (2009). Fully homomorphic encryption using ideal lattices. *ACM symposium on theory of computing STOC'09* (pp. 169–178).

Hellmann, W., & Eble, S. (2009). Ambulante und Sektoren übergreifende Behandlungspfade: Konzepte/Umsetzung/Praxisbeispiele.

Helms, T., Pelleter, J., & Ronneberger, D. (2007). Telemedizinische Betreuung chronisch herzinsuffizienter Patienten am Beispiel des telemedizinischen Patientenbetreuungs- und -schulungsprogramms "Telemedizin fürs Herz". *Herz, 32*(8), 623–629.

HFA (2010). Überwachung der Herzinsuffizienz – Tabelle Für Die Kontrolle der Krankheitszeichen. Heart Failure Association of the European Society of Cardiology. http://www.heartfailurematters. org/DE/Documents/HFM_uberwachung_der_herzinsuffizienz.pdf [Last access 2011/07/01]

IOM. (2006). *Identifying and Preventing Medication Errors – Institute of Medicine*. Washington, DC: The National Academies Press.

Karette, J., Neumann, K., Kainzinger, F., & Henke, K. (2005). *Innovation und Wachstum im Gesundheitswesen*. München: Roland Berger Strategy Consultants.

Kartseva, V., Hulstijn, J., Gordijn, J., & Tan, Y. (2010). Control patterns in a healthcare network. *European Journal of Information Systems, 19*, 320–343.

Kempf, K., & Schulz, C. (2008). Telemedizin bei Diabetes: Höhere Therapiezufriedenheit, verbesserte Stoffwechselparameter. DiabetivaR Studie Monika Dienstle, WDGZ.

Krum, H., & Abraham, W. T. (2009). Heart failure. *The Lancet, 373*(9667), 941–955.

KVB. (2008). *Grunddaten zur vertragsärztlichen Versorgung in Deutschland*. Berlin: KVB.

Lappé, J. M., Muhlestein, J. B., Lappé, D. L., Badger, R. S., Bair, T. L., Brockman, R., French, T. K., Hofmann, L. C., Horne, B. D., Kralick-Goldberg, S., Nicponski, N., Orton, J. A., Pearson, R. R., Renlund, D. G., Rimmasch, H., Roberts, C., & Anderson, J. L. (2004). Improvements in 1-year cardiovascular clinical outcomes associated with a hospital-based discharge medication program. *Annals of Internal Medicine, 141*(6), 446–453.

Leimeister, J. M., & Krcmar, H. (2004). Revisiting the virtual community business model. In *Tenth Americas Conference on Information Systems (AMCIS)*, New York.

Lisac, M., Reimers, L., Henke, K.-D., & Schlette, S. (2010). Access and choice – Competition under the roof of solidarity in German health care: An analysis of health policy reforms since 2004. *Health Economics, Policy and Law, 5*(01), 31–52.

Malone, T. W., Yates, J., & Benjamin, R. I. (1987). Electronic markets and electronic hierarchies. *Communications of the ACM, 30*(6), 484–497.

Marschollek, M., & Demirbilek, E. (2006). Providing longitudinal health care information with the new German health card – A pilot system to track patient pathways. *Computer Methods and Programs in Biomedicine, 81*, 266–271.

Mauro, C., Sunyaev, A., Leimeister, J. M., & Krcmar, H. (2009). Service-orientierte integration medizinischer Geräte- eine state of the art analyse. In *Wirtschaftsinformatik* (pp. 119–128). Vienna.

Neumann, T., Biermann, J., Neumann, A., Wasem, J., Ertl, G., Dietz, R., & Erbel, R. (2009). Herzinsuffizienz: Häufigster Grund für Krankenhausaufenthalte. *Deutsches Ärzteblatt, 106*(16), 269–275.

OECD. (2010). *OECD health data 2010: Statistics and indicators*. Paris: RDES: OECD.

Shekelle, P., Morton, S. C., & Keeler, E. B. (2006). *Costs and benefits of health information technology. Evidence report – technology assessment.* http://www.heartfailurematters.org/DE/ Documents/HFM_uberwachung_der_herzinsuffizienz.pdf [Last access 2011/07/01]

Smith, P. C., Stepan, A., Valdmanis, V., & Verheyen, P. (1997). Principal-agent problems in health care systems: An international perspective. *Health Policy, 41*(1), 37–60.

Timmers, P. (1998). Business models for electronic markets. *Journal of Electronic Markets, 8*(2), 3–8.

Weinhardt, C., Schnizler, B., & Luckner, S. (2003). Market engineering. *WIRTSCHAFTSINFORMATIK, 45*(6), 635–640.

ZTG. (2009). Testregionen in Deutschland. http://www.telematik-modellregionen.de www. telematik-modellregionen.de [Last access 2011/04/15]

Chapter 19
Smart Objects in Healthcare: Impact on Clinical Logistics

Martin Sedlmayr and Ulli Münch

Abstract Hospitals are confronted today with a plethora of approaches for asset management with RFID and WLAN, cooling chain monitoring using sensor networks and RFID, and patient tracking using virtually any existing technology. The downside is that most approaches are not necessarily compatible let alone coordinated. Further, none of the technologies is really integrated into legacy systems or corresponding organizational structures and processes, thus the full power of innovative applications is not utilized. Introducing the concept of smart objects inspired by the Internet of Things can improve the situation by separating the capabilities and functions of an object from the implementing technology such as RFID or WLAN. Wireless tags become interchangeable, and business applications can be built independent from the underlying communication network. Supported by synchronized technological and business developments smart objects have the power to transform a hospital from an agglomeration of technologies into a smart environment.

Keywords Ambient intelligence • Asset management • Healthcare logistics • Internet of things • RFID • Smart objects • Wireless sensor networks

M. Sedlmayr (✉)
Lehrstuhl für Medizinische Informatik, Friedrich-Alexander-Universität, Erlangen-Nürnberg, Erlangen, Germany
e-mail: martin.sedlmayr@imi.med.uni-erlangen.de

U. Münch
Fraunhofer IIS-SCS, Fürth, Germany
e-mail: ulli.muench@scs.fraunhofer.de

N. Wickramasinghe et al. (eds.), *Critical Issues for the Development of Sustainable E-health Solutions*, Healthcare Delivery in the Information Age, DOI 10.1007/978-1-4614-1536-7_19, © Springer Science+Business Media, LLC 2012

19.1 Introduction

Innovative Automatic Identification and Data Capture (AIDC) technologies such as Radio Frequency Identification RFID have proven to be a key enabler of sustainable process improvements on many domains by synchronizing material and information flows, avoiding manual notation or keyboard data entry (Fleisch 2010). This is why stakeholders in the healthcare sector such as hospitals increasingly adopt these technologies optimizing especially their logistic processes for cost-effectiveness, quality and safety. Typical use cases are inventory management, temperature monitoring of blood bags and patient identification. Besides such AIDC technologies, other means of communication technologies such as GSM, DECT, Bluetooth and WLAN exist and are already in use.

This is why hospitals today are confronted with a wealth of technologies, which all seem to have typical scenarios but are used for other applications as well. However, interoperability of the systems is not guaranteed, as most applications are proprietary products. And several technologies might be used for implementing the same use case. For example, temperature monitoring of blood-bags might be realized by RFID, sensor networks or WLAN tags. The problem arises when care providers such as hospitals have to assess and decide between technologies. Most often, the decisions and investments are not coordinated among scenarios, technologies and departments.

However, to realize the full potential, innovative processes and organization will be required. There is a need for standardization and proven interoperability, not only for one product, but also among all AIDC technologies within the health sector. While most approaches today only address very specific scenarios, we propose a holistic view on looking at a hospital as an ecosystem inspired by the Internet of Things. The challenge is to create an ecosystem, which combines the different technologies available and develops business services in combination with the technological solution (hybrid services) (Schmitt-Rueth and Pflaum 2010). This is why we introduce the concept of smart objects. The goal is to separate the physical implementation of the tagging infrastructure from the functions. Thus it allows the development of services across technologies.

For the remainder of this contribution we define the properties of smart objects and highlight some technologies in use. The third section discusses application scenarios for clinical logistics. We then forward our concept of medical smart objects by relating it to the Internet of Things and a common vision. Chapter 5 describes the synchronization or developments required to bring the expected impact before the concluding section.

19.2 Smart Objects

The main concepts related to smart objects are Automatic Identification and Data Collection (AIDC) and integration platforms that serve both as enabler for business applications. Put together, they aim at identifying objects, knowing where they are and collect data without further manual efforts (Want 2006).

By combining a tag with sensors and actors thus enabling it to participate in its surrounding we call it a smart tag. And by pairing smart tags with real life objects such as mobile medical devices, blood bags and patients, the objects become "smart", i.e. a smart object. Smart objects typically meet following requirements (Pflaum 2007):

- An identity, which must be unique in its context or system
- Sensors to gather the actual status of the object and actuators to interact with the environment
- The ability to determine the current position
- Memory to store master data, to record past events and gathered data
- The ability to communicate with other objects
- The intelligence to act autonomously to reach a given goal

This allows synchronizing the real world with its virtual counterpart and therefore enables better process and decision support. Many keywords exist, that are related: Auto ID, real time locating systems (RTLS), Ubiquitous Computing, Ambient Assisted Living, Body Area Network, Near Field Communication, and Internet of Things. The building blocks of these are the individual technologies, among the most important:

- Barcodes are the oldest and most widely used AIDC technology. Barcode labels are very cheap, can hold up to a few kilobytes of information and printed on virtual any product, e.g. on blood bags to improve patient safety (Li et al. 2005).
- Radio-frequency Identification (RFID) (Want 2006) is often considered as a radio-based successor of barcodes. They can be categorized in passive, active and semi-active depending on the power source used for transmission. Their sending range varies from a few millimetres up to more than 10 m. In contrast to other radio-based technologies, RFID tags are extremely robust and solutions exist for deep-frozen bio probes, blood bags in a centrifuge or extreme heat while e.g. sterilizing surgical instruments. Recent developments in RFID labelling include printable tags (Preradovic and Karmakar 2009; Harrop 2007). Thus, the amount of labelled objects will probably increase, if printing RFID chips is as cheap and simple as printing barcode labels.
- Wireless Lan (WLAN) is well known from mobile computing and often infra-structures already exist in hospitals and can be reused. WLAN tags exist similar to sensor network tags but require more energy thus limiting long term use (Alemdar and Ersoy 2010).
- Ultrasound tags can be used as a replacement for radio-based tagging of patients and devices (Shahid et al. 2010) and even inside a patient (Davilis et al. 2010). A major advantage is the absence of electromagnetic interference; but communication is only on room level.
- Infrared waves allow for short-range communication similar to ultrasound (Shahid et al. 2010).
- Wireless sensor networks (WSN) are also radio-based, but build a communication network utilizing local intelligence (see below).

All of these technologies are available, already proving their value in application domains like consumer logistics or production control. In this respect smart object technologies like RFID and WLAN are established technologies in these domains. Wireless sensor networks (WSN) merge the concept of both and takes them even a step further creating ubiquitous, self-organizing networks of intelligent objects actively monitoring their environment.

19.2.1 Wireless Sensor Networks

A wireless sensor network consists of many spatially distributed devices called tags (also: nodes or motes). These devices use sensors to monitor conditions such as temperature, sound, vibration, pressure, motion, or pollutants. Tags are equipped with wireless communication capability so that they can communicate with other motes either directly or indirectly via multiple hops. The fast-growing research effort in academia and industry has resulted in many protocols and applications of wireless sensor networks (Akyildiz et al. 2002; Alemdar and Ersoy 2010) such as IEEE 802.15.4-2006 (http://www.ieee802.org/15/), ZigBee (http://www.zigbee. org/), s-net® (http://www.iis.fraunhofer.de/en/bf/ec/dk/sn/index.jsp), and DASH7 (http://www.dash7.org).

The main objective of a sensor network beyond being a simple communication network is to gather and pre-process sensor data. Sensor nodes are able to make decisions locally (depending on the application) using local intelligence (i.e. computing power). Also in many sensor network applications, the sensor nodes have the ability to work collaboratively to solve complex problems, including measurement, detection, classification, and tracking in the physical world.

For many wireless sensor network applications, sensor data is required to be associated with location information. Thus, a sensor network needs to provide a service to provide the sensor location information by some kind of positioning technology, e.g., triangulation, data routing latencies, etc. In certain cases, sensors or sensor nodes in a network have the ability to determine their own location, especially for mobile sensor nodes.

A common aspect of most sensor network standards is their focus on cable replacement for sensors and actuators in home and industrial control and automation, meaning that objects are supposed to be fixed and immobile. The Internet of Things on the other hand consists of a large number of devices that are mobile and roam through the network. A protocol that supports such applications needs to be flexible and dynamic enough to support the continuous changing of the network topology as nodes change location and wireless connections need to be re-established.

Another aspect is energy consumption. Most available technologies assume that the infrastructure nodes are active 100% of the time, which also includes the transceiver, the most important contributor to energy consumption. In contrast, infrastructure nodes in s-net follow the same duty cycle as mobile nodes, being active only within frame periods (every eight seconds default). This is a trade-off between latency and network capacity.

In comparison to RFID, sensor networks are much more expensive as they require local intelligence for processing complex protocols. On the other hand, meshing nodes can generate energy efficient communication networks for proactive services where RFID fails. The possible omission of a fixed infrastructure (e.g. gates with RFID) is another advantage in dynamic environments. Thus, sensor networks enable new and ambient application scenarios.

19.2.2 Integration Platforms (IP)

An integration platform (also: middleware) is the connection point of the technologies described above with the existing IT-landscape of a business. It serves as a facade or bridge and allows exchange of data between participants and the use of services. Beside the simple data exchange, typical integration functions comprise the filtering, aggregation and (pre-)processing of sensor data. This is why they often include a business rule engine and solutions for complex event processing (Black et al. 2004; Cook et al. 2009). Both can be used to detect relevant events or alarms (Lempert and Pflaum 2010).

An integration platform for diverse smart object technologies like RFID, WSN and WLAN unites these technologies with a shared technology abstraction layer, controls the interaction between these technologies and existing enterprise infrastructures, supports intra-corporate and cross-company integration, and aims at reducing integration costs significantly.

Especially the open source community provides a lot of solutions that could be considered when implementing a universal integration platform (Lempert and Pflaum 2010) such as Global Sensor Networks (Lempert and Pflaum 2010; Aberer et al. 2006), ASPIRE (Soldatos 2009), and the OGC standard Sensor Web Enablement (SWE).

However, most products concentrate on RFID-based solutions. One reason may be the existence of a broadly accepted international standard by EPCglobal. Often, RFID-based middleware are extended to cover the functional aspects of other technologies. However, non-functional requirements are often neglected or the smallest discriminator with RFID is build disregarding any extended possibilities.

But while approaches exist for expanding the possibilities for such a single technology (especially RFID), comprehensive solutions across technologies and networks are widely neglected (Black et al. 2004). There is not much development in integration platforms beyond RFID, e.g. for WSN and WLAN (Lempert and Pflaum 2010). Further, most integration platforms are developed by academic institutions focusing on the technical aspects such as coping with distributed data management, sensor fusion and event processing.

19.3   Applications

Barcodes are the omnipresent technology e.g. on wristbands, packages and documents to identify patients, drugs, lab samples and charts. But radio-based technologies such as RFID and sensor networks are already in use and under development in the healthcare domain. The number of reports clearly demonstrates the broad applicability of the technologies (Vilamovska et al. 2008). The trend is also rising: Fig. 19.1 shows an intense progress of RFID related patents in healthcare in the last 10 years (data for 2009 not yet complete). Assuming a temporal offset of the patent and the actual product, many new applications can be expected in the next years.

Four main functions of wireless AIDC technologies have been identified as beneficial in healthcare applications (Vilamovska et al. 2008): tracking, identification and authentication, automatic data collection and transfer, and sensing.

- Tracking: Identification and motion of a person or object including both real-time position tracking and tracking of motion through choke points. This may lead to process improvements and increased efficiency of resources.
- Identification and Authentication can increase e.g. patient safety, enable electronic medical record maintenance and be used for automatic drug identification and login security.
- Automatic data collection and transfer: reducing manual input by electronic data capturing, process automation and monitoring, audit, inventory and asset management.
- Sensing: telemedicine, staff hygiene compliance, perishable medication and blood product handling.

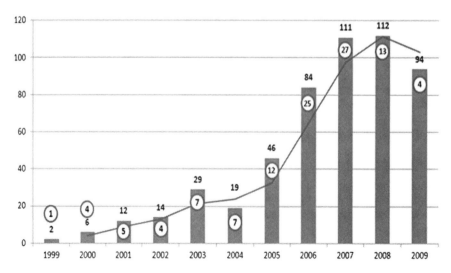

Fig. 19.1 Development of RFID and healthcare related patent in the triad (US, EU, JP) (Sedlmayr et al. 2010)

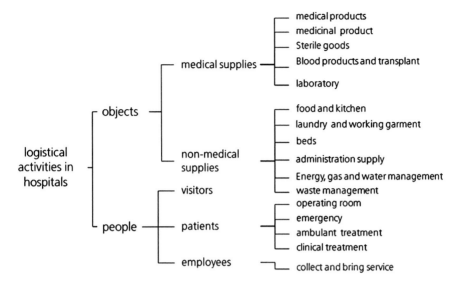

Fig. 19.2 Typical logistics activities in a hospital categorized by objects (Pflaum et al. 2010)

Looking at the published reports, it is apparent that some projects just use the wireless transmission capabilities of AIDC technologies in rather futuristic scenarios (e.g. toilet training using ZigBee tags in diapers and toilets (Chen 2010)). But many projects and products are already in productive use, especially for logistics scenarios (e.g. asset management).

19.3.1   Logistics Scenarios

Because of external and internal pressure, hospitals need to optimize processes and utilization of resources to increase efficiency and cost-effectiveness while maintaining high quality care. A basic requirement for optimization is transparency of the whereabouts of material and automatic capture and transfer of data about their environment (e.g. temperature). A huge potential to increase efficiency lies especially in logistics, which takes a major share of the processes in a hospital (Fig. 19.2).

Accordingly, the types of objects tagged so far are either persons (42%) or objects, such as drugs and laboratory samples (29%), medical devices (17%), and blood (6%) (von Eiff et al. 2007).

A typical example is the cooling chain of blood bags that be secured by active sensors continuously monitoring the temperature and even proactively raising an alarm in case of exceedance (Dzik 2007). RFID is also a viable alternative to bar codes in the bedside matching process, which are susceptible to dirt and wrinkles (Sandler et al. 2006), because it is extremely important to clearly identify the recipient to give the right blood to the right patient. Stationary RFID readers may even be built into operating tables to match the RFID-wristband of a patient with a blood bag tag (Dzik 2007).

Another is asset management where expensive medical devices are tagged to prevent theft, but also common goods are tagged to improve inventory management and material logistics (http://diuf.unifr.ch/drupal/sites/diuf.unifr.ch.drupal.softeng/files/file/publications/internal/rfidehealth.pdf). Another effect is the reduction of searching time, which sums up to half an hour per shift and ward (Glabman 2004). Most asset scenarios however are restricted to inventory control as further information such as the usage for a certain patient are not yet monitored (Frisch et al. 2010).

One project combining both – the blood bag monitoring and matching as well as asset management – based on wireless sensor networks is OPAL Health.

19.3.2   Case Report OPAL Health

One example of a system combining both scenarios on one platform is OPAL Health, which has developed a generic communication platform for clinical use (Sedlmayr et al. 2009). Based on the same hardware, completely different scenarios have been built and are under evaluation at the University Hospital Erlangen. Operating some mobile 300 tags for asset management and 230 tags for transfusion safety make OPAL one of the largest sensor network installations in the world.

The OPAL smart tag consists of a small embedded microcontroller, a wireless transceiver, an antenna, a battery and different sensors and actuators equipment. The layout is based on the S3 hardware reference design by Fraunhofer IIS (http://www.iis.fraunhofer.de/en/bf/ec/dk/sn/index.jsp), but has been extended towards a flexible clinical communication platform. The microcontroller executes the wireless MAC- and networking protocol, the drivers for the sensors and actuators including signal processing and all local services (such as matching algorithms). The wireless transceiver is used to transmit user and signalling information between nodes.

While the sensors and actuators are different for each target application scenario and sensor tag, the basic hardware remains the same among all types of tags, i.e. in OPAL: a device tag submitting its position, a blood bag tag to measure the temperature and to match it with a patient tag identifying a patient. Each of these mobile tags mainly varies in software configuration and the surrounding cases (square-cut for devices, soft edges and a wrist band for patients). Additionally so-called anchor nodes are installed at fixed positions as basic infrastructure to support the positioning of nodes and routing of messages. Gateway nodes allow access to the smart object network on an IP-level and IP-WSN crossover (Fig. 19.3)

The software on each sensor node is based on the s-net® protocol (http://www.iis.fraunhofer.de/en/bf/ec/dk/sn/index.jsp), which offers a platform for the implementation of application specific smart object network solutions.

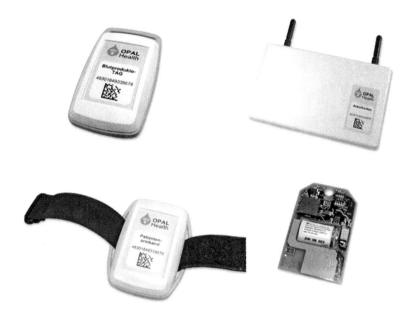

Fig. 19.3 OPAL Health tags (blood bag and patient wristband on the left) and a stationary anchor tag

One problem arises when tagging mobile medical devices is caused by the size of a tag. While larger ventilators offer enough space to put a tag on the back, very small infusion pumps within a rack offer no free space at all. Therefore on the one hand, a compromise between using a generic (and thus cheap) case design versus a device-specific (and thus expensive one) has to be found. On the other hand, it is already clear that without support from vendors a solution for tagging will be impossible.

Any new communication technology will only come to its full potential when being seamlessly integrated into clinical legacy systems. On the one hand, data about devices and other material (e.g. inventory numbers patient case identifiers, maintenance intervals) are required to initialize the object tags used for monitoring and identifying patients and objects. On the other hand, the network generates a wealth of important information on e.g. locations (tracking), usage (identification) and sensor readings (monitoring), which should be fed, back into clinical systems (Fig. 19.4). OPAL uses a webservice-oriented approach for flexible integration into the clinical IT-landscape. Hence, interfaces to the corresponding applications have been built using SAP-BAPI connections (device data), HL7 messages (patient data) and direct database access (blood bag data).

The data scheme used stores all sensor network generated events such as position events, temperature events and matching events. The logic to detect broken cold chains or unexpected movement of devices is calculated based on the event data. Information about alarming events such as missing tags, false matching events and the like is escalated through email and via DECT-based SMS (specific to the University Hospital Erlangen).

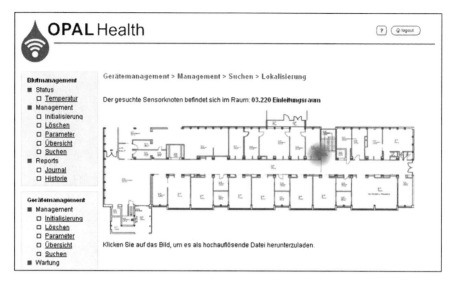

Fig. 19.4 Front end showing the current location of a certain medical device

19.3.3 Assessing the Costs and Benefits

The advantages of using smart object technologies in healthcare is the direct linkage of the objects, or more precise the data generated from them, and the other systems (back-end or legacy systems) (Chang et al. 2008): Large quantities of data can be communicated without manual intervention in higher quality over greater distances. Smart objects, seamlessly integrated with networks of medical devices, computers and systems, enable pro-active services and data intensive services. Another advantage is, that especially RFID-based systems are affordable (Alemdar and Ersoy 2010). This allows for generous use, creating pervasive healthcare systems, which monitor the surrounding in real-time and identify the context and potentially critical issues.

In general, the added value of using functions of smart object technologies in business applications can be expressed using the dimensions of time, quality and cost (Seitz et al. 2010):

- Time: The data generated by the system are more recent than manually entered data.
- Quality: By automating data elicitation, more and more detailed data is generated; further, by avoiding manual input the risk for errors is reduced.
- Cost: As the data is already generated electronically, it can easily be communicated among systems and actors and relieve personnel from manual tasks (time) and allows for further process optimization.

Especially for asset and inventory management, radio-based technologies have already proven their advantage over barcodes (Michael and McCathie 2005). The

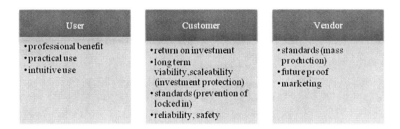

User	Customer	Vendor

• professional benefit
• practical use
• intuitive use
	• return on investment
	• long term
	  viability, scaleability
	  (investment protection)
	• standards (prevention of
	  locked in)
	• reliability, safety
		• standards (mass
		  production)
		• future proof
		• marketing

Fig. 19.5 Direct stakeholders and their concerns

time-consuming searching for medical instruments, which can sum up to 30 min per ward and working shift, can be significantly reduced with the help of the active tracking (Glabman 2004).

But many factors exist beyond monetary effects that hinder the assessment of smart objects concept. One is the number of stakeholders/actors in the healthcare sector and their relationships (Fig. 19.5).

- Users such as doctors and nurses expect professional benefits. Usability and ease of use have to be considered most to increase acceptance. But it is important to note, that there are major differences in the user groups and their involvement: nurses, doctors, technicians, administration, and others.
- Customers are the hospitals as business partner. The economic benefit and return on invest has to be demonstrated. Customers are interested in scalable and reliable solutions and protections of investments. Ideally solutions from different vendors are interoperable so that lock-in can be prevented.
- Commercial vendors and solution providers also require standards that allow for mass production. Fragmentation of the healthcare market requires customization to each customer and user.

However, there are many other parties involved in providing health services. These may benefit from advanced solutions but are not initially sharing the cost. For example service technicians and technical inspection authorities have faster access to devices located by an RTLS. But as long as service contracts are based on a lump sum per device instead of per-call maintenance they do not share the cost. Even within a hospital, tagging patients is an effort by the wards, while the benefit (monitoring blood transfusions) might only be on the blood bank's side. This is why solutions require consideration of the whole value chain. For example blood bags should be traceable from the donor to the recipient and proper disposal. This requires standardisation and interoperability across administrations, organisations, and IT services.

But innovative smart object solutions have more than just monetary effects. For example near miss events during blood transfusion are immediately reported in an active system. This will increase the detection rate and traceability of errors that will improve process quality and patient safety.

Interestingly, while many projects claim the technically universal application of their approach, hardly any proof exists. Especially the more powerful technologies such as sensor networks have not yet proven the "infrastructure effect", i.e. the deployment of additional services on top of an existing installation. Only a few examples exist that have started implementing different services on top of a common hardware platform (Sedlmayr et al. 2009). As for WLAN, the infrastructure effect is apparent – one network where everybody can hook up – while AIDC/RTLS applications in medical scenarios are still considered as an island.

However, the infrastructure effect is important to justify investments in relatively expensive yet more powerful technologies: while RFID tags may cost from 10ct to 2 Euros, sensor tags cost easily 20 times more per piece. Therefore, WSN tags may not compete in a single scenario e.g. temperature monitoring – even if an active communication is desired the cost may be too high.

19.4 Forwarding the Concept

Making objects smart is only a first step. Knowing the identity of an object ("what is") should be complemented by "where is", "when is", and "in what condition" (Michael et al. 2010). As can easily be seen, these properties are met by most of the wireless AIDC technologies. But the concept of smart objects goes beyond the application of a single technology; there will be no one-size-fits-all solution based on RFID or WLAN. We believe in heterogeneous networks of smart objects, each with its own advantage in a single scenario, but complemented in functionality by other concepts: RFID labels can be centrifugalized and deep-frozen, sensor networks are active systems and WLAN has a huge communication capacity. But all contribute to a single information cloud. Large networks of smart objects will enable new types of applications and new ways of service engineering and management.

It should be noted, that many types of smart objects exist, depending on the objects to which a smart label is attached, the functional requirements and the extent to which the smart object participates with its surrounding. Four different categories can be characterized (Fujinami 2010):

- A wearable (carriable) object typically accompanies its user closely for a longer time of the day, so continuous monitoring of physiological parameters becomes possible. GSM, WLAN, and Bluetooth are often used in these scenarios.
- An instrumental object is directly related to a task, such as a switch, and its state indicates the state of use. RFID allows for storing data with objects and travelling with them (tagging documents); but also sensor networks are used.
- A workspace object is not directly related to a specific task, but has a generic role such as a surgical table, which sets the stage for other objects. Especially passive RFID labels are in use e.g. to tag disposable materials.
- An architectural element (object) such as a building or room has no direct task associated, but builds the environment in which others operate; it might be associated with properties such as room temperature. This is where protocols like ZigBee aim at.

This is why development comes from various application areas each focussing on different communications aspects, sensors and use cases:

- Implantable and wearable sensors for monitoring vital signs of patients: wireless communication is used to transmit data across tissues or just as matter of comfort (omission of cables) (Frehill and Chambers 2007).
- Telemonitoring and teletherapy applications often combine different communication standards to establish a chain from wearable sensors (RFID, Bluetooth) over local networks (e.g. WLAN) to remote stations over the Internet (Ferguson et al. 2010).
- "Networked medical devices" is a recent buzzword dedicated to the growing intelligence of traditionally self-contained devices, which has even led to a new standard (ISO: IEC 80001 2010).
- Smart environment solution for home automation such as security, access control, smart metering and the like (Florentino et al. 2008).
- Logistic scenarios improving material flow within an institution including smart cabinets, blood bag surveillance, quality documentation and asset management (Kim et al. 2006, Kumar et al. 2009).

Overcoming these mostly segregated developments with only sporadic interconnections is the main vision of the Internet of Things (Zouganeli and Svinnset 2009). The Internet of Things is based on the idea that every object (person, machine, system) participates and communicates in a universal network. Often cited examples are the fridge that orders replacements when something is removed and the grocery store, which the customer can leave and money is deducted automatically based on the goods in the cart (http://ec.europa.eu/information_society/policy/rfid/documents/commiot2009.pdf).

From a more technological viewpoint, the Future Internet investigates the network and service infrastructures required by the Internet of Things. Concepts beyond the classical Internet are required to integrate networking with service development and advanced concepts of optical networks, autonomic network and service capabilities, trust and security and well as new architectures for distributed, adaptive and "intelligent" systems (National Intelligence Council).

Of course this requires new ways of designing and operating the complex work systems. Smart environments are envisioned as adaptive and learning systems (Streitz et al. 2007). The vision of ambient intelligence is based on blurred borders across technologies, dedicated sensor tags, traditional devices and backend information systems. This is where the concept of simply connected objects ends and the Internet of Things begins (Zouganeli and Svinnset 2009).

We believe the Internet of Things has advantages also in the healthcare setting, enabling the building of smart environments supporting many medical and logistics scenarios. There should be a common vision on what hospitals of the future could look like to help coordinating the individual development efforts (Fig. 19.6).

Many different technologies, each with its own capabilities and restrictions are available. There is also an enormous speed in innovation and evolution, making technology affordable, smaller, faster, more energy efficient. Yet, there is still a lack in integration on a technical as well as a business level.

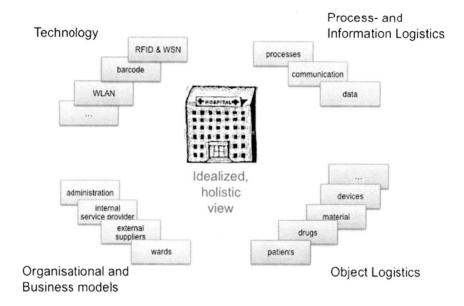

Fig. 19.6 Holistic view on a hospital as a smart environment enabled by smart object technologies

Introducing the technologies into the healthcare sector by tagging people, material, and buildings for identification, tracking and monitoring will increase transparency and will allow better process- and information logistics. This is where the concept of smart object will help to overcome technological barriers by separating the implementation of the infrastructure from the development of smart object based business services.

In the end, new and modified processes require new business models and models for operation. Many partners cooperate in the healthcare sector. Determining the return on investment is only possible, if all participants along a value chain share investments and receive benefits.

19.5 Synchronizing Developments

RFID technology has started its way into the hospital market due to its superiority to barcodes; wireless sensor networks even go beyond this by enabling pro-active services. But both are still in their infancy in clinical use with little empirical research (Tzeng et al. 2008). Hence, there is hardly any experience which could guide developers yet alone managers in developing and introducing it in the clinical daily routine besides promising case studies (Vilamovska et al. 2008).

A major problem is the rapid development of the technology. New generations of better, cheaper and more powerful sensor chips become available. Within the first

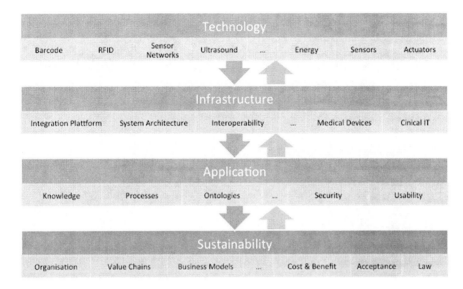

Fig. 19.7 Synchronizing developments

year of the OPAL Health project, the price calculated for one tag dropped by almost 30% while the processor capacity increased by 400% (Sedlmayr et al. 2009). Next generations of chips will integrate the microprocessor and the transceiver thus reducing the size of a smart tag. Strong cryptography will once become available on chip thus enabling high security features required to transmit patient related data. Applications not feasible today will be standard of the future.

On the other hand, technology enables services that will require organizational changes. It is not without reason, why hospitals as high-dependency environments are reluctant to organizational changes. Therefore, only proven applications with a clear return on invest might be accepted.

This is why intentional synchronization of the technical and business developments is needed: to improve the technology according to user needs building new types of applications and at the same time allow the user and organizations to adjust to the new possibilities (Fig. 19.7).

Concerning the technology the integration of different AIDC technologies (bar code, RFID, sensor nets) into holistic systems represents the largest challenge. Pushing the limits of restricted hardware by making the hardware smaller, faster and cheaper will improve adoption. Efficient energy management and harvesting capabilities and the development of new hardware components including sensors and actuators will make new employment scenarios possible.

But only integration the hardware with its operational environment delivers a full benefit. While current integrations platforms are just a façade or gateway for simple networks, future developments will allow for seamless services across technological, geographic and other borders. This will require new ways of designing systems and services. Especially governance of large and heterogeneous networks is still an open research issue (http://ec.europa.eu/information_society/policy/rfid/documents/commiot2009.pdf). Trends in networking medical devices (Cohen 2004) and of convergence of clinical IT with medical devices and AIDC should be fostered.

For the application, focussing on promising areas of application with a high or fast ROI may convince users to quickly adapt the new technologies (e.g. asset management, personnel or patient tracking, patient safety). Finally, however, a generalisation of the assigned technologies must take place to cover as many scenarios as possible (infrastructure effect). A strong research focus is on building ontologies to enable system interoperability and reuse of clinical data (Cimino and Ayres 2010). The Internet of Things and Future Internet initiatives also foster convergence of developments by focussing the integration and interoperability of services (http://ec.europa.eu/information_society/policy/rfid/documents/commiot2009.pdf). It is supported by the standardisation of healthcare through processes such as guidelines and pathways.

Of course, security is a major concern whenever data are transmitted and stored electronically. For the applications, security of individual components as well as for the entire system has to be ensured, for complex systems even across manufacturers and application borders. The analysis of the interference and mutual disturbance is just as important as the development of cryptography techniques for sensor communication. And while most developments are technology driven, a stronger focus should be put on usability to improve effectiveness of the systems and increase user acceptance (Zwicker 2009).

But in the end, new developments will only stay, if a real benefit is perceived. Business models along the whole value chain have to be found so that cost can be minimized or split among stakeholders, and benefits exist. However, this will require organisational changes beyond short-witted replacement of one technology with another. Telemedicine is a well-discussed example where organisational, legal and financial prevents technology to come to use, e.g. (Leung and Kaplan 2009; Klar and Pelikan 2009). RFID is often seen as successor to bar-code and simply replaces the striped label by a radio-enabled one not utilizing the possibilities of ambient technology (Michael et al. 2010).

19.6   Conclusion

Wireless sensor networks have demonstrated their ability to communicate data in an energy efficient way. They adapt to different application scenarios in dynamic topologies and can be equipped with sensors and actuators. Paired with real world objects they become smart objects synchronizing the physical world with its virtual representation, thus enabling new dimensions of process management, decision support, and novel services. By using their local intelligence, smart objects potentially become first class citizens in the Internet of Things.

Above all, the concept of smart objects is technologically not limited to sensor networks. Other technologies such as RFID and WLAN are being already used for similar and complementary purposes such as object tracking and monitoring. Visions of ambient intelligence such as for assisted living (AAL) and smart environments are based on blurred borders across technologies, dedicated sensor tags, traditional devices and backend information systems.

However, a conglomerate of technologies/products/concepts exists but hardly any attempts to integrate those into a (virtual) single platform have been made. Hospitals are confronted today with a plethora of approaches for asset management with RFID and WLAN, cooling chain monitoring using sensor networks and RFID, and patient tracking using virtually any existing technology. The downside is that most approaches are not necessarily compatible let alone coordinated. Further, none of the technologies is really integrated into legacy systems thus the full power of innovative AIDC and RTLS applications is not utilized.

Introducing the concept of smart objects inspired by the Internet of Things will improve the situation. Smart objects are using smart tags attached to an object or person to identify or locate it, or to enable further functions of sensing and acting. Smart objects communicate freely in a network and via gateways into the Internet. By separating the concept of a smart object from an implementing technology such as RFID or WLAN, they become interchangeable, and business applications are separated from the communication network.

Some approaches to smart object networks use integration platforms that serve as gateways between the different sensor networks and the business applications. However, integration platforms are simply a facade to (otherwise unrelated) separate sensor networks. Smart object networks should be interoperable by design allowing the user to purchase or replace a smart tag according to functional requirements not what else is installed.

Advancing the smart object concept requires on one side work on the technological solution, making the hardware smaller, cheaper and more energy efficient; making the protocols more reliable and secure; designing services that last. On the other side, integration and interoperability is still neglected. To unleash the full potential, smart object networks require interchange of data and services across technologies and locations.

Acknowledgement Research on OPAL Health was funded in part by the Federal Ministry of Economics and Technology.

References

Aberer, K., Hauswirth, M., & Salehi, A. (2006). Global sensor networks. Ecole Polytechnique Fdrale de Lausanne (EPFL), Tech. Rep. LSIR-REPORT-2006-001.

Akyildiz, I., Su, W., Sankarasubramaniam, Y., & Cayirci, E. (2002). Wireless sensor networks: a survey. *Computer Networks: The International Journal of Computer and Telecommunications Networking, 38*, 393–422.

Alemdar, H., & Ersoy, C. (2010). Wireless sensor networks for healthcare: A survey. *Computer Networks: The International Journal of Computer and Telecommunications Networking, 54*, 2688–2710.

Black, J., Segmuller, W., Cohen, N., Leiba, B., Misra, A., Ebling, M. R., & Stern, E. (2004). Pervasive computing in health care: Smart spaces and enterprise information systems. MobiSys 2004 workshop on Context Awareness, Boston, MA.

Chang, S.-I., Ou, C.-S., Ku, C.-Y., & Yang, M. (2008). A study of RFID application impacts on medical safety. *International Journal of Electronic Healthcare, 4*, 1–23.

Chen, Y.-C. (2010). ZigAlert: A zigbee alert for toileting training children with developmental delay in a public school setting. In *ASSETS'10: Proceedings of the 12th international ACM SIGACCESS conference on computers and accessibility*. Orlando, Florida doi: 10.1145/1878803.1878896

Cimino, J. J., & Ayres, E. J. (2010). The clinical research data repository of the US National Institutes of Health. *Studies in Health Technology and Informatics, 160*, 1299–1303.

Cohen, T. (2004). Medical and information technologies converge. *Engineering in Medicine and Biology Magazine, 23*(3), 59–65.

Cook, D., Augusto, J., & Jakkula, V. (2009). Review: ambient intelligence: Technologies, applications, and opportunities. *Pervasive and Mobile Computing, 5*, 277–298.

Davilis, Y., Kalis, A., & Ifantis, A. (2010). On the use of ultrasonic waves as a communications medium in biosensor networks. *IEEE Transactions on Information Technology in Biomedicine, 14*, F650–F656.

Dzik, W. H. (2007). New technology for transfusion safety. *British Journal of Haematology, 136*, 181–190.

Ferguson, G., Quinn, J., Horwitz, C., Swift, M., Allen, J., & Galescu, L. (2010). Towards a personal health management assistant. *Journal of Biomedical Informatics, 43*, S13–S16.

Fleisch, E. (2010). What is the internet of things? When things add value. Auto-ID labs white paper.

Florentino, G. H. P., Paz de Araujo, C. A., Bezerra, H. U., Junior, H. B. A., Xavier, M. A., de Souza, V. S. V., de M Valentim, R. A. A., Morais, A. H. F., Guerreiro, A. M. G., & Brandao, G. B. (2008). Hospital automation system RFID-based: technology embedded in smart devices (cards, tags and bracelets). Conf Proc IEEE Eng Med Biol Soc, 2008, 1455-1458. doi:10.1109/IEMBS.2008.4649441, Vancouver, BC.

Frehill, P., Chambers, D., & Rotariu, C. (2007). Using Zigbee to integrate medical devices. Conf Proc IEEE Eng Med Biol Soc, 2007, 6718-6721. doi:10.1109/IEMBS.2007.4353902.

Frisch, P.H., Booth, P., & Miodownik, S. (2010). Beyond inventory control: understanding RFID and its applications. *Biomedical Instrumentation & Technology Supplement*, 39–48. Busan, doi: 10.1109/FUTURETECH.2010.5482711 http://www.aami.org/publications/ITHorizons it is the 2010 edition.

Fujinami, K. (2010). Interaction design issues in smart home environments. In *5th international conference on future information technology (FutureTech)* (pp. 1–8).

Glabman, M. (2004). Room for tracking. RFID technology finds the way. *Materials Management in Health Care 13*, 26–28, 31–24, 36 passim.

Harrop, P. (2007). Printed Electronics-The Big Picture. Ink Maker,. Retrieved from http://www.onboard-technology.com/pdf_settembre2007/090706.pdf

http://diuf.unifr.ch/drupal/sites/diuf.unifr.ch.drupal.softeng/files/file/publications/internal/rfide-health.pdf

http://ec.europa.eu/information_society/policy/rfid/documents/commiot2009.pdf

http://www.dash7.org/

http://www.ieee802.org/15/

http://www.iis.fraunhofer.de/en/bf/ec/dk/sn/index.jsp

http://www.zigbee.org/

ISO: IEC 80001. (2010). Application of risk management for IT-networks incorporating medical devices.

Kim, S.-J., Yoo, S., Kim, H.-O., Bae, H.-S., Park, J.-J., Seo, K.-J., & Chang, B.-C. (2006). Smart Blood Bag Management System in a Hospital Environment Personal Wireless Communications. In P. Cuenca & L. Orozco-Barbosa (Eds.), 4217 (pp. 506–517). Springer Berlin / Heidelberg.

Klar, R., & Pelikan, E. (2009). Telemedicine in Germany: status, chances and limits. *Bundesgesundheitsblatt, Gesundheitsforschung, Gesundheitsschutz, 52*, 263–269.

Kumar, S., Swanson, E., & Tran, T. (2009). RFID in the healthcare supply chain: usage and application. *International Journal of Health Care Quality Assurance, 22*, 67–81.

Lempert, S., & Pflaum, A. (2010). Über die Notwendigkeit einer Integrationsplattform für unterschiedliche Smart Object Technologien. In *Conference Über die Notwendigkeit einer Integrationsplattform für unterschiedliche Smart Object Technologien* (pp. 71–74). Universität Würzburg, Institut für Informatik.

Lempert, S., Pflaum, A. (2010). Towards a reference architecture for an integration platform for diverse smart object technologies. In *Conference towards a reference architecture for an integration platform for diverse smart object technologies*. In Höpfner, H., & Specht, G. (Eds.). (2011). MMS 2011: Mobile und ubiquitäre Informations systeme. Proceedings der 6. Konferenz, 28. Februar 2011 in Kaiserslautern (Vol. 185). GI.

Leung, S. T., & Kaplan, K. J. (2009). Medicolegal aspects of telepathology. *Human Pathology, 40*, 1137–1142.

Li, B.-N., Dong, M.-C., & Vai, M. (2005). From codabar to ISBT 128: Implementing barcode technology in blood bank automation system. In *Proceedings of 27th annual international conference of the IEEE-EMBS* (pp. 542–545). New York.

Michael, K., & McCathie, L. (2005). The Pros and Cons of RFID in Supply Chain Management. In Proceedings of the International Conference on Mobile Business (ICMB '05). Sidney. IEEE Computer Society, Washington, DC, USA, 623-629. DOI=10.1109/ICMB.2005.103 http://dx.doi.org/10.1109/ICMB.2005.103.

Michael, K., Roussos, G., Huang, G. Q., Chattopadhyay, A., Gadh, R., Prabhu, B. S., & Chu, P. (2010). Planetary-Scale RFID Services in an Age of Uberveillance. Proceedings of the IEEE, 98(9), 1663–1671.

National Intelligence Council. Appendix F- background: The internet of things. In *Conference Appendix F- Background: The Internet of Things.*

Pflaum, A. (2007). *Theft prevention system based on networked active Tags (sensor networks).* Boston: RFID Smart Labels.

Pflaum, A., Meier, F., Muench, U., Fluegel, C., Gehrmann, V., Hupp, J., & Sedlmayr, M. (2010). Deployment of a wireless sensor network to support and optimize logistical processes in a clinical environment. RFID Systech 2010, Ciudad, Spain.

Preradovic, S., & Karmakar, N. (2009). Design of fully printable planar chipless RFID transponder with 35-bit data capacity. In *European microwave conference*, (pp. 013–016). Rome.

Sandler, S. G., Langeberg, A., Carty, K., & Dohnalek, L. J. (2006). Bar code and radio-frequency technologies can increase safety and efficiency of blood transfusions. *Labmedicine, 37*, 436–439.

Schmitt-Rueth, S., & Pflaum, A. (2010). Service engineering as a concept to develop hybrid services in health care. In *Fifteenth annual international meeting and exposition of the American telemedicine association.* Liebert, New York/San Antonio.

Sedlmayr, M., Becker, A., Muench, U., Meier, F., Prokosch, H. U., & Ganslandt, T. (2009). Towards a smart object network for clinical services. AMIA Annu Symp Proc, 2009, 578–582.

Sedlmayr, M., Becker, A., Prokosch, H.-U., Flügel, C., & Meier, F. (2010). OPAL health – A smart object network for hospital logistics. In S. Kirn (Ed.). *Process of change in organisations through eHealth, Proceedings of the 2nd international eHealth symposium*, Stuttgart.

Seitz, M., Meier, F., Münch, U., Ma, T., & Niemann, C. (2010). Das drahtlose Sensornetzwerk als Schattenbild der Patientenlogistik. fg-mocomed.gi-ev.de.

Shahid, B., Kannan, A., Lovell, N., & Redmond, S. (2010). Ultrasound user-identification for wireless sensor networks. In *Annual international conference of the IEEE engineering in medicine and biology society (EMBC)* (pp. 5756–5759).

Soldatos, J. (2009). AspireRfid Can Lower Deployment Costs. RFID Journal,. Retrieved from http://www.rfidjournal.com/article/view/4661.

Streitz, N. A., Kameas, A., & Mavrommati, I. (2007). *The disappearing computer : Interaction design, system infrastructures and applications for smart environments.* Berlin/Heidelberg: Springer-Verlag.

Tzeng, S.-F., Chen, W.-H., & Pai, F.-Y. (2008). Evaluating the business value of RFID: evidence from five case studies. *International Journal of Production Economics, 112*, 601–613.

Vilamovska, A.-M., Hatziandreu, E., Schindler, R., van Oranje, C., de Vries, H., & Krapels, J. (2008). Deliverable 1: scoping and identifying areas for RFID deployment in healthcare delivery. Study on the requirements and options for RFID application in healthcare, vol. TR-608-EC. RAND Europe, Brussels.

von Eiff, W., Hagen, A., & Prangenberg, A. (2007). Radio Frequency Identification – Instrument des Klinischen Risikomanagements. infomedis.ch.

Want, R. (2006). An introduction to RFID technology. *IEEE Pervasive Computing, 5*, 25–33.

Zouganeli, E., & Svinnset, I. E. Connected objects and the internet of things — A paradigm shift. In *Conference Connected Objects and the Internet of Things — A Paradigm Shift* (pp. 1–4).

Zwicker, F. (2009). *Ubiquitous Computing im Krankenhaus: Eine fallstudienbasierte Analyse betriebswirtschaftlicher Potenziale*. Gabler.

Chapter 20
Agency Theory in E-Healthcare and Telemedicine: A Literature Study

Joerg Leukel, Julia Fernandes, Anna Heidebrecht, and Simone Schillings

Abstract The agency theory is concerned with agency relationships between two or more parties involved in an economic transaction. IS research has attributed this theory with being helpful for describing and explaining effects of ICT usage. The healthcare domain is subject of both agency relationships and the adoption of various ICT. While IS research has applied agency theory to a lot of different domains already, often with very useful results, a broader view of the particular role of agency theory in e-health research does not exist yet. This chapter thus analyses (1) to which extent agency relationships have been considered in e-health research, and (2) to which extent e-health research explicitly makes use of the insights, and results of agency theory. For this purpose, we report the process and results of a two-step literature review. The first step covers IS journals in general and identifies research that employs an agency theory perspective. The second step studies a specific e-health application, telemedicine, and unfolds the consideration of agency relationships.

Keywords Hidden action • Hidden characteristics • Hidden information • IS adoption • New Institutional Economics • Transaction

20.1 Introduction

During the last years great importance has been placed on innovative information and communication technology (ICT) in the healthcare sector. In particular, optimizing patient processes and minimizing avoidable, costly diagnostics is still a

J. Leukel (✉) • J. Fernandes • A. Heidebrecht • S. Schillings
Information Systems 2, University of Hohenheim, Stuttgart, Germany
e-mail: joerg.leukel@uni-hohenheim.de

N. Wickramasinghe et al. (eds.), *Critical Issues for the Development*   313
of Sustainable E-health Solutions, Healthcare Delivery in the Information Age,
DOI 10.1007/978-1-4614-1536-7_20, © Springer Science+Business Media, LLC 2012

central topic. For instance, information systems can help hospital management to better assess and control physicians' service delivery. In this way, ICT can help reducing costs (Kohli and Kettinger 2004). Nowadays, the healthcare domain is considered as a value system consisting of various participants that contribute their specific resources and skills to delivering healthcare services to the final customer, the patient. In such a value system, diverse bilateral relationships exist between participants. A particular type of relationship is that between a principal and an agent, e.g., patient and physician, or hospital management and physician. Introducing ICT into such a value system affects necessarily its relationships, and thus these agency relationships.

Looking at the relationship between hospital and physicians, the problem of hidden actions leading to the risk of moral hazard can occur. The hospital management as the principal cannot directly estimate whether a physician, for instance, accesses and makes use of the latest relevant information when examining a patient or devising a treatment plan. The reason is that these decision making processes are subject of the physician; their inherent complexity hinders the documentation of all considerations taken and the supervision by a third party. . The cause of problems associated with agency relationships is information asymmetry. Since ICT adoption in healthcare very often aims at improving information delivery, exchange, and integration, some effects of this adoption on the value system can be described and explained by agency theory very well.

IS research has applied agency theory to a lot of different domains already, often with very useful results. The problem is, however, that a broader view of the role of agency theory in e-health research is still lacking. The objective of our research is thus to analyze (1) to which extent agency relationships have been considered in e-health research so far, and (2) to which extent e-health research explicitly makes use of the insights, and results of agency theory. For this purpose, we report the process and results of a two-step literature review. A barrier to reaching this objective is that most researchers describe, more or less, some characteristics of relationships between healthcare actors, but without giving explicit references to agency theory, its terminology, concepts, and insights. Therefore, we need to determine a matching of such descriptions to constructs of this theory. For this purpose, we conduct a two-step literature review: First, we search IS journals for work that takes a dedicated agency theory perspective to study domain phenomena. Second, we provide a more detailed analysis of a particular e-health application, which is telemedicine. This step unfolds the consideration of agency relationships in this domain.

The remainder is structured as follows: Sect. 20.2 introduces the theoretical background of agency relationships and healthcare. Section 20.3 describes the design of our research. Section 20.4 reports the main findings. The final section draws conclusions and points to further research.

20.2 Theoretical Background

20.2.1 Agency Theory

The epistemological object of the agency theory is the relationship between the principal and the agent. The theory deals with an efficient delegation of tasks between principal and agent. Referring to Ross (1973, p. 134) "an agency relationship has arisen between two (or more) parties when one, designated as the agent, acts for, on behalf of, or as representative for the other, designated the principal, in a particular domain of decision problems". Agency relationships exist in many occurrences such as buyer/supplier, employer/employee, and stock holder/top executives. The objective of the agency theory is to explain problems associated with agency relationship, and finally to determine the optimal institution for regulating this relationship, i.e., by a contract. Figure 20.1 visualizes the main constructs of the theory (Eisenhardt 1989; Arrow 1986; Jensen and Meckling 1976; Ross 1973; Picot et al. 2008).

The basic assumptions of the agency theory say that the involved parties behave under bounded rationality, pursue different objectives, have different risk preferences, and maximize their self-utility. In addition to these assumptions, an asymmetric information distribution between the principal and the agent can be stated. Different types of information asymmetries (hidden action, hidden information, hidden characteristics) cause different problems: moral hazard and adverse selection.

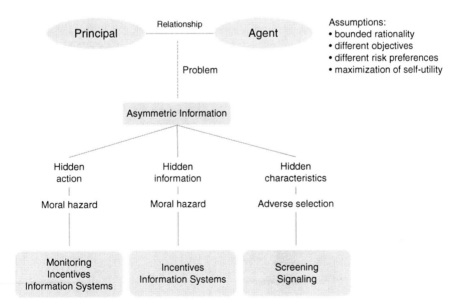

Fig. 20.1 The agency theory

Moral hazard occurs after a contract (agreement) has been closed between the principal and the agent; it is caused by hidden information and hidden action.

Hidden information means that the principal can watch the result of the agent's actions, but not the action itself: on the other hand, the agent has exclusive access to information unavailable for the principal. Using this information, the agent may execute the task with less effort than the principal expects and pays for. As in the case of unobservable performance this leads to the problem of moral hazard. Approaches to reduce this asymmetric information are the design of incentives or information systems as mentioned before.

Hidden action illustrates the situation *after* the agreement between principal and agent, where the principal cannot directly observe the performance of the agent so that the principal cannot assess the result of the agent's action objectively. For instance, the agent could explain her own bad results in performing a task by exogenous factors rather than admitting her failure (self-utility maximizing agent). In this case, the risk for the principal is her lack of information. The agent may choose a behaviour that is not conform to the principal's interests. This problem is called moral hazard. The intention of the principal is to reduce the risk of moral hazard. By monitoring the agent, the principal has the possibility to directly monitor the actions of the agent. It should be noted that monitoring may lead to costs that are out of all proportion to the effort. Another solution is to create incentives in a way that the agent's goal is in congruence with the principle's goal. Furthermore information systems can be used to close the lack of information of the principal about the external disturbance. It should be ensured that the additional information is verifiable.

Adverse selection occurs *before* an agreement is closed; it is caused by characteristics hidden to the principal. That is, the principal can observe the performance of the agent but she cannot assess the reliability of the agent's offer. Usually the agent is better informed about her personal characteristics than the principal. This situation leads to the problem of adverse selection: if the principal offers for example a contract tailored to the average type of agent, she must fear that an agent with bad characteristics will hide them and will copy an agent with good characteristics. So the principal chooses the agent with bad characteristics. The agent with good characteristics does not accept the conditions of the contract because they are not adequate to her preferences. To make the lack of information of the principal smaller she can screen the agent regarding relevant personal attributes to make a statement about the agent's characteristics. This is called screening. A different possibility for the agent would be to highlight her characteristics ex ante to make them transparent for the principal; this is called signaling. Though a signal will only be sent, if it is worth for the agent to discover her characteristics. A signal is reliable for the principal, if it causes costs for the agent.

20.2.2 Agency Theory and e-Health

The patient-physician relationship is often regarded as a typical example for a principal–agent relationship "in many respects, the physician-patient relation exemplifies the principal-agent relation almost perfectly. The principal (the patient) is certainly unable to monitor the efforts of the agent (the physician)." (Arrow 1986, p. 1193). In this context, the use of ICT to reducing information asymmetries seems to be appropriate and of particular interest for the IS discipline.

Hidden characteristics as an information asymmetry prior to the agreement can occur, for instance, during the selection of an appropriate physician or hospital. Patients often cannot evaluate the actual skills of the healthcare providers. In such a case, a web-based infomediary may help with the search and provide additional relevant information on the provider's service quality, reliability, reputation etc. Providers can improve their reputation by participating in a quality audit of a certification authority. The certification will support the faith of customer in providers' characteristics.

20.3 Research Design

20.3.1 Framework and Selection

For describing the relevant IS literature in a systematic way, we defined the framework shown in Fig. 20.2. It consists of two components that represents constructs of the underlying theory (agency relationship, problem) and two other parts that serve for selecting literature and classifying it with regard to a canon of IS research methods.

The literature survey took place in two subsequent steps:

1. Survey of IS research that adopts an agency theory perspective on the healthcare domain. The research question is to which extent does IS research actually use this theory as an analytical lens to describe and explain domain phenomena?
2. Survey of telemedicine research that studies relationships between actors of the healthcare value system. The research question is to which extent does telemedicine research consider the existence and nature of agency relationships?

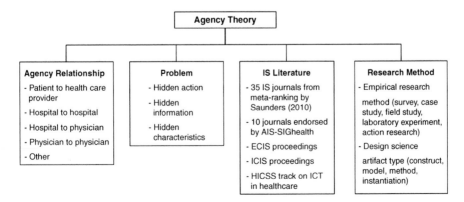

Fig. 20.2 Framework of the literature review

The rationale of these steps is twofold: First, the search for journal papers addressing ICT-related themes in the healthcare domain that explicitly reference agency theory in their title, abstract or list of keywords yielded a surprisingly low number of articles. This could be attributed to the fact that all major IS outlets cover a broad range of domains, hence coverage of the healthcare domain is relatively small. Another conjecture may be that IS research in this domain is still mainly concerned with issues in which relationships between actors are less important. However, this would contradict the shift towards value systems, increased competition between healthcare providers as well as fragmentation, specialization, and cooperation – and seems thus not to be a valid explanation. Another, potentially much more relevant, supposition is that the proven descriptive, analytical, and prognostic strength of the agency theory has not been employed sufficiently in the healthcare / healthcare ICT domain so far.

The second step focuses thus on telemedicine as an application that necessarily includes two or more actors, and which can thus be seen as a suitable example application of ICT in healthcare.

20.3.2   Survey of IS Research in Healthcare

The first step was to identify relevant outlets. The choice of journals was based on the meta-analysis by Saunders (2010) that evaluated nine IS journal rankings. From this initial list of 110 journals we removed those that were covered by one ranking only (37). Then we removed all ACM and IEEE transactions (6), since they originate from computer science not IS. From the remaining list of 67 journals we took the top-10, and added 15 more journals from the top-40 (randomized selection). The final list thus contains 25 IS journals. Next, we enriched the list by a set of domain-specific journals. These were taken from journals that are endorsed by AIS's special interest group on health information management research (AIS-SIGhealth). We selected 10 out of 44 journals randomly. Finally, we ended up with 35 outlets. Table 20.1 lists these journals.

A literature review should initially define the 'key variables and set the boundaries on your work' (Webster and Watson 2002, p. XV), we defined terms that represent constructs of the agency theory and terms that reflect the domain of discourse. We used these terms for retrieving the respective publication databases. The search query was thus as follows: ("agent" OR "agency theory" OR "principal-agent theory" OR "new institutionalism" OR "new institutional" OR "asymmetric information" OR "hidden information" OR "hidden characteristics" OR "incentive" OR "adverse selection" OR "moral hazard" OR "hold up" OR "signalling") AND ("health" OR "hospital" OR "telemedicine" OR "clinic" OR "clinical" OR "medic" OR "medical" OR "medicine").

The search query covered title, abstract, and keywords. We limited the survey to the period of 1999–2009. All identified papers were then reviewed individually by the authors to exclude papers that are a result of the search, but do not respond to

Table 20.1 Journals covered by the survey of IS research [no. in square brackets indicates rank as of Saunders (2010)]

Top-10	Selection from top-40	Selection of e-health journals
1. MISQ [1]	11. SMR [19]	26. Artificial Intelligence in Medicine
2. ISR [2]	12. CAIS [20]	27. BMC Medical Informatics and Decision Making
3. CACM [3]	13. ACS [22]	28. Computers in Biology and Medicine
4. MS [4]	14. JAIS [26]	29. International Journal of Medical Informatics
5. JMIS [5]	15. JMS [29]	30. Journal of Clinical Monitoring and Computing
6. DSI [7]	16. OS [30]	31. Journal of Medical Internet Research
7. HBR [8]	17. ISJ [32]	32. Journal of Medical Systems
8. EJIS [11]	18. ASQ [33]	33. Journal of the American Medical Informatics
9. DSS [12]	19. IS [37]	Association
10. I&M [14]	20. AMR [39]	34. Medical Decision Making
	21. JACM [40]	35. Online Journal of Nursing Informatics
	22. HCI [42]	
	23. JSIS [45]	
	24. JCIS [51]	
	25. WIRT [61]	

Table 20.2 Classification of relevant IS articles

	Liang et al. (2005)	Kohli and Kettinger (2004)	Zahedi and Song (2008)
Agency relationship	Patient – pharmacy	Hospital – physician	Web customer – infomediary
Agency problem	Hidden information	Hidden action	Hidden information
Application	Online prescriptions	Physician's profiling	Health infomediaries
Research method	Survey	Action research	Laboratory experiment

the research question. Surprisingly, the entire search returned only three relevant articles (one each from MISQ, JMIS, and CAIS). Obviously, this results list does also not include those papers that involved elements from agency theory but did not refer to them in their title, abstract, or keyword list.

Each article was coded as follows: agency relationship, addresses problem (i.e., hidden action, hidden information, hidden characteristics), application, and research method (see Table 20.2).

20.3.3 Survey of Telemedicine Research

20.3.3.1 Methodology

The survey of telemedicine research was conducted similarly to the first survey, with narrowing the scope to a particular application. At the same time, we extended the research question to consideration of agency problems, instead of dedicated research that applies the agency theory. We focused on one particular outlet that can be regarded as a representative source for e-health research. The HICSS conference series maintains a track on ICT in the healthcare sector since 1999. We selected the proceedings from 1999 to 2010. A preliminary search yielded a significant number of articles on telemedicine from this interval.

Telemedicine is defined as "the use of electronic information and communication technologies to provide and support health care when distance separates the participants" (Field 1996). It is important to stress "distance" in this definition, so that intra-organizational applications do not belong to telemedicine. For this reason, two articles that use the term telemedicine had to be removed from the initial list of 45 papers. One article was added, because it was listed in the collaboration systems and technologies track of 2010.

We applied the same theoretical framework and coded all articles respectively. Since we are interested in whether researchers acknowledge the existence and relevance of agency relationships, it was necessary to read each article carefully. The classification was done by a group of seven researchers. Each article was classified by two persons independently, followed by a review and discussion lead by a third person. We paid in particular attention to assumptions, model elements, organizational settings of reported cases, and conclusions.

20.3.3.2 Results

The main group of results relates directly to agency problems. First, the principal agent relationship is of interest. The set of actors includes patient (individual person in need of care and acting on its own), health care provider (HCP, umbrella for different types of providers such as hospital, healthcare centre, clinic, healthcare professional), hospital (larger organizational entity), and physician (professional acting independently from a hospital). Following these definitions, we subsume all physicians employed by a hospital under hospital. Second, we studied which agency problem was considered by the article's authors. The results are shown in Table 20.3.

None of the articles qualified the relationship between telemedicine actors as that of principle-agent relationship. This finding also means that no article used the agency theory to study telemedicine. We thus mapped elements found in descriptions, characterizations, and reported problems of telemedicine relationships to constructs of the theory.

Principal–agent relationship: The most frequently covered relationship is clearly that of hospital to hospital (35 articles, thus 79.5%), followed by patient to HCP (36.4%) (Fig. 20.3). The former could be explained by the fact that telemedicine is about accessing specific, sparse professional expertise from remote locations. Such expertise is most often found at larger healthcare providers, e.g., University hospitals. The patient's role of principal has emerged first in 2001 and since then received an increasing backup by research, with reaching a coverage of 61.5% for the period of 2005–2010, compared to 69.2% for hospital to hospital.

Table 20.3 Classification of relevant telemedicine research

Article #	Authors	Year	Principal–agent relationship					Consideration of agency problem		
			Patient to HCP	Hospital to hospital	Hospital to physician	Physician to hospital	Physician to physician	Hidden action	Hidden information	Hidden chara-cteristics
1.	Bangert et al. (Introducing…)	1999		x				No	No	No
2.	Bangert et al. (Evaluating…)	1999		x				No	No	No
3.	Dardelet	1999		x				No	No	No
4.	Floro et al.	1999		x				No	No	No
5.	Garshnek and Burkle Jr.	1999		x				No	No	No
6.	Hu et al.	1999		x				No	No	No
7.	Nguyen et al.	1999		x	x			No	No	No
8.	Paul	1999		x	x			Yes	No	Yes
9.	Rasberry and Garshnek	1999		x				No	No	No
10.	Tanriverdi and Venkatraman	1999		x	x			No	No	No
11.	Hu et al.	2000		x				No	No	No
12.	Sankaran and Bui	2000		x				No	No	No
13.	Tiwana and Ramesh	2000		x				No	No	No
14.	Hu et al.	2001		x				Yes	No	No
15.	Klecun-Dabrowska and Cornford	2001		x				No	No	No

(continued)

Table 20.3 (continued)

Article #	Authors	Year	Principal–agent relationship					Consideration of agency problem		
			Patient to HCP	Hospital to hospital	Hospital to physician	Physician to hospital	Physician to physician	Hidden action	Hidden information	Hidden characteristics
16.	Scheideman-Miller et al.	2001		x				No	No	No
17.	Tyler	2001	x					No	No	Yes
18.	Croteau et al.	2002		x				No	No	No
19.	Hu et al.	2002		x				No	No	No
20.	LeRouge et al.	2002	x	x				No	No	Yes
21.	Linderoth	2002		x				Yes	No	No
22.	Scheidemann-Miller et al.	2002	x					No	No	No
23.	Brown et al.	2003	x	x				No	No	No
24.	Deng and Poole	2003		x		x		No	No	No
25.	Hu	2003	x	x				No	No	No
26.	Mbarika and Okoli	2003		x				No	No	No
27.	Scheidemann-Miller et al.	2003	x					No	No	No
28.	Gagnon et al.	2004		x				Yes	No	No
29.	LeRouge et al.	2004	x					No	No	No
30.	Poole et al.	2004				x		No	No	No
31.	Ramani	2004	x	x				Yes	No	No
32.	Fontelo et al.	2005		x				No	no	No
33.	Fruhling et al.	2005		x				No	No	No
34.	LeRouge and Hevner	2005	x					No	No	Yes

#	Author	Year								
36.	Tulu and Chatterjee	2005	x	x	x	x	x	No	No	No
37.	Dhillon and Forducey	2006	x					No	No	No
38.	Cho et al.	2008		x				No	No	No
39.	Kifle et al.	2008		x				No	No	No
40.	Nwabueze et al.	2009	x	x				No	No	No
41.	Pare et al.	2009	x					No	No	No
42.	Topacan et al.	2009	x					No	No	No
43.	Kijl and Nieuwenhuis	2010	X	X				No	No	No
44.	Paul	2010	x	x				No	No	No
		Sum:	16	35	4	3	1	6	0	4

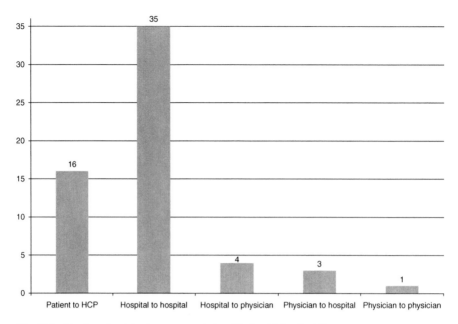

Fig. 20.3 Number of articles by agency relationship (multiple, N = 44)

All other relationships have a relative low coverage over the entire period for study (between 2.3% and 9.1%).

Agency problems: The researchers of nine articles considered agency problems in telemedicine (20.5%). Concretely, hidden actions were found in 6 articles and hidden characteristics in 4 articles. Thus only 1 article contains indications of both problems. Since the number of articles is not sufficient for further statistical analysis, we report about the nature and appearance of these agency problems by referring to selected articles.

Table 20.4 lists 4 quotes from articles that consider *hidden actions*. In Paul (1999) and Linderoth (2002), physicians that act as principals describe experiences made during teleconsultations. In Paul (2005), a physician that acts as an agent reflects his own behaviour. These empirical observations provide important insights into effects that telemedicine may have on the hidden action problem; these concern not only better monitoring the agent (Paul 1999), but also potential dangers to the principal because of new forms of hidden action, e.g., pretending expertise (Paul 2005), and loose of control due to distance (Hu et al. 2001; Linderoth 2002). We characterize these effects in the right most column of Table 20.4.

In Table 20.5, we list quotes from all four articles that consider *hidden characteristics*. In Paul (1999), the principal-agent roles are inverted as follows: physician A (principal) consults another physician B (agent). In the course of the consultation, B asks A to observe and report a particular physical or medical state of the patient. Thus B becomes the principal and A the agent. Here, telemedicine is in danger of hiding a relevant characteristic of A (qualification, expertise).

Table 20.4 Consideration of hidden actions

Article reference	Quote	Effect on the hidden action problem
Paul (1999)	(principal/physician says) "I like [teleconsultations] because I can see the other individual and if they're acting smart alec or in a way that doesn't enhance trust, it doesn't enhance the ability, doesn't really help me a whole lot, I can cut it short."	Telemedicine enables the principle to monitor the agent's action by means of real-time video transmission (here: revealing the action of smart alec).
Hu et al. (2001)	"In spite of the implicit concerns from several neurosurgeons, the department did not implement any monitoring or evaluation systems for its teleconsultation services."	Telemedicine enables hidden actions if no monitoring means are implemented.
Linderoth (2002)	(principal/physician says) "we don't know if we can trust the answers, while the system is not scientifically validated"	
Paul (2005)	(agent/physician says) "And it's one of those things that you don't want to admit you really don't know much about it. So you kind of read up on it a little bit and it's not something that you can just read up on it a little bit."	Telemedicine enables hidden action of pretending medical expertise due to the agent's professional pride.

Table 20.5 Consideration of hidden characteristics

Article reference	Quote	Effect on the hidden characteristics problem
Paul (1999)	(principal/physician says) "You really do have to rely on the expertise of the person on the other end. [..] So if you can't actually touch the patient yourself, you have to rely on the person at the other end. And if that person is a pediatrician, chances are they are going to do an okay job. If they are nurses, they may well do a great job, but you just don't know."	Telemedicine hides characteristics of the remote professional qualification for executing the transaction successfully.
Tyler (2001)	"From the patient's point-of-view, a remotely located radiologist may seem to have less professional liability than the local physician."	Telemedicine reduces the patient's ability to assess the physician's personal characteristics due to distance, nonpersonal atmosphere, and anonymity.
LeRouge et al. (2002)	(expert about the agent's environment) "There should be a desk, or a bookcase with some books in it, or perhaps some diplomas on the wall behind the physician. So that it has the feeling of a physician's office."	Telemedicine does not release the agent from sending trustable signals about his professionalism.
LeRouge and Hevner (2005)	"[..] the patient may not be able to readily determine whether the consulting provider has access to relevant records."	Telemedicine reduces the patient's ability to assess the physician's technical infrastructure due to not perceiving the existing organizational boundaries.

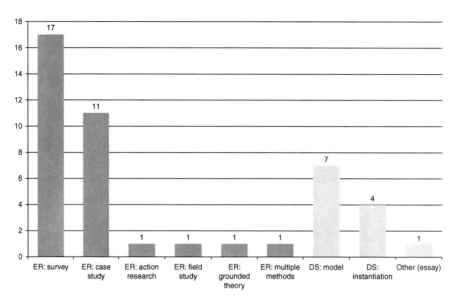

Fig. 20.4 Number of articles by research method (single, N = 44) (ER: empirical research, DS: design science)

The remaining articles describe three distinctive problems that occur in patient to HCP relationships. These all relate to the way patients perceive and assess the remote physician. Tyler (2001) is concerned with professional liability (LeRouge et al. 2002) with signs of professionalism, and (LeRouge and Hevner 2005) with the physician's technical infrastructure. The findings from these articles suggest that telemedicine may increase hidden characteristics when compared to delivering on-site healthcare services.

Research method: This dimension distinguishes articles that develop artifacts (design science) and articles that capture the essence of research by relying on observation (empirical research). In case of design science, the artifact type is of further interest (construct, model, method, instantiation). Empirical research is subdivided into specific empirical methods such as case study, survey, and action research. The results are shown in Fig. 20.4. Empirical research accounts for 72.7% and design science for 25.0% of all articles (one article turned out to be an essay and thus does not belong to any category of the classification). The most used empirical research methods are survey (53.1%) and case study (34.4%). In design science, models represent 63.6% of all artifacts (instantiations: 36.7%). The relative high number of both case studies and instantiations are indications that telemedicine in IS research was and is still concerned quite often with single applications and experiences, rather than models, frameworks, and theories of broader validity.

When looking at those articles that consider one or more agency problems, the picture gets clearer (Table 20.6): 8 out of 9 articles belong to empirical research,

Table 20.6 Consideration of agency problems by research method

Article No.	Article reference	Year	Consideration of agency problem				If design science: artifact type	If empirical research: method
			Hidden action	Hidden information	Hidden characteristics			
8	Paul (1999)	1999	Yes	No	Yes		–	Grounded theory
14	Hu et al. (2001)	2001	Yes	No	No		–	Case study
16	Tyler (2001)	2001	No	No	Yes		Model	–
20	LeRouge et al. (2002)	2002	No	No	Yes		–	Multiple
21	Linderoth (2002)	2002	Yes	No	No		–	Case study
27	Gagnon et al. (2004)	2004	Yes	No	No		–	Survey
30	Ramani (2004)	2004	Yes	No	No		–	Case study
33	LeRouge and Hevner (2005)	2005	No	No	Yes		–	Multiple
34	Paul (2005)	2005	Yes	No	No		–	Survey

which ranges from case studies to surveys and multiple methods employed. In other words, 8 out of 32 empirical works consider the existence of agency problems (25.0%), whereas this is true for only 1 out of 11 design science papers (9.1%).

20.4   Conclusions

This chapter analyzed to which extent agency relationships have been considered in e-health research and to which extent e-health research explicitly makes use of the insights, and results of agency theory. The literature survey yields a number of important findings.

First, the survey of 25 IS journals and 10 domain-specific journals over the period of 1999–2009 yielded only three articles that employ agency theory as an analytical lens. This number is surprisingly low, in particular compared to other areas such as manufacturing or IT outsourcing; past research in these areas has used this theory successfully for explaining, e.g., make-or-buy decisions and effects of IT adoption. Our finding indicates that e-healthcare research, while exhaustive in coverage and quantity, still lacks theoretically grounded constructs and models for describing, analyzing, explaining, predicting, and designing an empirically highly relevant phenomena – the relationship between healthcare service provider and service consumer (ultimately, the patient).

Second, the survey of telemedicine research, covering the respective HICSS track over the period of 1999–2010, found nine articles that describe agency-induced problems; this number represents 20.5% of all articles. Telemedicine was chosen since it can be regarded as a prime example of principal–agent relationship in the healthcare domain by placing a healthcare service provider as the agent who delivers his expertise to another remote service provider (here: 79.5% of all relationships) or to the patient (here: 36.4%) via an electronic network. Again, agency theory is not used explicitly by any researcher for unfolding agency problems. 8 out of 9 identified problems are reported by empirical research, in particular surveys and case studies. We observed that 25.0% of all empirical research reported such problems, whereas design science researchers consider these problems to a less extent (9.1%). This difference is significant and suggests that empirical researchers are able to identify those problems better. At the same time, design science researchers neglect these problems by, e.g., focusing on technical aspects of telemedicine, while abstracting from social and economic determinants of the telemedicine environment. With regard to agency problems, hidden actions (9.1%) and hidden characteristics (13.7%) were considered, whereas hidden actions were not reported.

Our findings have implications for IS research. A major stream of research studies *adoption* of telemedicine systems. Researchers still report a lack of approaches that are explanatory and can be used for assessing and predicting the success or failure of telemedicine projects. Our findings suggest that an important factor of the organizational setting has not been considered in studying adoption, which is the existence and nature of agency relationships.

Another important implication is that on how IS research perceives relationships between healthcare actors. Our survey of telemedicine yielded a set of qualifications of these relationships, of which most can be aggregated to "collaborative". For instance, Deng and Poole make it explicit by stating "we conceptualize telemedicine as an integrated IT-enabled health care network of collaborative relationships" (Deng and Poole 2003). Paul extends it to the entire domain, i.e., "health care delivery is fundamentally a collaborative process" (Paul 2005). This qualification emphasizes that actors share the goal of delivering the right care to the patient in need. However, it is in danger of neglecting or underestimating the fact that actors are also governed by their organizational objectives and settings, which are potentially conflicting to those of other actors.

We found only one explicit indication of agency in telemedicine, i.e., "the contractual relationship between doctor and patient" in Tyler (2001). An explanation could be that many IS researcher studied telemedicine projects funded by government or research agencies, whereas these settings differ from other healthcare service delivery, because they minimize "liability issues" and personal risks of physicians (Paul 1999), let it be the principal or agent. By acknowledging the existence and relevance of agency relationships and its associated problems, IS research in e-healthcare could both benefit from a valid theory (agency theory) and enrich its coverage of relevant empirical phenomena.

Acknowledgement   We wish to thank Stefan Kirn and Marcus Mueller for their helpful comments on an earlier version of this chapter. We thank Ansger Jacob, Marcus Mueller, Andreas Scheuermann and Daniel Weiss for contributing to the classification and coding of telemedicine articles.

References

Arrow, K. J. (1986). Agency and the market. In *Handbook of mathematical economics* (Vol. 3, pp. 1183–1195). Amsterdam: Elsevier.

Deng L., & Poole, M. S. (2003). Learning through telemedicine networks. In *HICSS '03 Proceedings of the 36th annual Hawaii international conference on system sciences (HICSS'03)* (Vol. 6 p. 174).

Eisenhardt, K. M. (1989). Agency theory: An assessment and review. *Academy of Management Review, 14*(1), 57–74.

Field, M. J. (Ed.). (1996). *Telemedicine: A guide to assessing telecommunication in health care.* Washington DC: National Academy Press.

Gagnon, M.-P., Lamothe, L., Fortin, J.-P., Cloutier, A., Godin, G., Gagné, C., & Reinharz, D. (2004). The impact of organizational characteristics on telehealth adoption by hospitals. In Proceedings of the 37th annual Hawaii international conference on system sciences (Vol. 6, p. 60142b).

Hu, P., Chau, P. Y. K., Chan, Y. K., & Kwok, J. (2001). Investigating technology implementation in a neurosurgical teleconsultation program: A case study in Hong Kong. In *Annual Hawaii international conference on system sciences (HICSS-34)*.

Jensen, M. C., & Meckling, W. H. (1976). Theory of the firm: Managerial behavior, agency costs and ownership structure. *Journal of Financial Economics, 3*, 305–360.

Kohli, R., & Kettinger, W. J. (2004). Informating the clan: Controlling physicians' costs and outcomes. *Management Information Systems Quarterly, 28*(3), 363–394.

LeRouge, C., & Hevner, A. R. (2005). It's more than just use: An investigation of telemedicine use quality. In *Proceedings of the 38th annual Hawaii international conference on systems sciences* (Vol. 6, p. 150b).

LeRouge, C., Garfield, M. J., & Hevner, A. R. (2002). Quality attributes in telemedicine video conferencing. In *Proceedings of the 35th annual Hawaii international conference on systems sciences* (Vol. 6, p. 159).

Liang, H., Laosethakul, K., Lloyd, S. J., & Xue, Y. (2005). Information systems and health care-I: Trust, uncertainty, and online prescription filling. *Communications of the AIS, 15*(1), 41–60.

Linderoth, H. C. J. (2002). Implementation and evaluation of telemedicine – A catch 22?. In *Proceedings of the 35th annual Hawaii international conference on systems sciences* (Vol. 6, p. 160).

Paul, D. L. (1999). Wicked decision problems in remote health care: Telemedicine as a tool for sensemaking. In *Proceedings of the 32nd annual Hawaii international conference on systems sciences*.

Paul, D. L. (2005). Collaborative activities in virtual settings: Case studies of telemedicine. In *Proceedings of the 38th annual Hawaii international conference on systems sciences*. (Vol. 6, p. 147a).

Picot, A., Reichwald, R., & Wigand, R. (2008). *Information, organization and management*. Heidelberg: Springer.

Ramani, K.V. (2004). IT enabled applications in government hospitals in India: Illustrations of telemedicine, e-governance, and BPR. In Proceedings of the 37th annual Hawaii international conference on system sciences (Vol. 6, p. 60156b).

Ross, S. A. (1973). The economic theory of agency: The principal's problem. *The American Economic Review, 63*(2), 134–139.

Saunders, C. (2010). MIS journal rankings, http://ais.affiniscape.com/displaycommon.cfm?an=1&subarticlenbr=432. Cited 19 Oct 2010.

Tyler, J. L. (2001). The healthcare information technology context: A framework for viewing legal aspects of telemedicine and teleradiology. In *Proceedings of the 34th annual Hawaii international conference on systems sciences*.

Webster, J., & Watson, R. T. (2002). Analyzing the past to prepare for the future: Writing a literature review. *Management Information Systems Quarterly, 26*(2), XIII–XXII.

Zahedi, F. M., & Song, J. (2008). Dynamics of trust revision: Using health infomediaries. *Journal of Management Information Systems, 24*(4), 225–248.

Chapter 21
Cost Accounting and Decision Support for Healthcare Institutions

L. Waehlert, A. Wagner, and H. Czap

Abstract In the healthcare sector a growing dynamic in terms of social and economic challenges can be observed. Against this background, healthcare institutions are required to develop business tools and models for analysis, calculation and planning of activities and their costs in relation to the revenue. This requires a meaningful cost and performance accounting system that supports operational and strategic decisions. Amazingly, there are no appropriate decision support systems that provide automated metrics and the relevant data.

The intention of this paper is to present the background information, the technical and conceptual design as well as the implementation requirements of a prototype software solution for managing and controlling the relevant costs and performance of business operations in healthcare institutions. The developed cost and activity accounting model and the corresponding software solution complies with the specific requirements and supports the planning of activities or staff capacities, as well as strategic decisions like co-operations or make or buy. Finally, this model significantly contributes to meeting today's challenges.

Keywords Decision support system for healthcare institutions • Management of healthcare institutions • Clnical pathways • Past cost accounting

L. Waehlert (✉) • A. Wagner • H. Czap
Department of Business Information Systems, University of Trier, Trier, Germany
e-mail: lilia.waehlert@uni.trier.de; andreea.wagner@uni-trier.de; hans.czap@uni-trier.de

N. Wickramasinghe et al. (eds.), *Critical Issues for the Development* 331
of Sustainable E-health Solutions, Healthcare Delivery in the Information Age,
DOI 10.1007/978-1-4614-1536-7_21, © Springer Science+Business Media, LLC 2012

21.1 Background Information: Necessity and Objectives of Cost and Activity Accounting for Healthcare Institutions

In the health sector a growing dynamic in terms of performance and cost structures can be observed. Demographic developments, scarce financial resources, the introduction of federal or national DRG and changes of billing practices,[1] increase the cost and quality pressure on healthcare providers (von Schulenburg 2007, Noweski 2008, Krier et al. 2006, Straub 1997). In addition, the national healthcare expenditures have increased continuously (Statistisches Bundesamt 2008). This trend is reinforced by structural changes, as indicated by an increase in the importance of partnerships between service providers, like cross-sectoral partnerships, mergers and acquisitions or medical centers.

Partnerships in healthcare pursue the idea to optimize patient pathways in terms of quality and costs and lay a focus on integrated care structures. In this context, the concept of clinical pathways is currently discussed in science and practice. Clinical pathways represent a standardized treatment scheme, which includes all relevant activities (Eckardt 2006, Czap 2010). The classical organization structure of hospitals is the departmental structure resulting out of the medical disciplines and the dominance of medical issues over economic ones. In connection with high specialization of these departments and highly specialized computing and information systems the information flow between departments in general is very poor. This situation is increased regarding the inter-sectoral information flow. Typically, the treatment of any disease will combine different departments or different medical sectors. Therefore, patients moving from one department to the next or from one sector to the other will encounter avoidable waiting times and doubled examinations or treatments due to the insufficient information flow. Optimizing patient pathways carries an enormous economic potential and will substantially contribute to greater efficiency and medical quality. Last but not least, for any service provider, joining a network of providers and concentrating on selected activities within this network results in scale effects allowing increased profit margins (Güssow 2007, Roeder et al. 2003). Therefore, the objective of integrated care structures lies in the coordination of activities and processes offered by different service providers and the necessity for specific medical treatments of patients. The ultimate goal of clinical pathways is to increase efficiency and quality.

Optimization of the treatment process implies the selection of those service providers, which are most suited to perform a needed activity at its best. This shortens the treatment process and therefore the patient faster can be re-integrated into working life. From the viewpoint of health insurances, integrated care structures lead to economic benefits by decreasing social security costs. For the patients, double

---

[1] The German DRG-system is described in Thiexe-Kreye and von Collas (2005). In Germany, a change to rehabilitation and ambulant flat-rates is under discussion or has been introduced (Güssow 2007, Without author 2008).

examinations can be avoided by better communication and high quality treatments can be assured by a higher specialization level. Cooperation can thus help reducing the dynamics of cost increase in healthcare and limiting the need of additional financial resources.

Any decision about co-operations, personnel resources or services offered to patients has to be based on a most realistic and accurate knowledge of the underlying costs of activities. In most Western countries general hospitals have to offer an all-round service. Since in many countries medical treatments are paid by diagnosis related flat rates per case, based on diagnosis related groups DRGs, the unit of payment is not the specific treatment activity. Rather it's the set of all activities and treatments necessary for the patient's recovery. This is a strong economic reason to concentrate on the costs of clinical pathways. Also, due to scale effects the received payments for particular DRGs, respectively for all cases of a specific kind of disease, do not always cover the overall costs of these DRGs. Therefore, to allow positioning of the healthcare provider in the long run, management at least needs to know, which departments respectively treatments generate profits respectively losses.

Since medical services and treatments are not directly comparable to industry services, the standard calculation methods developed for industrial purposes are not applicable to the healthcare sector. One needs a cost and activity accounting model tailored to the specific needs of medical services and based on clinical pathways. Only this will offer the necessary support for a rational decision about medical services and the classical question of make or buy.

Despite the long and enduring discussion of cost accounting and clinical pathways in practice and sciences, there is at time no system available, which uses the concept of clinical pathways from an economic point of view, and therefore supports operational and strategic decisions. This is where the concept of the developed system, called *d*ecision *s*upport *s*ystem for *h*ealthcare *i*nstitutions DSSHI, starts. DSSHI is based on a model of path costs measuring costs of activities or clinical pathways at different levels of aggregation and supporting the cost calculation of clinical pathways.

Against this background the paper first describes the calculation of the contribution margin of DRGs. Second, the use of the developed instrument for decision support will be demonstrated.

21.2   The Concept "Expected Costs of Clinical Pathways"

There is a strong worldwide tendency to pay case based flat rates for clinical services, like DRG flat rates.[2] Figure 21.1 illustrates the consequences connected to this paying scheme.

---

[2] In Germany, for example, this flat rate is determined by InEK for each year. The base are the cost accounting data from hospitals that voluntarily participate in the calculation.

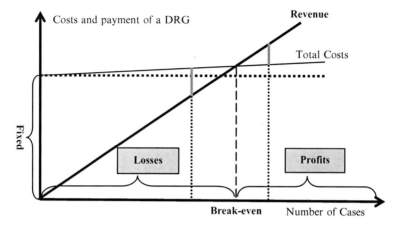

Fig. 21.1 Contribution margin as a function of costs, payment and number of cases (Czap 2010)

First, the total revenue generated by a specific DRG is proportional to the number of cases of this DRG, see the bold line "revenue" of Fig. 21.1. On the opposite side, due to the overwhelming personal costs, in any hospital there is a large block of fixed costs and comparably low variable costs, which is demonstrated in Fig. 21.1 by the line "Total costs". At the number of cases, where both lines intersect, the break-even point is given. If the number of cases for a specific DRG treated by a hospital is below break-even, losses with respect to this specific DRG are generated and, vice versa, if the number of cases is above the break-even point profits will result. Clearly, in the short run, general hospitals have to cross-subsidize DRGs generating losses by other DRGs (Czap 2010) since they are obliged to offer all basic services. But in the long run, management could think of co-operations with other service providers or look for more cost-effective ways of providing these services.

Second, if payment is based on a full treatment case, the details of how cost-efficient the service is provided become essential. Therefore, the concept of Clinical Pathways becomes very relevant. The term "clinical pathway", generally, is understood very differently. Literature uses the terms (clinical) care pathways, clinical pathways, standardized treatment protocols, integrated care pathways, treatment guidelines, etc. (Roeder et al. 2003, Salfeld et al. 2008).[3] Here, the focus is on the idea of a standardized flow for treatments based on a specific diagnosis, enabling the control of activities under optimization criteria. It is essential, that clinical pathways represent no binding flow of treatments. Activities and flow may vary from patient to patient. Standardization thus does not affect medical aspects, but describes an idealized sequence of treatments, which reflects the recommended procedure and activities with respect to a specific diagnosis.

---

[3] In the following we use the term clinical pathways.

Since a clinical pathway in this paper is an abstract scheme, it does not make sense to look only on pathway costs. Rather, one has to consider the concrete cases of real patients. For them one can calculate the actual costs of treatments and in addition one may ask how likely this specific treatment and correspondingly these actual costs will happen during the planning period. The combination of these individual treatments makes up the (abstract) clinical pathway. For planning purposes it's necessary to have a figure expressing the planned costs of a clinical pathway, which, in a straight forward manner, turns out to be the expected costs of the possible treatment variations.

The term "costs of a DRG" needs some differentiation: Talking about an actual case, which always relates to exactly one DRG, one may sum up all the activity-costs of this concrete case yielding the actual costs of this case. Considering any time period, one may sum up all the costs of the specific cases related to the DRG in question in order to end up with the (actual) period costs. But asking for the costs of any DRG for planning purposes, one has to take the concept of the expected DRG costs, i.e. the expected value of the costs of all related pathways.

In summary, if the abstract treatment scheme is addressed, one has to talk about planned costs. It draws on historical or estimated data. If concrete treatment cases are addressed, one has to talk about the actual costs of a clinical pathway. They result from the assignment of actually provided services and their costs incurred.

The following section describes the concept of expected costs in detail.

21.3 Conceptual Details

21.3.1 Clinical Pathways and Their Calculation

Medical services are influenced by a variety of factors. For example the health status varies from patient to patient and consequently the questions, whether complications arise during treatment or not, which precautions have to be taken etc., influence treatments, costs, and outcome. The comparison of cases in the medical service delivery process is therefore not possible (Czap 2010, Zapp 2005). These facts have implications for the definition of possible *cost objects* and the development of a cost accounting model.

Cost objects are variously defined in the literature and practice. Usually the patient respectively the "case" is taken as cost object (Güssow 2007, Zapp 2005). However, as shown above, uniqueness of cases and their treatments do not allow comparisons. This violates the essential property of any cost-object, which requires comparability of cost figures relating to the same issue (Czap 2010).

In order to observe this *law of comparability*, cost objects must be reasonably uniform and standardized. Therefore a new accounting model was developed, the path cost accounting model (Czech and Güssow 2006, Hellmann and Rieben 2003). It uses patient pathways as cost objects (Hellmann and Rieben 2003, Güssow 2007). The path cost accounting model relies on the assumption that pathways are similar and thus can act as cost objects.[4] Accordingly, patient pathways are considered to be the optimal form of treatment having the character of a standard (Hellmann and Rieben 2003). This makes it possible to match treatment procedures with this standard and thus to ensure optimal care. Costs are calculated as average in order to account for the variations related to each pathway.

The "MIPP" model for example offers a way to address cost fluctuations and handle cost accounting (Hellmann and Rieben 2003). The developed clinical pathways within the "MIPP" model involve standardized activity categories to which different types of activities are assigned. Accordingly, the MIPP model distinguishes particular characteristics of different performances.[5]

This method is only suitable for the accounting of standard costs, as the determination of costs depends on planned treatment durations. But it cannot reflect the actual cost of a treatment. Moreover, it is not possible to take into account the differences of costs related to individual services, which occur for example with respect to different salaries, or in the case of different costs per minute resulting from differences in productive time. As a consequence, we don´t accept the underlying assumption of the past cost accounting model that individual pathways related to the same DRG have a standard character and therefore are comparable. Insofar, the cost model presented in this paper follows a different approach. The cost model of DSSHI relies on the following principal considerations:

First, looking at the diversity of cases (e.g. the individuality of each patient pathway respectively individuality of each case) and observing the principle of cause-based cost distribution, it seems appropriate to calculate the cost rates on an individual base respectively for groups of persons having similar characteristics in order to take into account cost differences like different salaries.

Second, since personnel costs make up the major cost item in healthcare, the accurate measurement respectively estimation of durations of treatments is of great importance.

Third, the identification and analysis of superfluous resources respectively of bottlenecks is a key starting point for the optimization of clinical pathways.

Taking these considerations into account, DSSHI focuses on the classical process-cost accounting procedure but combines it with the idea of clinical pathways.[6] Single activities make up the starting point of the cost model of DSSHI. This is similar to the "MIPP" model, but the approach here regards the versatile nature of single activities being a component of several pathways. Single activities as cost objects are defined by considering the principle that cost objects must be standardized

---

[4] See the model "MIPP" of the Swiss hospital Aarau, which is based on a path cost accounting model for cost objects. This approach was developed by Hellmann and Rieben (2003).

[5] For example, Hellmann and Rieben set different time periods related to single activities (Hellmann and Rieben 2003).

[6] The concept presented in this paper builds on a traditional cost element and cost center accounting. See for example Horvath (2006). All regulations for cost accounting in hospitals can be integrated. For further information about the basics of cost accounting in healthcare see Kehres (1998).

Table 21.1 Relationship of activities, activity types, categories, catalogs and processes (own creation)

Structural reasons			Cost accounting reasons	
Process	Activity catalog	Activity category	Activity	Activity type
Operation	Operation	Bypass	Sew on bypass	Normal
				High

and thus comparable to similar ones. For example, the activity "provide a computer tomogram of the head" cannot be standardized, since the necessary effort depends on the state of consciousness of the patient. Thus, standardization requires a fine granular definition of activities, e.g. "provision of a computer tomogram of the head in the case of an unconscious patient at regular working times". As a consequence, clinical pathways are not cost objects in the usual sense. Rather they are *cost association objects*, establishing a layer above conventional cost accounting.

21.3.2   Definition of Activities, Activity Types and Cost Objects

The example above, "provision of a computer tomogram of the head in the case of an unconscious patient at regular working times" had been characterized as an activity since it observes the principle of comparability. In concrete implementations this requirement will lead to an enormous amount of activities showing slightly differences only. Therefore the management has to decide which level of detail is necessary for taking precise decisions. In the DSSHI-system the activities are divided in at most three activity types according to their effort, for example one may differentiate in "normal", "medium" and "high". These activity types form the smallest cost unit and represent the most concrete expression of an activity.

Also, for the purpose of navigation and structuring, the activities occurring in healthcare institutions are grouped into activity categories. They bundle activities and activity types and thus represent a higher level of aggregation. In addition, by matter of subject, activity types are combined to listings called activity catalogs.

Clinical pathways had been characterized above as an abstract, standardized flow of treatments based on a specific diagnosis. Consequently, any pathway as an abstract scheme consists of activities. But the concrete treatments of patients are made up of activity types, i.e. activities that are more closely characterized by the needed effort "normal", "medium" or "high".

Table 21.1 gives an example of the relationship of activities, activity types, categories, catalogs and processes.

Activity types serves as cost units. Therefore, in order to define these costs one has to measure respectively estimate the time, amount and qualification of persons that are required for their performance including their salary level. Clearly, input of material must be registered as well.

21.3.3 Personnel Cost Calculation

The staff cost rate is, as usual for service companies, the largest cost factor in health-care companies (Haas 1999).[7] In particular, the cost of medical and nursing staff plays a major role and should be considered separately.[8]

Known cost accounting practices in healthcare often do not differentiate between different personnel functions and positions and work with average minutes rates for each cost center (Zapp 2005, Greiling et al. 2004) or professional group (Hellmann and Rieben 2003). However, it makes a significant difference for the accuracy of the cost determination, whether average costs or a differentiated view of the cost rates per minute are calculated. A chief doctor gets a higher salary than an assistant doctor resulting in different cost rates (Zapp 2005). For this reason, DSSHI separates the staff in groups with similar cost rates. In general, each cost center therefore consists of different staff groups formed by qualification and cost rates.

Beyond that, determining the minute rates one has to differentiate the time any person is directly involved in service provision (productive time) from the time the person is busy with other activities (further time), like time for management activities or meetings. While the productive time can be charged directly to the cost objects, the further time will be charged as overhead costs to the cost centers and in a subsequent step will be distributed as indirect costs to the activity types.

Immediately after the introduction of the cost model of DSSHI, generally, productive time of staff will not be available. In this case, as preliminary calculation one can take estimated values, which at the end of the accounting period should be replaced by actual data (costing) in order to charge all costs incurred.[9]

In some cases, the accurate recording of activities and the nuanced determination of the cost objects economically does not make sense. This can be the case if the activities are similar regardless of the particular case. For example, certain administrative services differ little from each other so that a differentiated analysis does not make sense. In order to offer economical efficient procedures for cost determination DSSHI contains the possibility to determine flat rate cost of cost units like minute rates, daily rates or rates per case.

However, flat rates do not allow a differentiated cost- and performance analysis. For this reason, in each case one must weigh the pros and cons of a differentiated analysis of activities and cost object definition.

---

[7] Staff costs make up 75% of the operating costs (Hellmann and Rieben 2003).

[8] In Germany, for 2007 medical and nursing staff costs in hospitals amount to nearly 84% of total staff costs and 50,6% of total costs (Statistisches Bundesamt 2008).

[9] For a more detailed description see Wagner et al. (2010).

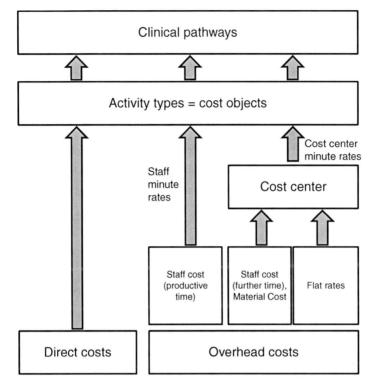

Fig. 21.2 Summarized cost and activity accounting model (own creation)

21.3.4 Summarized Cost and Activity Accounting Model

As shown, in the presented cost and activity accounting model the defined activity types act as cost objects. Figure 21.2 summarizes the described interrelations.[10]

21.4 Structure and Functionality of the Decisions Support System for Healthcare Institutions (DSSHI)

In order to give relevant cost- and performance information for the management of healthcare institutions, appropriate software is essential. The following section deals with the description of architecture and implementation needs of DSSHI and gives an overview about its capability.

---

[10] For more details see also Waehlert et al. (2010).

Fig. 21.3 Architecture of
DSSHI (own creation)

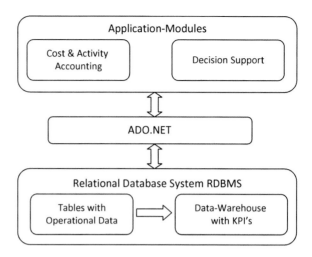

21.4.1 Architecture and Implementation Requirements

21.4.1.1 Basic Considerations

The software is divided into two modules: the cost and activity accounting and the decision support system. The cost and activity accounting tool allows the definition, documentation and administration of activities, activity types and cost objects as well as clinical pathways and their costs based on the described minute rates. The decision support tool provides key performance indicators related to capacities, activities, costs and quality of clinical pathways. It offers management reports on different aggregation levels.

When programming the software special attention was given to a layered object-oriented approach and a functional separation of the different modules (Fig. 21.3). These architectural elements ensure high adaptability allowing future modifications and developments. Programming was done with MS Visual Studio using C#.

As seen in Fig. 21.3 data are stored in a relational database management system (RDBMS). The implementation at time uses the database system MySQL with the InnoDB-Engine, which allows the checking of constraints of the database.

Separation between the application system and the database is realized by using ADO.NET.[11] ADO.NET stores external tables internally in corresponding tables of DataSets and realizes synchronization of these tables. Since, with ADO.NET the application only accesses data from internal memory, response times to any user interactions are very short.

---

[11] See Microsoft Corporation, http://msdn.microsoft.com/de-de/library/e80y5yhx.aspx (status from 05.09.2010).

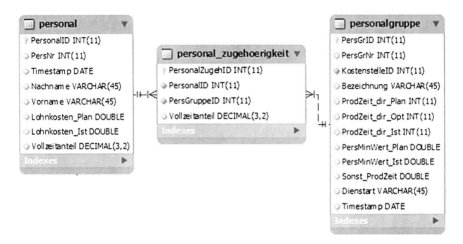

Fig. 21.4   Representation of staff and staff groups (own creation)

The application modules themselves are based on the model-view-controller paradigm (Reenskaug et al. 2010, Waehlert et al. 2010), where the controller encapsulates user interactions, the view component shows the presentations and the model component realizes the application logics.

The classes and objects of the application modules correspond to the tables of the database system. These architectural considerations ensure high modularity and ease understanding of program structures.

In the following sections more details of the implementations are shown.

21.4.1.2   Entities and Relations in the Cost and Activity Accounting Module

Figure 21.4, based on the Extended Entity-Relationship-Model, gives an example of how staff and the grouping of staff had been realized.

The shown attributes have the following meaning: staff number (*PersonalID*), first name (*Vorname*), last name (Nachname), the planned labor costs (*Lohnkosten_Plan*), the actual labor costs (*Lohnkosten_Ist*) and an indication of full-time or part-time as a number between 0 and 1 (*Vollzeitanteil*). Because of the fact that a person can belong to more than one staff group (*personalgruppe*), you need an own table for the assignment of person to staff group (*personal_zugehoerigkeit*) showing for each person and staff group the assigned full- or part-time factor.

Similarly, Fig. 21.5 shows the structure of all data concerning activity types (*Leistungsart*), activities (*Leistung*), activity categories (*Leistungskategorie*) and activity catalogs (*Leistungskatalog*).

As it is seen, the table *leistung* contains the attribute *StandardLeistungsart*. Resources shown for this attribute correspond to the expected value of the different specifications, normal, medium and high, of activity types. It allows the creation of

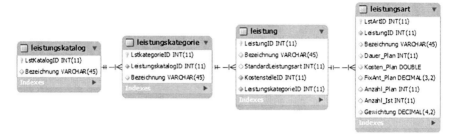

Fig. 21.5 Representation of activities, groups and catalogs of activities (own creation)

standardized clinical pathways, which can then be generated automatically and be compared with specific patient pathways. The attribute weighting (*Gewichtung*) in the table *Leistungsart* reflects the effort that is necessary for the fulfillment of an activity type.

21.4.2 Storage Scheme in the Decision Support Module

A typical requirement for data warehousing is the so called data-cube. It offers the usual operations drill down, slice and dice that correspond to the possibilities to group any performance indicator by different dimensions, to aggregate figures along the given dimensions or fix specific dimensions while varying others. For example, one wants to know how many cases of a specific diagnosis were treated on a monthly base or during last year and how all the cases of different DRGs sum up to the MDC, the major disease category. In order to realize these possibilities within DSSHI a star-scheme is used. A typical example is shown in Fig. 21.6.

21.4.3 Information Categories of Cost and Activity Accounting Module: User Interface

Figure 21.7 shows the relevant data of the Cost and Accounting Module and their relationships.

The cost and accounting module differentiates into two user groups having different rights[12]: Administrators are allowed to define, integrate and create all relevant cost and activity data. Moreover, they can use the tool to create and change stan-

---

[12] This division is only a first, basic division. More detailed differentiation, for example a differentiation between the clinical path managers, can be made afterwards. In that way the different path managers can obtain write and change permissions for their particular paths.

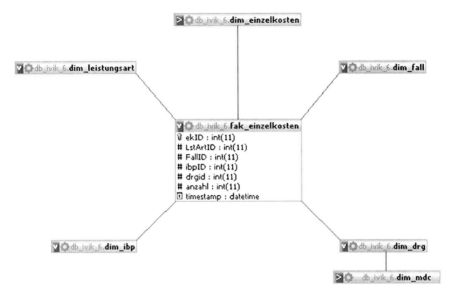

Fig. 21.6 Star scheme showing facts and dimensions of cost units (own creation)

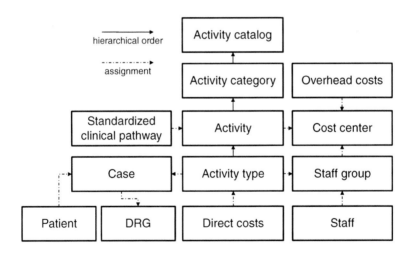

Fig. 21.7 Information categories of the cost and accounting module (own creation)

dardized clinical pathways. The resulting data model is the base for the planning of clinical pathways and their respective details. Clearly, application personnel, like physicians or nurses should not be able to change these definitions.

As an example of how the user interface of DSSHI looks like, consider the screen shot showing all relevant personnel data (Fig. 21.8).

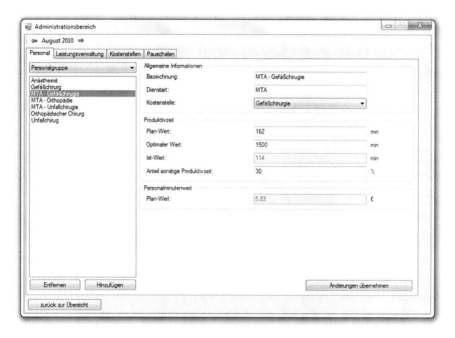

Fig. 21.8 Staff groups (own creation)

The staff group (*Personalgruppe*) includes general information such as the job type (e.g. medial technical assistant, doctor in chief) and associated cost center. There are also information about the productive time (e.g. the time that is needed for the fulfillment of the activity) of the staff group, which is differentiated in a planned productive time and an optimum productive time. While the plan value is based on realistic estimates, the optimum value (*Optimaler Wert*) records the optimal utilization of the staff group. These values are subsequently used to determine the staff capacity and can after combination with the actual value of the productive time (calculated automatically) be used for optimizing the working balance. The slot *Anteil sonstige Produktivzeit* allows the entry of further productive time. *Personalminutenwert* is the average cost of a person from the clicked staff group.

The recording of activities, activity types, categories and catalogs is implemented in a tree structure. If you click on a specific activity (here: sew bypass – single = *Bypass annähen – einfach*), general information, like planning values (e.g. the typical time for fulfilling the activity, amount of activity), structural information (assignment to the next aggregation level), definition of standard activity type or not and the underlying personal use appear on the right side of the screen (Fig. 21.9).

The cost center management integrates required regulations. The assignment of cost centers and new cost centers is possible. Furthermore, the planning values (e.g. cost center minute rates, overhead costs) are calculated automatically and cannot be changed.

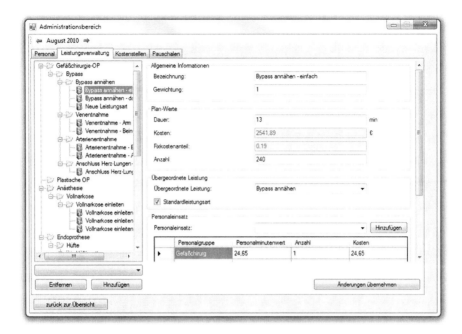

Fig. 21.9 Activities and their structuring (own creation)

A very important part of the module is the possibility to create and plan clinical pathways. Therefore it is necessary to fix a standardized path. It is used as a template into which a current patient or case can be entered. This has the advantage that the path will not be re-created for each new case. At the same time it serves to identify deviations from the standard and supports the further optimization (Fig. 21.10).

With removal (*Entfernen*) or addition (*Hinzufügen*), new standardized pathways are created or deleted. By the right field the required activities can be selected and their order can be determined using the arrow buttons. The button *Änderungen übernehmen* fixes the changes.

In the user's view (*Benutzerbereich*) the recording of actual data has to take place. All relevant data referring to specific cases and patients are entered and managed. Furthermore, each case or patient can be assigned to a DRG and a standardized clinical pathway. There is also the possibility to create an entirely new case. For this reason, activities and activity types can be added through a drop down menu (Fig. 21.11).

21.4.4   *Reporting with the Decision Support Module*

The Decision Support Module contains an evaluation tool which meets the requirements of the different management levels of healthcare institutions. This module therefore, is not only helpful for the top management but also for the lower management

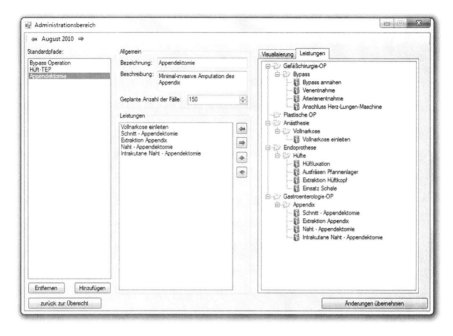

Fig. 21.10 Standardized pathways (own creation)

starting with group leaders and process managers for the different clinical pathways by providing specialized reports on different aggregation levels.

This decisions support module uses external data like DRG-tables as well as the data from the up streamed Cost and Activity Accounting Tool and transfers it into a data warehouse-system which is isolated from the operative data system. The included evaluation software processes the collected data and creates reports with different focuses on different aggregation levels.

The analyzing-reports are structured by three main focuses. The Decision Support Module first contains reports with regard to costs and earnings, besides this are reports, which focus on processes and quality aspects of data and personnel reports. The following sub items describe the three main reports in detail.

21.4.5   Reports with Regard to Costs and Revenues

One of the most important services of the decision support module is the analysis of cost data and the comparison of actual data, goals, cost figures and revenues. By means of these reports profitable departments and pathways as well as loss making ones can be identified. Figure 21.12 illustrates how a non profitable DRG can be distinguished by using a cost/revenue comparison report.

The knowledge of the profitability of divisions or DRG's enables management to focus on strategies for strengthening profitable ones and reduce unprofitable ones.

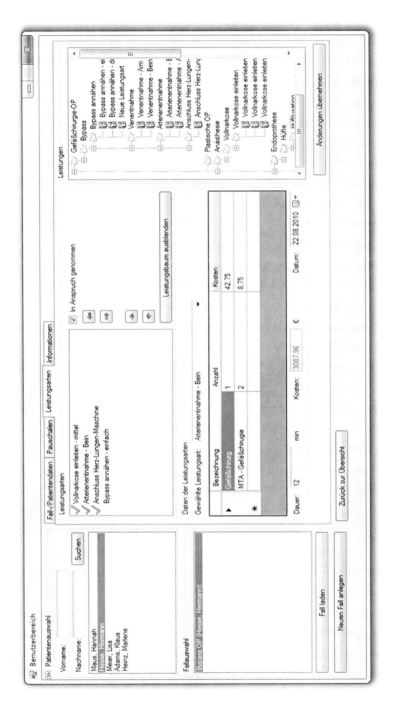

Fig. 21.11 Recording patient specific data (own creation)

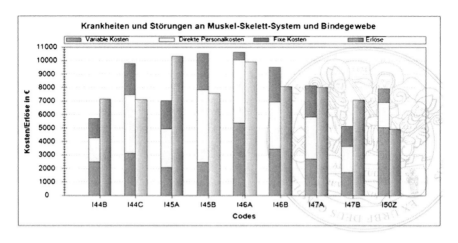

Fig. 21.12 Report showing cost and revenues of DRGs (own creation)

For example for unprofitable parts one may develop outsourcing strategies by entering co operations. Other strategies would be to improve revenues by increasing the number of specific cases.

Besides the classical cost/revenue comparison most reports also define the profit contribution of each DRG, which is the difference between the revenue and the variable costs. This information determinates whether the respective DRG has the potential to become profitable or not. A possibility to increase profitability of any DRG consists in raising the number of cases, since the fixed costs per unit usually decrease proportionally. However the fixed costs of medical care contain also the direct staff costs, which occur during the service provision and increase proportional to the number of cases. Therefore these costs have to be filtered out of the fixed costs. They act like variable costs and cannot be reduced by raising the number of cases. Correspondingly only the DRG with profit contributions that are higher than the direct staff costs can become profitable through strategic interventions focused on raising the number of cases. Therefore the cost and revenue reports of the developed Decision Support Module show the amount of direct staff, the other fixed and also the variable costs of each DRG or diagnose and thus enable the identification of profitable DRGs.

The cost/revenue comparison can be realized only on DRG or case-level because of the current compensation system in the German healthcare sector.[13] Other cost reports are available also on lower aggregation levels like cost units or activities.

In addition the cost reports contain an actual/target/budget-cost comparison (see Fig. 21.13) which enables the management to identify discrepancies and cost reduction

---

[13] Currently most of the hospital treatments are compensated by case based flat rates (DRG-flat rates). The treatments within the rehabilitation sector are still compensated by day rates; a change to rehabilitation DRG-flat rates is currently under discussion.

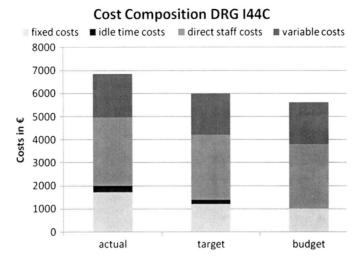

Fig. 21.13 Report showing personnel costs (own creation)

potentials. Such cost reports are generated by the Decision Support Module for all the different aggregation levels.

Besides the actual/target/budget-cost comparison the amount of idle time costs within the overall costs is important for taking management decisions. Idle time costs accrue when the staff is underemployed and therefore the available productive time is not fully used within patient's treatment. This report values the staff utilization rates in monetary units. High idle time costs are a signal for low staff utilization rates, they can be seen as a cost reduction potential which can be taped by approaching the optimal staff utilization rate. Negative idle time costs, on the other hand stand for a too high utilization rate which, in the short run, has positive impact on the cost situation, but in the long run negative impact on the motivation of personnel and quality of the treatments. Observing negative idle time costs the management has to take action in order to disburden the staff members concerned.

Further information regarding the staff utilization rates can be extracted from the personnel reports presented in the following.

21.4.6   Reports with Regard to Processes and Quality

Within the presented system the clinical pathways not only indicate the recommended treatment process for the medical staff and have the role of cost association objects, but rather they support the registration of activities for each patient. Thus, they represent the most important planning unit. All the cases assigned to one of the clinical pathways receive the pathway activities as a preregistration in their electronic health record. The nursing or medical personnel have to confirm the performed services by mouse click only. In opposite, clinical path variations have to be registered explicitly. The registration time, thus, considerably is reduced and the cost and activity accounting tool in the background is enabled to gather all the relevant management information without any supplementary effort.

The decision support module generates reports containing the treatment deviations of cases from the defined clinical pathways within a certain period which can be freely fixed. This information is on the one hand useful for the further development of the clinical pathways and on the other hand helpful for the revision and evaluation of internal processes.

21.4.7 Staff Reports

In addition to the cost/revenue and process reports the Decision Support Module offers also the possibility to control some personnel ratios by disposing staff reports. The evaluation and monitoring of these data are decisive, insofar, as the human resource is the most important factor of healthcare institutions.

The staff reports contain the earlier mentioned staff utilization rates for the different predefined personnel groups, but also an aggregation of these rates up to section and house level. The utilization rates can be calculated by using the registered adduced types of activities and their durations. This information is highly important for the manpower requirement planning process as it reveals the bottlenecks of the treatment processes, as well as the domains with personnel abundance.

Personnel dissatisfaction can occur either because of overwork or under challenge and should be avoided or at least reduced through management decisions. A too high or too low staff utilization rate can be interpreted like an early indicator for personnel dissatisfaction and the management has to act against it for example by hiring new personnel or raising the number of cases.

An important aspect of the calculation of the staff utilization rate is to consider that the highly educated and specialized personnel needs enough time for important further education activities. Therefore the amount of time dedicated to direct patient care should not be too high. This aspect can also be controlled by using the personnel reports. Having enough free space for further education not only raises the personnel satisfaction but also helps rising the institutional reputation and therefore raising the number of cases.

In summary, the personnel data cannot be seen as an indicator for the personnel job satisfaction only, but also as a helpful information for the economical handling of human resources.

21.5 Summary and Outlook

The illustrated cost and activity accounting model and the software solution enables the management of healthcare institutions to take decisions based on relevant cost and performance information. It is essential that the delivered information are not only with respect to financial data, but in the same way about activities, cases and clinical pathways. Deviations from the defined standardized clinical pathway can be detected and thus can drive forward process optimization. In addition, all case activities are recorded. This leads to more transparency of the business operations. By defining standardized activity types as cost objects, it is possible to assign the costs accurately. This enables a differentiated analysis of costs and revenues on different levels of aggregation. In particular, staff capacity can be shown and bottlenecks can be identified. This in turn can lead to a better distribution of tasks. In addition, costs, revenues and activities can be planned on the base of previous periods and can be compared with actual values. For this reason DSSHI supports the planning responsibilities of the management. It thus provides the basic information, for example, for make or buy decisions, for scope and depth of the treatment spectrum or alliances.

However, the significance of DSSHI is limited predominantly to the economic aspects of clinical pathways. To support strategic decisions in the future it will become increasingly important to integrate other, qualitative factors. In light of the existing demographic and financial trends, particularly the consideration of the interests and objectives of different stakeholders will play a major role in the positioning and viability of healthcare institutions. Yet there is a lack of appropriate business instruments that provide the management with strategic information. In the development of strategic business tools lays, especially for healthcare institutions, a great potential.

Acknowledgement This work partly had been supported by "Foundation Rhineland-Palatinate for Innovation". Programming was done by students majoring in business information systems at University of Trier. Especially we have to thank H. Jung, S. Müller, S. Schneider, S. Stadlbauer, J. Stass, C. Süßmeier, K. Walter and S. Zonker.

References

Czap, H. (2010). Erwartete Deckungsbeiträge von DRGs und Pfaden. In J. Hentze, B. Huch, & E. Kehres (Eds.), *Krankenhaus-Controlling – Konzepte, Methoden und Erfahrungen aus der Krankenhauspraxis* (4th ed., pp. 201–211). Stuttgart: Kohlhammer.

Czech, M., & Güssow, J. (2006). Pfadcontrolling – Pfadkostenrechnung. In J. Eckardt & B. Sens (Eds.), *Praxishandbuch Integrierte Behandlungspfade – Intersektorale und sektorale Prozesse professionell gestalten* (pp. 167–198). Heidelberg: Economica.

Eckardt, J. (2006). Was sind integrierte Behandlungspfade (IBP)? In J. Eckardt & B. Sens (Eds.), *Praxishandbuch Integrierte Behandlungspfade – Intersektorale und sektorale Prozesse professionell gestalten* (pp. 9–37). Heidelberg: Economica.

Greiling, M., Buddendick, H., & Molter, S. (2004). *Klinische Pfade in der Praxis – Workflow-Management von Krankenhaus-Prozessen*. Bamberg: Baumann Fachverlag.

Güssow, J. (2007). *Vergütung Integrierter Versorgungsstrukturen*. Wiesbaden: Deutscher Universitäts.

Haas, J. (1999). *Flexible, prozeßkonforme Plankosten- und Leistungsrechnung auf Teil- und Vollkostenbasis für Krankenhausunternehmen*. Aachen: Shaker.

Hellmann, W., & Rieben, E. (2003). *Pfadkostenrechnung als Kostenträgerrechnung*. Augsburg: Ecomed.

Horvath, P. (2006). *Controlling* (10th ed.). München: Vahlen.

Kehres, E. (1998). Kosten- und Leistungsrechnung im Krankenhaus. In J. Hentze, B. Huch, & E. Kehres (Eds.), *Krankenhaus-Controlling. Konzepte, Methoden und Erfahrungen aus der Krankenhauspraxis* (pp. 61–92). Stuttgart/Berlin/Köln: Kohlhammer.

Krier, C., Bublitz, R., & Töpfer, A. (2006). Explorative Einführung und Auswirkung von klinischen Pfaden. In A. Töpfer & D. M. Albrecht (Eds.), *Erfolgreiches Changemanagement im Krankenhaus* (pp. 135–164). Berlin/Heidelberg: Springer.

Noweski, M. (2008). *Der Gesundheitsmarkt. Liberalisierung und Reregulierung als Resultat politischer Koalitionen*. Berlin: Köster.

Reenskaug, T., Wold, P., Lehne, O. A. (2010). Working with objects. The OOram software engineering method. http://heim.ifi.uio.no/trygver/1996/book/WorkingWithObjects.pdf. Accessed 11 Dec 2010.

Roeder, N., et al. (2003). Frischer Wind mit klinischen Behandlungspfaden (I): Instrumente zur Verbesserung der Organisation klinischer Prozesse. *Das Krankenhaus, 1*, 20–27.

Salfeld, R., Hehner, S., & Wichels, R. (2008). *Modernes Krankenhausmanagement – Konzepte und Lösungen*. Berlin/Heidelberg: Springer.

Statistisches Bundesamt (2008). Gesundheit: Kostennachweis der Krankenhäuser, 12, 6.3 (2007). Wiesbaden

Straub, S. (1997). *Controlling für das wirkungsorientierte Krankenhausmanagement: ein Value-Chain basierter Ansatz, Schriftenreihe zur Gesundheitsökonomie*. Bayreuth: Verlag PCO.

Thiexe-Kreye, M., & von Collas, T. (2005). Interne Budgetierungssysteme im DRG-Zeitalter - Beispielhafte Darstellung einer praxiserprobten Methode. In A.J.W. Goldschmidt & M. Kalbitzer & J. Eckardt (Eds.), *Praxishandbuch Medizincontrolling* (pp. 141–166). Heidelberg: Economica.

von J-M, Schulenburg. (2007). Die Entwicklung der Gesundheitsökonomie. In O. Schöffski & J.-M. von Schulenburg (Eds.), *Gesundheitsökonomische Evaluationen* (3rd ed., pp. 13–22). Berlin/Heidelberg: Springer.

Waehlert, L., Wagner, A., & Czap, H. (2010). Potenziale und Nutzen einer Pfadkostenrechnung auf Basis von Behandlungspfaden für Einrichtungen im Gesundheitswesen. *Zeitschrift für öffentliche und gemeinwirtschaftliche Unternehmen (ZögU), 33*(4), 368–380.

Wagner, A., Waehlert, L., & Czap, H. (2010). Pfadkostenrechnung für Behandlungspfade – Ein Instrument zur Entscheidungsunterstützung für Einrichtungen im Gesundheitswesen. *Gesundheitsökonomie und Qualitätsmanagement, 6*, 299–304.

Without author (2008). EBM 2008: Ein Meilenstein für die Zukunft. In KBV (Ed.), *Beilagen Deutsches Ärzteblatt*. (21.11.2008), http://www.kbv.de/publikationen/2435.html. Accessed 22 June 2010.

Zapp, W. (2005). *Kostenrechnung und Controllinginstrumente in Reha-Kliniken*. Lohmar-Köln: Eul.

Chapter 22
A Comprehensive Approach to the IT: Clinical Practice Interface

David Zakim and Mark Dominik Alscher

Abstract Medicine in the twenty-first Century is beset with two fundamental problems. Everyday care is poor quality care. And clinical research programs do not provide consistent answers to pressing clinical questions. Both problems affect individual lives and contribute to a system of health care that is not sustainable financially. Poor quality health care drives cost because most health care expenditures are for treating expensive, hard-to-reverse complications of disease we know how to prevent. Inefficient clinical research develops clinical scenarios for which one treatment fits all instead of defining populations that will benefit from individualized treatment. Deficiencies in quality of care and clinical research have a common etiology in the inability of physicians to collect detailed clinical data about their patients and to translate medical knowledge to evidence-based clinical decisions. These problems can be solved simultaneously with expert system software that makes computing the central element for collecting clinical data, for translating knowledge to evidence-based clinical decisions, and for collecting population-based, observational databases on the longitudinal behavior of disease to empower robust clinical research programs. CLEOS® is a prototype of this approach.

Keywords History-taking • Phenotype • Information technology • Expert-system • Computing • Cognitive overload

D. Zakim (✉)
Institute for Digital Medicine, Stuttgart, Germany
e-mail: dzakim@pacbell.net

M.D. Alscher
Institute for Digital Medicine, Stuttgart, Germany

Robert Bosch Krankenhaus, Stuttgart, Germany

N. Wickramasinghe et al. (eds.), *Critical Issues for the Development of Sustainable E-health Solutions*, Healthcare Delivery in the Information Age, DOI 10.1007/978-1-4614-1536-7_22, © Springer Science+Business Media, LLC 2012

22.1   Introduction

Information technology (IT) holds the promise of making health care more efficient and affordable. But current applications of IT to the clinical side of medical practice are unlikely to have either effect because IT to improve efficiency is founded on the false assumption that medical practice is fundamentally sound but needs tweaking around the edges. Health care, however, does not deliver the value of which it is capable because physicians cannot achieve clinical outcomes with levels of accuracy in diagnosis and efficacy of treatment that it is possible to reach by applying existing medical knowledge (Institute of Medicine 2001; McGlynn et al. 2003; Gandhi et al. 2006; Ramsey et al. 1998a; Enright et al. 1999; Altman 1994). This failure in the effective use of medical knowledge produces a health care system in which the majority of resources are used to treat illnesses and complications of illnesses we have the know-how to prevent (Wolff et al. 2002). Creating a system that uses existing medical knowledge effectively – that makes health care efficient and affordable – requires more than tweaks at the edges.

22.2   The Root Cause of Poor Quality Health Care

The key to understanding and doing something to improve the quality of health care is to acknowledge that human cognitive capacity is finite and limits of long- and short-term memory were exceeded long ago by the scope (exceeds capacity of long-term memory) and complexity (exceeds capacity of short-term memory) of medical knowledge. No one can learn and remember more than a minute fraction of the knowledge represented in the books and journals in Fig. 22.1 let alone in the three-fold to fourfold greater volume of information in the complete library. And learning and remembering the content in Fig. 22.1 does not insure rational use for decision-making because the number of variables factored into common clinical decisions exceeds the capacity of human short-term memory (Miller 1956; Tversky and

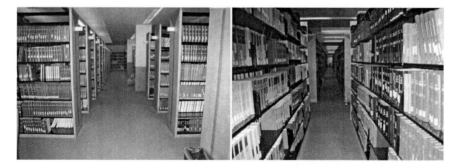

Fig. 22.1 One row (*left*) and 1 column of the row at the University of California San Francisco medical library. The library has three floors of these stacks, 1 floor of newly arrived journals, and no longer stores print copies of the most popular journals

Kahneman 1964). Yet the medical community persists in promoting the myth that medical knowledge can be translated to evidence-based decision-making by teaching every physician all he/she needs to know. The problem of a dysfunctional health care system is as "simple" to fix, therefore, as addressing the obvious mismatch between what is known and what humans can learn, can remember and can use rationally. IT can solve the limitations of human cognition as they affect medical practice; but to do so the IT approach must address the pervasiveness of the cognitive limits.

22.3 Everyday Medical Practice is a Rational, Rules-Based Activity

The knowledge in Fig. 22.1 is a distillation of clinical observations into sets of empirical rules for collecting clinical data in a way that fits symptoms (what a patient feels is awry) and signs (what is discovered as abnormal by physical and laboratory examination) with diseases, which is the process of diagnosis. There is a further set of rules for correlating diagnoses with ultimate causes of disease in specific organs and for selecting best modalities of treatment. The diagnosis "hepatitis," for example, identifies liver as the site of a disease process but is insufficient for determining a course of treatment, which depends on the specific cause of hepatitis in a given patient. Treatment for hepatitis caused by an adverse reaction to a medication will be different from treatment of hepatitis due to hepatitis B virus or say alcohol abuse. There are further sets of rules for finding and quantifying risk for disease in people not overtly sick.

Figure 22.2 represents graphically the rules for organizing the processes for delivering care from doctor to patient and how medical knowledge should be used. Each box encompasses a knowledge- and time-intensive task related to collecting and

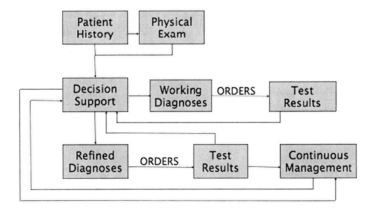

Fig. 22.2 Graphic depiction of the clinical method to illustrate data elements and flow of clinical information during evaluation and on-going management of patients. Information flows between tasks in the directions of the *arrows*. Note that flow is iterative. Working diagnoses are tested; test results and effects of treatment regimes feed-back to the decision support to refine prior decisions. Ideally, decisions are informed by the most recent, applicable evidence

evaluating the significance of clinical information according to established sets of rules separate from organization of the processes of care. But the organization and individual processes depicted in Fig. 22.2 are directed by the knowledge represented in Fig. 22.1. The physician today stands as the only link between the knowledge base in Fig. 22.1, the rules for organizing practice in Fig. 22.2 and the patient.

Delivery of clinical care begins with the patient's medical history. This set of data remains the sine qua non for an outcome that will match what it is possible to achieve given the current knowledge base relating to a specific set of problems in a specific patient. The facts of a medical history are the basis for almost all subsequent, evidence-based clinical decisions. Diagnoses can be made more than 80% of the time, for example, from history alone; and the history defines co-morbid states, significant past medical events, environmental risks and family history. Nothing in the foreseeable future will diminish the clinical value of detailed history-taking. Historical data and findings from a physical examination are integrated in the box labeled "Decision Support" to generate rank-ordered diagnostic possibilities (Working Diagnoses) to be confirmed or excluded with results from laboratory tests (Refined Diagnosis). The processes of data collection, evaluation and testing are iterated until an acute medical problem is resolved satisfactorily. In the case of chronic disease, these are life-long processes in which results from "Continuous Management" feed-back to "Decision Support" for constant assessment of therapeutic efficacy.

22.4   The Complexity of Clinical Decision-Making

To illustrate the cognitive challenges of decision-making in the context of Fig. 22.2, consider the common clinical problem of prescribing a medication to control blood sugar in an adult with the new diagnosis of type 2 diabetes. The problem is common because type 2 diabetes affects about 8% of the population. It is important because control of blood sugar reduces the incidence of complications that limit quality of life and life-span and that are expensive-to-treat, e.g., kidney failure, heart attack and stroke. There is a clearly defined target level for blood sugar arrived at by the balance between treatment that simultaneously minimizes the occurrence of long-term complications and the chance of serious side effects from low levels of blood sugar. The task of controlling blood sugar is performed poorly. Most diabetics do not attain target levels for blood sugar even though diagnosing diabetes is not difficult. Diagnosis can be made when a patient's blood sugar in the fasting state exceeds 126 mg/100 mL blood. Cognitive difficulties arise once the diagnosis is made and treatment for blood sugar must be prescribed. This task has 2 complex components. The first is determining a patient's clinical attributes besides the diagnosis of diabetes to define the patient's phenotype of diabetes and one or more co-morbid states. The second task is matching the patient's phenotype with medications that lower blood sugar.

On the patient side of the decision, NIH and European Endocrine Society guidelines specify a set of 13 clinical attributes to define phenotype in a manner that will maximize therapeutic effect and minimize adverse reactions to medications (ICSI 2010). The physician must acquire and interpret the data relevant to defining phenotype. Some of these attributes are simple to define, e.g., age, body weight, level of blood sugar. Others depend on knowledge- and time-intensive tasks to determine by history and physical examination whether or not the patient has, for example, chronic lung disease and/or chronic kidney disease and/or chronic diarrheal disease and so on. Assuming the 13 attributes are properly defined, the next step is to factor the combination of attributes to determine which of 2^{13} unique combinations of diabetes and the 13 attributes, i.e. 8,192 phenotypes of diabetes plus co-morbid states, describes a specific patient. Then comes the decision of which drug or combination of drugs matches best to the patient's phenotype.

On the medication side, there are two classes of oral agents that stimulate insulin release from the pancreas. There are two classes of oral agents that increase sensitivity to insulin. There is a class of agents that inhibits absorption of glucose from the intestine. There are several classes of agents within a group referred to as peptide analogs. There are multiple specific drugs with different contraindications and side effects within each class. Treatment can be initiated with one or more oral agent; one or more oral agents can be co-administered with one or more types of insulin, which is still another large class of drugs. So the almost common-place decision of what to prescribe to control blood sugar is a formidable cognitive task and far more difficult than diagnosing diabetes.

There is a still further level of cognitive difficulty in managing blood sugar. Diabetics typically have high blood pressure, levels of LDL-cholesterol ("bad" cholesterol) that are abnormally high and levels of HDL-cholesterol ("good" cholesterol) that are abnormally low. Each of these is as complex a management problem as blood sugar. So it is not surprising to find that only 1 in 20 diabetics has a blood sugar, a blood pressure and an LDL-cholesterol that meet therapeutic targets (Saddine et al. 2002). Nor is it surprising that doctors fail to change treatment in a majority of diabetics with blood sugars (assessed by the test HbA1c), blood pressures and/or blood cholesterols that exceed a therapeutic target (Phillips et al. 2001a; Shah et al. 2005; Grant et al. 2005). Doctors facing uncertainty do what everyone else does in this setting. They decide not to decide (Tversky and Kahneman 1981). Doctors "get away" with this behavior in patients with type 2 diabetes, and many other chronic diseases, because their failures do not damage patients acutely. Complications like kidney failure and heart attack are long-term complications of diabetes and occur only after years of therapeutic neglect.

22.5   Using Short- and Long-Term Computer Memory to Overcome Limits to Human Cognition

It is possible to assign to computing all the tasks just outlined for diagnosing type 2 diabetes and then for selecting the best agent to control blood sugar in the affected patient because the tasks are rules-based. Indeed, we can generalize from the example of diabetes just given. Thus, to the extent that the rules directing processes in Fig. 22.2 are known, medical practice is a rational activity. All the known rules for implementing the processes in Fig. 22.2, with regard to any disease, can be formalized as machine-readable code to enable computers to "read" and "understand" the rules for practice and to take patient-specific, rules-based actions, e.g. ask a patient a set of questions designed to collect a medical history, acquire a context-specific, interim history at a later encounter, interpret the data collected according to rules for diagnosis and treatment to generate, without direct human intervention, diagnoses and recommendations for treatments. Computers can be programmed to perform these functions iteratively in order to follow patients longitudinally in the context of their specific medical problems. In other words, it is possible to embed computers within the processes of Fig. 22.2 and thereby to substitute the essentially unlimited short-term and long-term memory of computers for the limited cognitive capacity of humans to insure that the knowledge in Fig. 22.1 is translated to rules-based decisions during every clinical encounter. Computers can undertake the knowledge-intensive and time-intensive tasks now solely within the purview of health care providers. There is no other way to deal with the quality problem in delivering health care.

22.6 The Extraordinary Power of Computing Applied to Medicine

22.6.1 Consequences for Everyday Medical Practice

The advantages of properly designed and executed IT applied to implementing the processes in Fig. 22.2 are extraordinary. For example, whereas, as mentioned, the patient's life-long medical history is the starting point and sine qua non for a quality medical outcome, physician-acquired histories are known to be incomplete, inaccurate, biased by the physician's lack of knowledge in specific areas of medicine and unreliable for defining clinical phenotype (Bentsen 1976; Romm and Putnam 1981; Ramsey et al. 1998b; Cox et al. 2003). In addition, physician-acquired medical histories are collections of unstructured data and are useless for building a global database of "clinical experience" across populations and time. By contrast with physicians as history-takers, a properly programmed computer can insure that every medical history is based on a complete understanding of the signs and symptoms with which disease and risk for disease present or manifest clinically, that every patient's medical history is complete and that every medical history is acquired according to a single, standardized protocol so that differences in clinical data between patients with identical diagnoses are reliable for defining clinical phenotype. And beyond the issue of collecting clinical data directly from primary sources, computing can analyze the data collected in the context of best available current knowledge to output diagnoses, protocols for confirming diagnoses and recommendations for treatment based on identifying specific causes for disease, i.e., alcoholic hepatitis not a non-specific diagnosis "hepatitis." The computer can perform these functions iteratively whenever new data are added to a patient's clinical record. A further advantage of substituting computing for human cognition in Fig. 22.2 occurs for finding and correcting medical errors and adding new knowledge as medical research expands. In regard to error-correction, a properly programmed computer will leave an indelible record of how data were collected and how data were interpreted. This record can be searched to pin-point errors of omission, e.g. errors of data collection, and errors reflecting incorrect interpretations of data. Once found, correcting a single copy of software permanently removes a specific error from the system. And, obviously, up-dating a single copy of software permanently incorporates new knowledge into the program, which can be applied immediately, as needed, to medical issues in patients or people at risk world-wide.

22.6.2 Consequences for Clinical Research

There is a still further important advantage in substituting computers for physicians as the primary engine for collecting clinical data from primary sources. This approach can revolutionize the way in which existing rules for practice can be extended and new ones discovered. These activities comprise, of course, the domain of clinical research, which, as currently constituted, is inadequate to the tasks of improving on current rules for practice and discovery of new ones (Ioannidis et al. 2001; Begg 2004; Chan et al. 2004; Adams and White 2005; Ioannidis 2006; Gormley et al. 2007; Luce et al. 2009; Hennekens and DeMets 2009; Buchanan et al. 2009; Boutron et al. 2010; Institute of Medicine 2010; Tzoulaki et al. 2009). The evidence for this judgment is that results from controlled clinical trials often do not apply when extended to a broad population of patients and often are not confirmed when the clinical issue of interest is restudied with new cohorts of patients. Moreover, even validated clinical research provides less information than is needed for efficient treatment decisions. An example of what we mean here is provided by data for mitigating the risk of heart attacks (coronary events) by lowering levels of LDL-cholesterol ("bad cholesterol") in blood. Adherence to current guidelines for identifying and quantifying level of risk in relation to levels of LDL-cholesterol are effective in reducing the incidence of coronary events. But the guideline is inefficient: 200 people must be treated to prevent one coronary event (Pletcher et al. 2009).

Just as little energy has been expended to analyze why everyday medical practice delivers poor outcomes, not much thinking focuses on the idea that the clinical research enterprise is seriously flawed and needs to be reenergized. Substituting computing for human cognitive power to drive the processes in Fig. 22.2 can do this at an affordable cost by creating a convergence between the now separate components of clinical practice and clinical research. These activities should not be but largely are independent of each other. Practitioners, as noted already, are ineffective in translating research results to evidence-based clinical decisions; and the clinical research enterprise sees no value in the observational data that can be collected during routine medical care. Obviously, we want the benefits of validated clinical research to accrue to patients. It is equally desirable that results from prior research are used in an evidence-based manner in practice to determine true efficacy and safety so that new protocols or reanalysis of data can be built on real-world results from prior research. The absence of feed-back from everyday practice to clinical research interdicts building an evidentiary foundation for designing new experiments to extend prior results. Another consequence of separating clinical practice from clinical research is reliance of the latter on controlled, prospective, clinical trials, which are less controlled than their proponents will admit and too expensive to cover the myriad of unresolved clinical issues.

There is considerable phenotypic heterogeneity within single cohorts of patients enrolled in trials on the basis of identical diagnoses. "Controlled trials" do not control adequately for this phenotypic variability. Results from clinical trials do not apply generally and/or cannot be duplicated because the phenotypes of the broad public and/or phenotypes in a new cohort of study patients do not match those for patients in the original study. But better definition of phenotypic differences within a study cohort will increase the number of patient cohorts needed for a study, which increases the cost of the work. Since there is insufficient money to expand clinical trials in this way, trials compromise the criteria for enrolling patients. The realistic option for mounting a clinical research program that avoids this kind of compromise is convergence of clinical practice and clinical research. This can be done by capturing the observational data from everyday medical practice in a manner that is useful for clinical research, which has the power to expand enrollment in trials from a few thousand patients in the largest trials to millions of patients. There are 300,000,000 out-patient visits a year in the U.S. There probably is a similar number in the E.U. The clinical records for these patients are irrelevant for clinical research at present because the data in these charts are incomplete, inaccurate and not structured. A program that standardizes collection of clinical data for all patients in all practices in routine care and that extends the range of data collected to all fields bearing on health for every patient interacting with the health care system will create convergence between delivery of care day-to-day and the clinical research enterprise by utilizing clinical data from as many as 600,000,000 patient visits a year (in the U.S. plus E.U.) as a basis for the clinical research program.

22.7 Implementation of Autonomous Software Programs That "Practice" Medicine

We mentioned that dysfunctional health care is as "simple" to fix as formalizing the rules for medical practice. This is a straight-forward but not trivial task because of the scope and complexity of the knowledge to formalize. The task becomes tractable by narrowing the focus of an initial set of formalizations to generate a program that is useful even if not complete. A program to interview patients to acquire complete medical histories is the natural starting point (Fig. 22.2). A further way to focus the huge problem of formalizing medical knowledge is to concentrate at the outset on diseases that use the greatest fraction of medical resources, that affect large numbers of people and that are managed poorly. This is the strategy we used to develop an expert medical system called CLEOS® (Clinical Expert Operating

System) that deploys computing as the operating element in Fig. 22.2 for (1) collecting and managing clinical data; (2) translating existing knowledge to evidence-based diagnostic and treatment decisions; and (3) providing detailed clinical data to support an efficient program for clinical research. CLEOS® specifically has a knowledge base that applies to common, serious acute and chronic diseases of adults that account for more than 80% of physician visits and health care expenditures in developed countries and that are known to be managed poorly. The knowledge base formalized within CLEOS® drives history-taking at an initial encounter with the program, integrates laboratory data, analyzes the clinical significance of the data collected and outputs reports to physicians of findings, diagnoses, prevention issues needing follow-up, and recommendations for diagnosis and treatment. The program generates actionable orders coupled to interpretive outputs, e.g., an electronic order for lab tests to confirm a diagnosis or a prescription for a specific medication.

22.7.1 Description of CLEOS®

CLEOS® is accessed by out-patients from any computing device connected to the Internet. Inside the Robert–Bosch–Krankenhaus, Stuttgart, Germany, CLEOS® is accessed via wireless connection to the hospital intranet. The patient interface is textual (Fig. 22.3) and graphic (Fig. 22.4) but can use audio prompts when appropriate for helping patients interact with the computer. The patient interface could be audio primarily; but it is faster for patients to read text and use graphics than to interact via spoken words. We are programming selected voice responses from patients but believe voice recognition software is not sufficiently advanced for use in CLEOS®. An interview collects medically significant demographic data from the patient and initiates the medical interview by asking: "Why do you need medical care now?" The specific attributes of the patient's main complaint directs the patient to a next question. And subsequent questions are generated in the context of the chief complaint and continuous evaluation of the clinical significance of the sum of answers to any point in the interview. The patient experiences a seamless single program.

History-taking is directed by well-established, empirical rules that relate symptoms (what a patient experiences) to pathologic states. The CLEOS®-knowledge base is modular, where modules focus on organs and specific types of medical problems within organs. There is a module, for example, that centers on gastrointestinal problems; but there are in addition separate modules for abdominal pain, vomiting, and diarrhea, which open when any of these is the patient's main complaint. Modules are knit together by empirical medical knowledge so that the program operates as a single, seamless decision graph at the patient interface. Knowledge inside CLEOS® is represented by decision graphs (Fig. 22.5) and inferences in which arguments are data elements. Figure 22.5 is specifically one of several decision graphs that collect historical data about abdominal pain. A patient reaches this graph because they have a main complaint of pain that they locate somewhere in the abdomen or they indicate

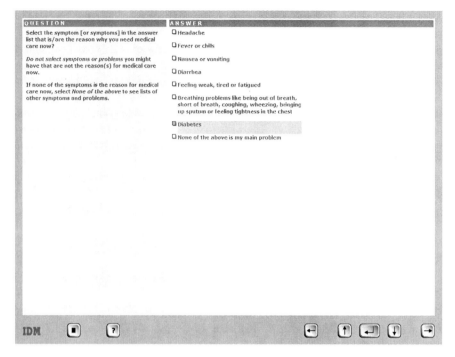

Fig. 22.3 Sample of textual interface by which patient enters historical data. This page represents a question in which multiple answers can be entered. The program also has question types allowing a single choice from multiple choice answers, selection of answers representing "Yes" or "No," selection of answers "Yes," "No" or "Cannot Decide" and entry of free text at the end of a string of questions to which the patient makes no definitive answer. The highlight shown on the answer "Diabetes" appears when the patient scrolls over an answer. Clicking anywhere on the highlight selects the answer. The patient moves to the next page by clicking the forward *arrow*. Clicking the back *arrow* erases answers to the preceding question and redisplays the page for this question. The patient may click the back *arrow* any number of times in succession to go backwards through the interview

with a graphic that they have pain in the abdominal region. The decision graph then works in the following ways. When a node is traversed by the path taken through the graph, the question represented by the node is presented to the patient. The subsequent path is determined by the patient's answer(s) to this question, which labels an arrow determining the path between nodes. ABDHIA167, for example, is a question posed to the patient with abdominal pain in the case that answers to prior questions direct the path across this node. If a traversed node is a question already asked, the prior answer directs the subsequent pathway. A node can be any kind of data element, as for example a laboratory test with values already known. A node also can be an inference in which the arguments are answers to a set of prior questions. ABDXC109 is an example of an inference for which the arguments are answers to some set of prior questions. Answer value *a* for ABDXC109 indicates the rule for the inference is satisfied, i.e., true, and *b* that it is not. Node MIT represents

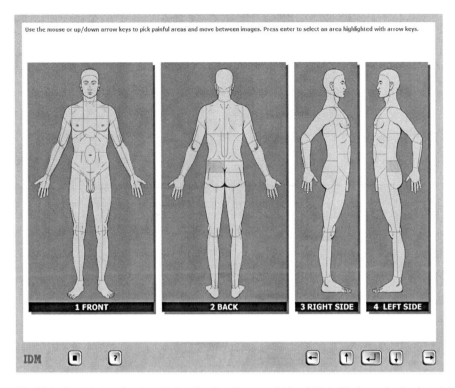

Fig. 22.4 Graphic interface by which patient localizes area(s) in which he/she has pain. A selected area becomes highlighted. Clicking a highlighted area removes the selection. Any number of areas may be selected

a set of decision graphs outside the module for abdominal pain. Note that the path from ABDXC160 through ABDHIA167 and crossing MIT, constitutes a rule for opening the set of graphs within MIT. This structure enables the program to emulate the "thinking" of a skilled clinician where "thinking" is the continuous evaluation of the differential diagnosis and changes to it as the clinical database expands during the interview.

CLEOS® collects all the components of a standard medical history: the chief complaint; history of the present illness, which is determined by the chief complaint; review of systems, which is a thorough search for symptoms of illness in every organ system outside the organ system probed in the present illness; history of significant past medical events as for example prior surgery, hospitalizations and so on; social history; and family history. A CLEOS® history-taking session can be quite long for patients with several chronic illnesses. But a complete history does not have to be obtained at a single session. The history can be interrupted and resumed at a later time at the point at which a session is stopped. We are using this feature in the emergency department. The program in this setting acquires a history of the present illness and completes history-taking after a patient is admitted to the hospital or after

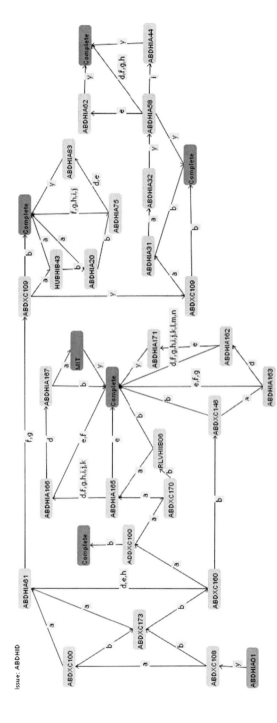

Fig. 22.5 One of several decision graphs for collecting historical data about abdominal pain by direct interview of the patient. *Arrows* are labeled with answer values for a question that determine the pathway through the graph. ABDHIA167 is a question posed to the patient with abdominal pain in the case that answers to prior questions direct the path across this node. ABDXC109 is an example of an inference for which the arguments are answers to some set of prior questions. Value *a* indicates the rule is satisfied and *b* it is not. MIT is an example of a node representing a set of decision graphs outside the module for abdominal pain

it is clear the patient will be discharged from the emergency department. The knowledge base of the current version of CLEOS® is represented by >14,400 decision nodes in 380 decision graphs that direct data collection to populate >27,000 data fields. All features of the knowledge base are infinitely expandable.

As noted above, CLEOS® uses inferences as nodes to analyze the clinical significance of data as data are collected in order to direct the line of questioning. CLEOS® also contains a large set of inferences that automatically analyze the clinical significance of all data at the conclusion of an interview and when new data are added to a completed interview as for example results of a lab test. The program uses these inferences to report diagnostic and therapeutic recommendations, organize data elements as clinical narratives for the physician, and generate orders for diagnostic tests and therapeutic interventions (Fig. 22.6). Rules analysis operates iteratively to refine diagnoses and adjust treatment as new clinical data feed-back from testing regimes, therapeutic results, interim histories and the natural course of the patient's illness. The current program has >6,000 explicit rules for interpreting and organizing the data it collects. Physicians access reports for a patient via any device connected to the Internet. Physicians inside the Robert–Bosch–Krankenhaus can access reports generated by CLEOS® in the same way as they access results for any lab test.

22.7.2 Clinical Performance of CLEOS®

CLEOS® has not been used as yet to provide routine health care. Outputs from the program have been tested in real clinical settings, however, by comparison with outputs of routine care provided by physicians. The program has been used by outpatients in sub-specialized medical practices, but formal comparison of routine care and CLEOS® has been made available only for in-patients on general medicine at the Robert–Bosch–Krankenhaus.

CLEOS® reports findings of fact as clinical narratives organized by concepts of pathophysiology not as statements of what was asked and answered. This introduces the possibility that CLEOS® collected a data element but failed to report it. We have found so far no significant omissions of fact from this sort of reporting error.

The main method of analysis to evaluate performance of CLEOS® was direct comparison of medically significant historical data and their clinical interpretations recorded in a patient's hospital chart with findings reported by CLEOS® after computer-based interview of the same patient. This work has shown that CLEOS® acquires and reports a more detailed and accurate medical history as compared with physicians (Zakim et al. 2008). CLEOS® found an average of 4.5 significant co-morbid states/patient that were not documented in charts from usual care. These problems occurred across a gamut of medical issues and involved all organ systems. CLEOS® also was far more effective as compared with usual care in identifying patients with significant histories of past adverse reactions to medications and documenting the nature of an adverse drug reaction; patients with significant side effects from current medications; patients under-medicated for diagnoses like heart failure

Office ID: **RBK081**	Hx Taken: 4/19/2006

Patient is Caucasian male born in 1948. Self-reported height: 1.7 m; weight: 60 kg. , BMI: <u>21</u>
Occupation: Human Resources

Present Illness:	Cough (10 -14 day duration) is only respiratory complaint. Cough started as part of a URI. Cough is in termittent. The cough is productive of sputum described as viscous. Patient has felt feverish and has had a highest recorded temperature of 38. 0. Has had one shaking chill. Patient has episodes of persistent cough on a regular basis at least yearly. Patient presents with cough that began about Onset cough was within the last month. Physical activity not limited by exacerbations. Cough provoked by tickling sensation in throat. Cough does not vary from day to night. Patient is not hoarse and does not have a sore throat from cough. Patient feels that coughing clears lungs. Cough does not worsen once it starts. No associated nasal stuffiness. The patient stopped smoking within the last year. Primary tobacco source: cigarettes. Typical habit is 1 pack/day. Years smoked: > 20 years. Symptoms triggered by lying down. Symptoms triggered by exercise. Taking no meds for persistent/recurring cough. Positive history pneumonia once. Event: 3 - 5 years ago. Hospitalized: no. No history TB. No history exposure to TB. Patient has not been skin tested for TB.

MEDICATIONS	**ALLERGIES**
Drugs Indication none	none

ACTIVE PROBLEMS	**PROCEDURES**
Cough of less than 4 weeks dur'n.	Thyroid nodule treated by surgical extirpation.

PAST HISTORY	**FAMILY HISTORY**
The patient is a former smoker (Typical habit is 1 pack/day for > 20 years). Stopped within the last year. History thyroid nodule.	No data entered.

Fig. 22.6 Sample page from a computer-generated report showing historical data from a patient interview are compiled as clinical narratives and that key items are highlighted in sets of tables. The figure shows only the first page of a sample report. Several tables of findings and narratives for the review of systems, social and family histories are not shown. The time-intensity of sound plots on the left hand side of the figure describe these features for all known systolic murmurs. The data on the right hand side of the figure contain all other data fields for characterizing a systolic murmur, e.g., where it is heard best and to whether it radiates to neck, back or axilla

and asthma; patients taking combinations of medications that are contraindicated; and patients unaware of how to monitor their medicines and responses to therapy. CLEOS® was more effective than routine care in identifying patients at risk for diabetes and breast cancer on the basis of family histories of these problems. It was highly unlikely that the superiority of CLEOS® as compared with routine care for identifying non-trivial medical problems reflects false positive findings by the computer program. Thus, diagnostic outputs from the CLEOS® program almost always depend on a constellation of findings not an answer to a single question. It is reasonable to conclude therefore that CLEOS® outperforms physicians in the primary task of history-taking, on which quality outcomes depend. We also have shown that CLEOS® can out-perform physicians in determining risk for coronary events and recommending treatment to mitigate this risk (Zakim et al. 2010). We examined this aspect of the program in detail because CLEOS® incorporates standard National Cholesterol Education Panel (NCEP) guidelines for quantifying risk and recommending therapy to reduce risk by treating levels of LDL-cholesterol. CLEOS® is designed to output a level of risk for coronary disease for every patient interviewed where risk is evaluated by automated analysis, according to NCEP guidelines, of clinical data collected. Review of more than 200 charts from routine care showed that physicians usually recorded insufficient data to stratify risk by NCEP guidelines; a level of risk was not stated explicitly in any chart; and treatment in usual care was not initiated or modified for the majority of patients needing initiation or modification of treatment. The review also showed that a majority of patients in whom treatment was initiated did not need it. It is known already that NCEP guidelines are ignored generally despite their effectiveness in preventing coronary events (Abookire et al. 2001; Wang et al. 2001; Phillips et al. 2001b; Yarzebski et al. 2002; Whincup et al. 2002). The new findings in the CLEOS® study were that the data included in medical histories from routine care were usually insufficient for applying NCEP guidelines but that CLEOS® solved the problem of data collection. In addition, CLEOS® interpreted its findings properly to assign risk according to NCEP guidelines and to indicate levels of LDL-cholesterol at which therapy should be instituted or modified according to principles of the guidelines (Fig. 22.7). CLEOS® was less than perfect, however; four errors made by the program in assigning level of risk in 213 patients were traced to an inference for interpreting data elements related to smoking history. This error was removed from the program permanently. By contrast, there was no trail from which to discern in charts from usual care why they were deficient and why incorrect clinical decisions were made.

Patient acceptance of CLEOS® is excellent. Almost all patients interviewed by CLEOS® report that no physician had ever interviewed them in the detail acquired by their interaction with the program. Patients believed for this reason alone that the program would be a significant positive factor for their health care. About half of all patients interviewed at Robert–Bosch–Krankenhaus had not previously used a computer. Their main problem in navigating the program was using a mouse, which no longer is necessary. A younger cohort of out-patients using the program in a physician's office uniformly believed the data collected by CLEOS® would be important for their health care.

> ˙ On the basis of historical data, the LDL-cholesterol <130 is minimal target in
> this patient because of age and active smoking. Further reduction of risk in
> patients with this risk profile is achieved with LDL-cholesterol <=100. Patient
> should stop smoking, but this will not alter current target value for LDL
> cholesterol. The patient's risk for CAD/stroke has to be stratified further by
> systolic BP, total cholesterol and HDL-cholesterol. Once these are entered, the
> program will calculate whether risk for CAD =>20% over 10 years, in which case
> maximum preventive benefit is achieved at LDL-cholesterol =<70.

Fig. 22.7 Sample text of output by the CLEOS® program for reporting stratification of risk for a
coronary event and target for treating LDL-cholesterol in a smoker

22.7.3 Intended Use of CLEOS®

We have discussed development of a program to substitute for human cognition at
the doctor-patient interface as if the intent were to replace physicians completely.
This is not the current goal for deploying CLEOS®. We propose that the program
will interact directly with primary sources of clinical data to collect, analyze and
store these data but that outputs from data analysis will be adjuncts to routine practice. Physicians will provide patients with access to CLEOS®. Patients will interact
with the program prior to a first or follow-up visit. Findings will be reported to physicians as a detailed clinical note that can be read prior to the patient's office visit.
The physician will have ultimate responsibility for following or rejecting actions
recommended in the analyzed outputs. CLEOS® can be seen in this way as a consult
note or a highly detailed referral note prepared by a panel of expert physicians, who
cover the full range of medical specialties. So whereas the technology described in
relation to implementing the clinical method in Fig. 22.2 could be interpreted as
disruptive, the technology works in a way that does not alter the work flow of routine medical practice. Indeed, it is fair to say that CLEOS® creates time in the clinical encounter for physicians to do what they say they most want to do – think about
their patients' problems and interrelate better with them.

22.7.4 Capture by Computer of Data from
Physical Examination of Patients

We have neglected until now the box in Fig. 22.2 for direct examination of patients.
An advisor early in the course of developing CLEOS® opined we should forget these
data because physical examinations are not done or done so poorly that no useful
clinical information comes from them. This assessment was not inaccurate (Reilly
et al. 2005); but the fact remains that physical examination data are useful for diagnosis and treatment decisions. In the long-term, computing will be configured to
conduct many of the observations of the physical exam, as for example examination
of heart and lungs through recording and interpreting heart sounds and breath
sounds. But physical examination by the doctor – the "laying on of hands" – will be

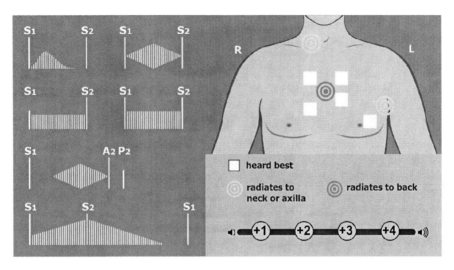

Fig. 22.8 Interface for physician entry of findings from the physical examination. This page is for entry of details of findings related to presence of a heart murmur during the systolic phase of heart action

increasingly important for bonding between patient and physician as computing takes over other cognitive tasks within the traditional doctor-patient relationship.

> What is so important in teaching medical students about the physical exam is instructing them not to perform it blindly and without thinking out the necessity for performing each step. The exam should never be performed mechanically. Students should understand they must have in most cases considered a differential diagnosis based on the history or previous findings and to understand with each step in the physical exam its value for identifying a diagnosis. (Bernstein 2010)

This quote encapsulates how we are dealing with collection of physical examination data. We have formalized the rules for physical examination where these rules are the indicators of abnormal findings in each organ system, and we have linked these rules to interpretive outputs from analysis of historical data. The purpose of the physical examination program is not just to capture findings but to guide physicians to those parts of the examination immediately relevant to the most pertinent clinical questions and to insure that these aspects of the exam are completed. The physician interface is a hand held device connected wirelessly to a local intranet. This makes it easy for users to enter findings contemporaneously during an exam. Pages for entering findings are arranged intuitively. The examiner does not search for data fields in which to enter findings but is prompted to enter findings in a step-wise manner. The page in Fig. 22.8 appears, for example, if the doctor finds a heart murmur during the systolic phase of cardiac action. This page contains not only all the data fields needed to characterize any systolic murmur. The page guides the user to enter findings according to standard, well established criteria. The time-intensity plots of different murmurs indicate the kinds of findings to which the user must be attuned. The user similarly is guided to look for and enter important characteristics such as where the murmur is heard best and to where the sound of the murmur radiates. Data from the physical examination can be used as arguments in an inference or as nodes in a decision graph so that physical exam data are fully integrated with all other clinical data.

22.8   Ownership of Autonomous Software Programs That "Practice" Medicine

It probably is no accident that programs like CLEOS® have not been developed so far by commercial entities, especially by start-ups. IT ventures must turn a profit quickly and on the back of the product for which a company is started. Vendors thus commit to products with narrow foci and short development times so that a global IT solution to the problem like limited human cognition, as it affects medical practice, is exactly what commercial enterprises want to avoid. We think it is a natural phenomenon that CLEOS® is owned by a charitable foundation, The Institute for Digital Medicine (IDM), and that development is directed by academic physicians. Once it is clear, however, what can be accomplished with programs like CLEOS®, commercial interest will be piqued because of the size of the market. Ownership of software programs that function as described for CLEOS® then will become a socially significant issue because the public interest will not be served by commercial ownership of CLEOS® and programs like it. It is clear from their past and present behavior that profit at any social cost is the only concern of commercial entities in health care (Yank et al. 2007; Moynihan 2009; Freudenheim 2009; Tanne 2009). Programs like CLEOS® are especially vulnerable to maximization of profit without concern for social cost. The medical content of such programs can be corrupted easily to further narrow commercial interests. Medical content could be formalized, for example, never to recommend inexpensive generic medications, always to recommend products of a single pharmaceutical manufacturer, to recommend devices that are not essential, to allow advertising coupled to patient-specific clinical information and in general to corrupt the intent of existing clinical guidelines in ways we cannot imagine. Commercial ownership of CLEOS® and similar IT could remove development of new knowledge from control by the medical community. A still further danger of commercial ownership of these kinds of IT programs relates to their importance for clinical research. Commercial ownership of the clinical databases collected by programs like CLEOS® would privatize clinical research, monetize development of new rules for medical practice and remove this development from professional direction.

22.9   Final Thoughts

CLEOS® and programs like it will be deployed widely with the passage of time because IT can substitute for and outperform physicians in carrying out complex, memory intensive cognitive tasks essential for efficient use of the medical knowledge base. There is no other mechanism, save rationing, to control escalating costs of care. But there will be resistance to adopting expert system software that substitutes computing for human intervention between patients and the medical knowledge base. While the public has a sense that something must be done to improve health care and will be more willing than the professional community to accept change, physicians will not embrace loss of their mythic power. They will have strong allies in right-wing politicians, especially in North America, and entrenched business interests that profit from the profligacy of health care spending. The argument we can expect from these forces is medical practice is not a rational activity but "art." We need therefore to keep in mind that artfulness in medical practice begins where knowledge ends. We strive continuously to narrow the "art" of medical practice by imposing on it ever more effective evidence-based rules. There is no evidence to the contrary that the benefits physicians bring to patients are derived from evidence-based, clinical decisions. Artfulness in medical practice not evidence-based decision-making has created the mess within current health care systems in the developed world.

References

Abookire, S. A., Karson, A. S., Fiskio, J., & Bates, D. W. (2001). Use and monitoring of "statin" lipid-lowering drugs compared with guidelines. *Archives of Internal Medicine, 161*, 53–58.

Adams, J., & White, M. (2005). When the population approach to prevention puts the health of individuals at risk. *International Journal of Epidemiology, 34*, 40–43.

Altman, A. G. (1994). The scandal of poor medical research. *British Medical Journal, 308*, 283–284.

Begg, C. B. (2004). On the use of familial aggregation in population based case probands for calculating penetrance. *Journal of the National Cancer Institute, 4*, 143–153.

Bentsen, B. G. (1976). The accuracy of recording patient problems in family practice. *Journal of Medical Education, 51*, 311–316.

Bernstein, M. (2010). www.medpedia.com/questions/1178-is-the-physical-examination-now-of-any-value. Accessed 31 Dec 2010.

Boutron, I., Dutton, S., Ravaud, P., et al. (2010). Reporting and interpretation of randomized controlled trials with statistically nonsignificant results for primary outcomes. *Journal of the American Medical Association, 303*, 2058–2064.

Buchanan, A. V., Sholtis, S., Richtsmeier, J., & Weiss, K. M. (2009). What are genes "for" or where are traits "from"? What is the question? *BioEssays, 31*, 198–208.

Chan, A. W., Hróbjartsson, A., Haahr, M. T., et al. (2004). Empirical evidence for selective reporting of outcomes in randomized trials: Comparison of protocols to published articles. *Journal of the American Medical Association, 291*, 2457–2465.

Cox, J. L., Zitner, D., Courtney, K. D., MacDonald, D. L., et al. (2003). Undocumented patient information: An impediment to quality of care. *The American Journal of Medicine, 114*, 211–216.

Enright, P. L., McClelland, R. L., Newman, A. B., Gottlieb, D. J., & Lebowitz, M. D. (1999). Under diagnosis and under treatment of asthma in the elderly. Cardiovascular Health Study Research Group. *Chest, 116*, 603–613.

Freudenheim, M. (2009). NY Times 9 Aug 2009, And you thought a prescription was private. www.nytimes.com/2009/08/09/business/09privacy.html?scp=1&sq=and you thought prescriptions were&st=cse. Accessed 31 Dec 2010.

Gandhi, T. K., Kachalia, A., Thomas, E. J., Puopolo, A. N., Yoon, C., Brennan, T. A., & Studdert, D. M. (2006). Missed and delayed diagnoses in the ambulatory setting: A study of closed malpractice claims. *Annals of Internal Medicine, 145,* 488–496.

Gormley, M., Dampier, W., Ertel, A., et al. (2007). Prediction potential of candidate biomarker sets identified and validated on gene expression data from multiple datasets. *BMC Bioinformatics, 8,* 415.

Grant, R. W., Buse, J. B., & Meigs, J. B. (2005). Quality of diabetes care in U.S. Academic medical centers low rates of medical regimen change. *Diabetes Care, 28,* 337–342.

Hennekens, C. H., & DeMets, D. (2009). The need for large-scale randomized evidence without undue emphasis on small trials, meta-analyses, or subgroup analyses. *Journal of the American Medical Association, 302,* 2361–2362.

ICSI. (2010). Management of type 2 diabetes mellitus. www.guideline.gov/content. aspx?id=14856&search=diabetes. Accessed 3 Dec 2010.

Institute of Medicine. (2001). *Crossing the quality chasm: A new health system for the 21st century.* Washington, DC: National Academies Press.

Institute of Medicine. (2010). *A national cancer clinical trials system for the 21st century: Reinvigorating the NCI Cooperative Group Program.* Washington, DC: National Academy Press.

Ioannidis, J. P. A. (2006). Commentary: Grading the credibility of molecular evidence for complex diseases. *International Journal of Epidemiology, 35,* 572–577.

Ioannidis, J. P. A., Haidich, A. B., Pappa, M., et al. (2001). Comparison of evidence of treatment effects in randomized and nonrandomized studies. *Journal of the American Medical Association, 286,* 821–830.

Luce, B. R., Kramer, J. M., Goodman, S. N., et al. (2009). Rethinking randomized clinical trials for comparative effectiveness research: The need for transformational change. *Annals of Internal Medicine, 151,* 206–209.

McGlynn, E. A., Asch, S. M., Adams, J., Keesey, J., Hicks, J., DeCristofaro, A., et al. (2003). The quality of healthcare delivered to adults in the United States. *New England Journal of Medicine, 348,* 2635–2645.

Miller, G. (1956). The magical number, seven plus or minus two: Limits on our capacity for processing information. *Psychological Review, 63,* 81–92.

Moynihan, R. (2009). Court hears how drug giant Merck tried to "neutralise" and "discredit" doctors critical of Vioxx. *British Medical Journal, 338,* b1432.

Phillips, L. S., Branch, W. T., Cook, C. B., Doyle, J. P., El-Kebbi, I. M., Gallina, D. L., Miller, C. D., Ziemer, D. C., & Barnes, C. S. (2001a). Clinical inertia. *Annals of Internal Medicine, 135,* 825–834.

Phillips, L. S., Branch, W. T., Cook, C. B., et al. (2001b). Clinical inertia. *Annals of Internal Medicine, 135,* 825–834.

Pletcher, M. J., Lazar, L., Bibbins-Domingo, K., et al. (2009). Comparing impact and cost-effectiveness of primary prevention strategies for lipid-lowering. *Annals of Internal Medicine, 150,* 243–254.

Ramsey, P. G., Curtis, J. R., Paauw, D. S., Carline, J. D., & Weinrich, M. D. (1998a). History taking and preventive medicine skills among primary care physicians: An assessment using standardized patients. *The American Journal of Medicine, 104,* 152–158.

Ramsey, P. G., Curtis, J. R., Paauw, D. S., Carline, J. D., & Weinrich, M. D. (1998b). History taking and preventive medicine skills among primary care physicians: An assessment using standardized patients. *The American Journal of Medicine, 104,* 152–158.

Reilly, B. M., Smith, C. A., & Lucas, B. P. (2005). Physical examination: Bewitched, bothered and bewildered. *The Medical journal of Australia, 182,* 375–376.

Romm, F. J., & Putnam, S. M. (1981). The validity of the medical record. *Medical Care, 19,* 310–315.

Saddine, J. B., Engelgau, M. M., Bechles, G. L., et al. (2002). A diabetes report card for the United States: Quality of care in the 1990s. *Annals of Internal Medicine, 136,* 565–574.

Shah, B. R., Hux, J. E., Laupacis, A., et al. (2005). Clinical inertia in response to inadequate control: Do specialists differ from primary care physicians? *Diabetes Care, 28,* 600–606.

Tanne, J. H. (2009). Pfizer pays record fine for off-label promotion of four drugs. *British Medical Journal, 338*, b3657.

Tversky, A., & Kahneman, D. (1964). Judgment under uncertainty: Heuristics and biases. *Science, 185*, 1124–1131.

Tversky, A., & Kahneman, D. (1981). The framing of decisions and the psychology of choice. *Science, 211*, 453–458.

Tzoulaki, I., Liberopoulos, G., & Ioannidis, J. P. A. (2009). Assessment of claims of improved prediction beyond the Framingham risk score. *Journal of the American Medical Association, 302*, 2345–2352.

Wang, T. J., Stafford, R. S., Ausiello, J. C., & Chaisson, C. E. (2001). Randomized clinical trials and recent patterns in the use of statins. *American Heart Journal, 141*, 957–963.

Whincup, P. H., Emberson, J. R., Walker, M., Papacosta, O., & Thompson, A. (2002). Low prevalence of lipid lowering drug use in older men with established coronary heart disease. *Heart, 88*, 25–29.

Wolff, J. L., Starfield, B., & Anderson, G. (2002). Prevalence, expenditures, and complications of multiple chronic conditions in the elderly. *Archives of Internal Medicine, 162*, 2269–2276.

Yank, V., Rennie, D., & Bero, L. A. (2007). Financial ties and concordance between results and conclusions in meta-analyses: retrospective cohort study. *British Medical Journal, 335*, 1202–1205.

Yarzebski, J., Bujor, C. F., Goldberg, R. J., Spencer, F., Lessard, D., & Gore, J. M. (2002). A community-wide survey of physician practices and attitudes toward cholesterol management in patients with recent acute myocardial infarction. *Archives of Internal Medicine, 162*, 797–804.

Zakim, D., Braun, N., Fritz, P., & Alscher, M. D. (2008). Underutilization of information and knowledge in everyday medical practice: Evaluation of a computer-based solution. *BMC Medical Informatics and Decision Making, 8*, 50.

Zakim, D., Fritz, C., Braun, N., Fritz, P., & Alscher, M. D. (2010). Computerized history-taking as a tool to manage LDL-cholesterol. *Vascular Health and Risk Management, 6*, 1139–1146.

Epilogue

Superior access, quality and value of healthcare services have become a global priority for healthcare to combat the exponentially increasing costs of healthcare expenditure. E-Health in its many forms and possibilities appears to offer a panacea for facilitating the necessary transformation for healthcare. However, while a plethora of e-health initiatives keep mushrooming both nationally and globally, healthcare is still yet to realise the full potential of e-health. This is due to a myriad of reasons including the fact that the healthcare industry is faced with many complex challenges in trying to deliver cost-effective, high-value, accessible healthcare and has traditionally been slow to embrace new business techniques and technologies.

Healthcare to date has predominantly been shaped by each nation's own set of cultures, traditions, payment mechanisms and patient expectations. Therefore, when looking at health systems throughout the world, it is useful to position them on a continuum ranging from high (essentially 100%) government involvement (i.e. a public healthcare system) at one extreme to little (essentially 0%) government involvement (i.e., private healthcare system) at the other extreme with many variations of a two tier system (i.e. mix of private and public) in between. However, given the common problem of exponentially increasing costs facing healthcare globally, irrespective of the particular health system one examines, the future of the healthcare industry will be partially shaped by commonalties such as this key unifying problem and the common forces of change including: (1) empowered consumers, (2) e-health adoption and adaptability and (3) shift to focus on the practice of preventative versus cure driven medicine, as well as four key implications, including: (1) health insurance changes, (2) workforce changes and changes in the roles of stakeholders within the health system, (3) organizational changes and standardization and (4) the need for healthcare providers and administrators to make difficult, yet necessary choices regarding practice management.

It is for these reasons that the preceding has served to present a miscellany of chapters written by respective experts on critical issues all vital for achieving successful e-health solutions. By having four sections of Innovation and Process, Design and Organisation, People and Information Systems and Information

N. Wickramasinghe et al. (eds.), *Critical Issues for the Development*
of Sustainable E-health Solutions, Healthcare Delivery in the Information Age,
DOI 10.1007/978-1-4614-1536-7, © Springer Science+Business Media, LLC 2012

Technology we hoped to emphasis the importance of considering all these aspects in formulating a particular e-health solution. Simply stated, just getting the technology right while clearly a necessary condition is not sufficient it one is to have superior e-health solutions.

The future for healthcare delivery is indeed challenging but we are confident that it is also bright. We believe that many of the key points raised throughout this book will serve to assist the realisation of the full potential of e-health so that we might all ultimately enjoy better healthcare delivery.

Nilmini, Raj, Reima & Stefan
The Editors, 2011

Index

CPSIA information can be obtained at www.ICGtesting.com
Printed in the USA
LVOW072123131112

307219LV00005B/37/P